Bariatric Surgery

Michael Korenkov

Editor

Bariatric Surgery

Technical Variations and Complications

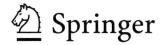 Springer

Editor
Assoc. Prof. Michael Korenkov
Abteilung für Allgemein- und Visceralchirurgie
Klinikum Werra-Meissner
Akademisches Lehrkrankenhaus der
Universität Göttingen
Elsa-Brendström-Straße 1, 37269 Eschwege
Germany
michael.korenkov@klinikum-wm.de

Originally published: Michael Korenkov: Adipositaschirurgie. Verfahren, Varianten und Komplikationen. © Verlag Hans Huber, 2010

ISBN 978-3-642-16244-2   e-ISBN 978-3-642-16245-9
DOI 10.1007/978-3-642-16245-9
Springer Heidelberg Dordrecht London New York

Library of Congress Control Number: 2011937717

© Springer-Verlag Berlin Heidelberg 2012

Springer is part of Springer Science+Business Media (www.springer.com)

Foreword

Let me have men about me that are fat!

Shakespeare: Julius Caesar 1.2

Adiposis or morbid obesity (BMI over 30) is or was made a topic of debate in society and medicine. Obesity has reached surgery!

Reasons for this might be rooted in evolution, when the survival strategy of increased food intake in times of shortage turned into a selection feature. It is a fact that man as a hunter and gatherer lived for millions of years competing for food, roaming the steppe to outrace or flee powerful rivals.

If he was lucky enough to find or capture food, he ate excessively as a precaution for the many hungry days and to survive.

Evolution, on the other hand, has also arranged circulation and metabolism to tone down automatically during the frequent periods of hunger.

As for Homo sapiens, i.e. for us and only for us, the situation is different now, but the ancient selection features still remain, this is the result: Not being hungry and not roaming the steppe, either, leads to obesity!

This connection, well known to science, explains the failure of so many diets and the often ridiculed yo-yo effect. It also provides the most sensible treatment option, which is: reasonable eating with regard to amount and type and physical activity!

But Homo sapiens is, as so often, incapable of being rational. Our present times show in many ways that man tends to be more irrational than sensible; great thinkers of all epochs have confirmed this.

With this connection in mind, it is a moral obligation to remember that the greater part of mankind is still fighting for food to survive and is literally still roaming the steppe. Only a minority is overeating, spending the day moving as little as possible – and is now consulting the surgeon….

Obesity in our society, as it is and as it is perceived, raises the following questions:

Is obesity a disease or merely a sociological problem due to the overemphasis on physical appearance today?

What about the maxim "voluntas aegroti suprema lex" – "The patient's wish is top priority" – if a teenager asks for surgical intervention?

Is surgery with its definitive character to be considered a treatment, even if it lowers body weight and improves comorbidities?

A life-long competent aftercare is required, which also means dependency and endangerment. I have given my view on these questions extensively in our Magazine "MIC". No 17/1 and 17/2 (2008).

Without pondering the very interesting question "What is a disease" too deeply, it remains a fact that obesity dramatically impairs a person's well being. A young mother cannot sit on the floor to play with her little children, another has difficulties maintaining personal hygiene, the car mechanic does not fit under the vehicles. The obese often hardly leave the house fearing ridicule and defamation. Adding the long list of comorbidities to this (diabetes, high blood pressure, joint pain), even the greatest skeptic will have to admit that obesity is a disease that justifies treatment.

This also makes it clear that psychotherapy with its theories yet again fails to solve the problem and can be ruled out as a treatment. For me, preoperative psychological consultations, as they are still regularly required, are a waste of time and often add to the patient's confusion.

This leaves us with surgery, which is problematic in its finality, although it fulfills the criteria of reducing body weight and improving comorbidities.

Surgical intervention is final; it can have dangerous long term effects, which lead to a life-long dependency on medical assistance.

This proves that the surgeon must assume utmost responsibility. Headlines and catch phrases such as "Bariatric Surgery – the greatest development in visceral surgery since the invention of MIC" or "Metabolic surgery will be as well established as bariatric surgery" need to be viewed very skeptically.

Remember the saying "Mehr Schein als Sein" (It is more illusion than reality), or, as André Comte-Sponville put it: "Shallow water will only seem deep if it is cloudy."

It is also undeniable, that many a self-acclaimed "bariatric surgeon" has bailed himself and his hospital out this way, not only financially.

For me it seems almost presumptuous to interfere with a physiological system with a scalpel. Surgery has seen many fatal aberrations, such as sympathectomy to cure diabetes, tuberculosis, or high blood pressure, or even more preposterous, the removal of endocrine glands to cure fatigue.

If this analysis is to treat the problem comprehensively, it is right, even important to describe current surgical procedure in detail. Endoscopy has heavily influenced bariatric surgery. This difficult technique has not become any easier, but more "pleasant" for the patient.

Michael Korenkov, who has occupied himself with these problems since the 1990s, knows the field. He has succeeded in bringing the bariatric elite from 12 countries worldwide together to complete this book. Gastric banding, for example, is described by six different authors. Five authors have portrayed the technically most demanding procedure, the biliopancreatic diversion with duodenal switch, and their preferred technique.

Michael Korenkov, who is well known for his brilliant analyses (Lancet. 2007; M.Korenkov et al., Clinical update; bariatric surgery) knows that the techniques featured here are not based on controlled studies. Comparison of the individual techniques as described by the expert surgeons makes the value of this book. All roads lead to Rome – this is not to serve as an excuse, but shows that the desired structured comparative trials are simply not available in reality, due to the number of different convictions and the lack of time. This happens frequently in surgery. A good example are the preferred reconstructions after gastrectomy.

This book is a "must" not only for bariatric surgeons. Security, the highest principle in surgery, has two basic conditions: choice of the right treatment (certainty) and complication-free execution (safety). This book complies with this principle in a way, as it gives detailed information.

I am convinced that this detailed description of surgical techniques will be a reference work for surgeons today and in the future, maybe even for surgery in general. Time will tell.

Haus Bucherhang, Germany   Hans Troidl

Preface

The last two decades have seen a rapid development of bariatric surgery from being an exotic outsider to becoming a new subspecialty in visceral surgery. Surgical as well as conservative therapy of obesity is not causal today. The objective of the surgical procedures is the reduction of calorie intake through changes within the gastrointestinal system. The repertoire of bariatric surgery has broadened considerably since the beginnings in the 1950s with small intestine resections and bypass. Some techniques are well established, others obsolete again and others are still being tested at the time.

Indications for surgical bariatric intervention are mainly based on the rule of thumb: "BMI over 40 or BMI over 35 + comorbidities."

Current procedures are classified as following:

Restrictive procedures:

Adjustable gastric banding (established)

Sleeve gastrectomy (trials currently under way)

Magenstrasse and Mill procedure (trials currently under way)

Gastroplasty (obsolete)

Malabsorptive procedures:

Small intestine bypass (obsolete)

Biliopancreatic diversion by Scopinaro (established)

Duodenal switch (established)

Combined procedures:

Gastric bypass (established)

Gastric pacing (trials currently under way)

In spite of the symptomatic character of surgical therapy, it is the only effective method of treatment for morbid obesity. Performance of the procedures is not the sole domain of a few highly specialized experts any more, but is routine in many hospitals or is established as a new offer. This development has many positive aspects, but the downside is the large number of difficulties that arise during the learning curve.

How can I perform my procedure safely and successfully? What do I do in case of complications? How can I avoid complications? Surgeons ponder these questions throughout their entire career. A peculiarity of modern bariatric surgery is the fact that although obese patients benefit very much from laparoscopy, this very method poses a great challenge for the surgeon because of obesity. It is undisputed that surgical technique has a great influence on the outcome of a procedure. Another surgical axiom is the rule: "The better a procedure is standardized, the safer it is."

Bariatric surgery is a "young" dynamic field with great potential for growth. But as in any developing discipline, there are many unanswered questions and among other aspects great variations in surgical technique. Numerous expert talks at national and international meetings, telephone calls and discussions with colleagues, and my experience with expert opinions have taught me that the technical and strategic aspects of bariatric surgery are viewed in many different ways. Even revision procedures and management of complications are discussed controversially.

These facts can be very confusing for the bariatric surgeon, especially at the beginning of his career. This is why surgeons, who have not reached the end of their learning curve yet, are the main target group for this book.

This book deliberately stresses the technical aspects of bariatric surgery. Each chapter begins with a description of the steps of the procedure, including possible intra- and postoperative difficulties. It is followed by statements by the experts, who present their own experiences with the particular bariatric technique. The same technical problem is sometimes presented similarly, but sometimes also very differently.

We present the current state of bariatric surgery and the many technical possibilities there are to achieve the surgical goal. We also show that a procedure does not necessarily have to be finished exactly the way it was planned beforehand. Facing intraoperative difficulties, it sometimes serves the patient better to discontinue the procedure or the next step and to proceed with another procedure or a different technical option. Guidelines and recommendations do not cover every single intra- or postoperative problem.

We have tried to improve the choice of individual treatment options beyond the official guidelines. We are aware that this book does not contain all possible procedures and technical tricks and pitfalls. Sleeve gastrectomy with ileal interposition for example is not included, because no expertise could be obtained.

In addition to the description of the surgical procedures, I included short chapters about the technical features of gastric balloon implantation, the possibilities of plastic surgery in obesity and anesthesiological particularities.

I am especially pleased to have won Mervyn Deitel, a pioneer of bariatric surgery and long-time chief editor of *Obesity Surgery* to write the fascinating and interesting chapter "History of Bariatric Surgery" for this book.

We hope we have succeeded in providing our readers with the current technical state of bariatric surgery. We welcome comments and critical remarks.

Eschwege, Germany   Michael Korenkov

Acknowledgments

We thank the authors who supported the idea of this book and whose contributions have significantly influenced its appearance. Thanks to PD Dr. Rudolf Steffen for his didactic suggestions we used for the concept of the book. We are especially indebted to Mirco Gundlach for his excellent drawings.

We also thank BBraun, Melsungen for their financial support in the making of the water color paintings and Dr. Klaus Reinhardt (Hans Huber Publishing) for being a sympathetic listener.

I would like to express my personal and special thanks to our dear doctor and author Markus Vieten, with whom we implemented the entire project step by step. His impressive expertise, strict discipline, clear ideas, and kind communicative skills guided me on the complicated path from the first idea up to the publishing of this book.

Michael Korenkov

Contents

Index of Authors

Editor

Michael Korenkov
Abteilung für Allgemein- und Visceralchirurgie
Klinikum Werra-Meissner, Akademisches Lehrkrankenhaus der
Universität Göttingen
Eschwege, Germany

Co-authors

S. Abegg-Zips
Leiter der Viszeralchirurgischen Sektion des
Medizinischen Competenz Centrum München GmbH, München
Germany

Rosaldo Allieta
Department of General Surgery
Regional Hospital "Umberto Parini"
Center of Excellence in Bariatric Surgery
Aosta, Italy

Gintaras Antanavicius, M.D.
Department of Surgery
University of Minnesota
Minneapolis, MN, USA

Guillaume Becouarn
Société de Chirurgie Viscérale
Angers, France

Ernesto Di Betta
Department of Surgery – 1° Chirurgia Generale
Spedali Civili, Brescia, Italy

Laurent Biertho, M.D.
Department of Surgery
Laparoscopic and Bariatric Surgery
Laval University, Hospital Laval
Quebec City, Quebec, Canada

Arthur Bohdjalian, M.D.
Department of Surgery
Medical University of Vienna
Wien, Austria

Wendy A. Brown
Australian Centre for Obesity Research
and Education
Monash University Clinical School
The Alfred Hospital
Prahran, VIC, Australia

Guy-Bernard Cadière
CHU Saint-Pierre
Clinique de Chirurgie Digestive
Bruxelles, Belgium

Matthias David
Klinik für Anästhesiologie
Universitätsmedizin der Johannes Gutenberg-Universität Mainz
Mainz, Germany

Mervyn Deitel, M.D., CRCSC, FACN, FICS
Editor-in-Chief Emeritus and Founding Editor, Obesity Surgery
Past President American Society for Bariatric Surgery
Founding Member and First Executive Director
The International Federation for the Surgery of Obesity
Toronto, Canada

Michael Gagner, FRCSC, FACS
Department of Surgery
Mount Sinai Medical Center
Miami Beach, FL, USA

M. Garcia-Caballero
Department of Surgery
University Malaga
Facultad de Medicina
Malaga, Spain

Hendrik W. Gervais
Klinik für Anästhesiologie
Universitätsmedizin der Johannes Gutenberg-Universität Mainz
Mainz, Germany

Kelvin D. Higa, M.D., FACS, FASMBS
Service de Chirurgie Digestive et Transplantation Hépatique
Hôpital Archet
Nice, Cedex

Faculté de Médecine
Université de Nice-Sophia-Antipolis
Nice

Centre Hospitalier Universitaire de Nice,
Pôle Digestif
Nice, France

Sayeed Ikramuddin, M.D.
Department of Surgery
University of Minnesota
Minneapolis, MN, USA

Ahad Khan, M.D.
USA

Leonid Lantsberg, M.D.
Surgical Unit
Chairman of Israeli Endoscopic Surgical Society
Soroka University Hospital
Beer-Sheva, Israel

Thomas Manger, M.D.
Department of General, Abdominal
and Paediatric Surgery
SRH Hospital Wald-Klinikum Gera GmbH
(Teaching Hospital of the Friedrich-Schiller-Universität at Jena)
Germany

Henrik Menke
Chefarzt der Klinik für Plastische
Ästhetische und Handchirurgie,- Zentrum für
Schwerbrandverletzte-
Klinikum Offenbach
Offenbach
Germany

Richard Merkle
Leiter der Viszeralchirurgischen Sektion des
Medizinischen Competenz Centrum München GmbH, München
Germany

Karl Miller, M.D., FACS
Surgical Department
Hallein Clinic
Hallein, Austria

Paolo Millo, M.D.
Department of General Surgery
Regional Hospital "Umberto Parini"
Center of Excellence in Bariatric Surgery
Aosta, Italy

Francesco Mittempergher
Department of General Surgery
Spedali Civili
Brescia, Italy

Philippe Mognol
Service de Chirurgie Générale A, Hôpital Bichat
Paris, Cedex, France

Mario Nardi Jr.
Department of General Surgery
Regional Hospital "Umberto Parini"
Center of Excellence in Bariatric Surgery
Aosta, Italy

David Nocca, M.D.
Department of Digestive Surgery Pr Fabre
Hopital Saint Eloi
University Hospital of Montpellier
Avenue Bertin SANS
Montpellier, France

G. Prager
Medical University of Vienna
Department of Surgery
Wien, Austria

Andrés Sánchez-Pernaute
Servicio de Cirugía 2
Hospital Clínico San Carlos
Madrid, Spain

Annette Schmidt
Klinik für Anästhesiologie
Universitätsmedizin der Johannes Gutenberg-Universität Mainz
Mainz, Germany

Rishi Singhal
Upper GI and Minimally Invasive Unit
Birmingham Heartlands Hospital
Birmingham, Great Britain

PD Dr. med. Rudolf Steffen
Facharzt FMH für Chirugie
Brunngasse 14
3011 Bern
Schweiz

Paul Super
Upper GI and Minimally Invasive Unit
Birmingham Heartlands Hospital
Birmingham, Great Britain

Philippe Topart, M.D.
Société de Chirurgie Viscérale
Angers, France

Hans Troidl, Membre Hon. AFC, Hon. FRCS (Eng.), M.D., FACS
Chirurgischen Klinik Köln-Merheim
"Haus Bucherhang"
Germany

R.A. Weiner
Head of the Department of Visceral- and bariatric Surgery
Krankenhaus Sachsenhausen
Frankfurt

Benno Wolcke
Klinik für Anästhesiologie
Universitätsmedizin der Johannes Gutenberg-Universität Mainz
Mainz, Germany

PD Stefanie Wolff
Klinik für Allgemein-Visceral- und Gefäßchirurgie
Otto-von-Guericke Universität Magdeburg
Magdeburg, Germany

All translations
Ulrike Falkenstein-Recht
Gartenstr. 8
50389 Wesseling
E-mail: u.Falkenstein-recht@t-online.de
Germany

Project management
Markus Vieten, Arzt und Autor
Ardennenstraße 73a
52076 Aachen
Germany
E-Mail: mv@markusvieten.de
Web: http://www.markusvieten.de

Drawings
2.1, 2.32, 3.1, 3.18–3.20, 3.22, 3.23, 3.26–3.29, 4.1, 5.1–5.3, 7.1:
Mirko Gundlach
Eschwege
Germany
2,43, 3.25, 3.60–3.62, 3.65, 3.75:
Lutz Kamieth (Dipl.Des.)

History of Bariatric Surgery

1

Mervyn Deitel

Introduction

Many thousand years ago, man suffered hunger and undernourishment. Our ancestors were hunters and gatherers, who worked hard and lived on a high protein diet. They developed "economy genes" to save energy for bad times efficiently. During the last 8,000 years, the development of an agricultural use of wild corn and cereals led to nutrition with more carbohydrates that stimulated the pancreas to secrete insulin regularly. With the industrialization in the twentieth century, the development of convenient fast food within the last 50 years, the overall abundance and the computer age with much sedentary work, the "economy genes" lead to obesity today. Obesity has since been spreading like an epidemic [1] and has been accompanied by the emergence of the metabolic syndrome.

Morbid obesity, i.e., obesity that is associated with serious, progressive, and disabling diseases, has proven to be a great and costly health problem that does not adequately respond to conservative measures [2, 3]. Bariatric surgery has turned out to be the only method to achieve significant and long-term weight loss. The indications for a bariatric procedure are listed in Table 1.1.

M. Deitel
Obesity Surgery Past President American
Society for Bariatric Surgery,
Founding Member and First Executive Director,
The International Federation for the Surgery of Obesity
Toronto, Canada
e-mail: book@obesitysurgery.com

Table 1.1 Indications for bariatric surgery [4, 5]

Severe obesity with a BMI over 40 or with a BMI over 35 and severe comorbidities
Written proof of a failure of dietary and pharmaceutical measures
Tolerably high surgical risk
Exclusion of endocrine causes (i.e., hypothyreoidism, Cushing's disease)
Availability of a multidisciplinary team with dietary, pharmacological, and psychological care
Exclusion of psychosis
Information of the patient before surgery
Cooperation for follow up and treatment
Experienced team of surgeons and anaesthesiologists, suitable clinic

Intestinal Bypass

The first operation to cure obesity was performed in the 1950s by Henrikson; it was an extensive small bowel resection, which led to malabsorptive weight loss [6]. This procedure was obviously irreversible, which led other surgeons to perform small bowel bypasses. Jejunocolic bypasses (Fig. 1.1) [7, 8] were tried first, but they led to a massive loss of liquid and electrolytes and severe liver dysfunction. Undoing the bypass in a revision procedure saved the patient's life.

Now jejunoileal bypass procedures were developed; Kremen et al. [9] from Minneapolis were the first to publish data. These procedures (with several variations) were popular in the 1970s for cases of severe obesity (Fig. 1.2a, b).

A jejunoileal bypass however could also lead to serious complications occasionally, such as a blind loop syndrome due to stasis and bacterial overgrowth or abdominal hemorrhage [13, 14]. Hypokalemia,

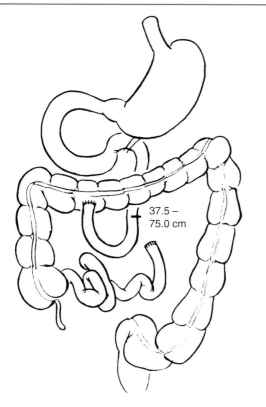

Fig. 1.1 Jejunocolic bypass: Payne et al. [7] connected the proximal 37.5 cm and Lewis et al. [8] the proximal 75 cm of the jejunum to the transverse colon

hypomagnesemia, floating arthralgia, urinary calculi, and liver dysfunction were possible even with adequate protein substitution, also electrolyte imbalance and a burning sensation around the anus due to diarrhea. All bariatric procedures required lifelong monitoring, especially the jejunoileal bypass; the surgeon had to be available at all times. The ensuing weight loss however also cured the associated diseases, such as diabetes, dyslipidemia, cardiovascular disease, sleep apnea syndrome, arthritis, and infertility [16, 17].

Modifications of the jejunoileal bypass were developed to avoid the blind loop syndrome. An ileogastrostomy drained the bypassed part of the small intestine into the stomach (Fig. 1.3) [18].

After a biliointestinal bypass, during which the gall bladder was connected to the end of the bypassed jejunum, bile flowed through the bypassed intestine; another effort to avoid the blind loop syndrome [19].

Gastric Bypass

In the 1960s, Edward E. Mason developed a new procedure to avoid the side effects of the jejunoileal bypass. He connected the jejunum to a proximal, horizontally, cut stomach pouch (Fig. 1.4a) [20].

Fig. 1.2 (**a**) Jejunoileal end-to-end bypass: Scott et al. (1977) [10]. Salmon [12, 11] and Scott drained the bypassed intestine into the transverse colon (A) or the sigmoid colon (B); [11] into the cecum (C). The lengths are indicated. (**b**) Jejunoileal end-to-side bypass (T-shaped anastomosis with the distal ileum by DeWind and Payne [13]. The appendix was removed in all cases. Some surgeons created a Y-shaped anastomosis to reduce reflux into the bypassed segment

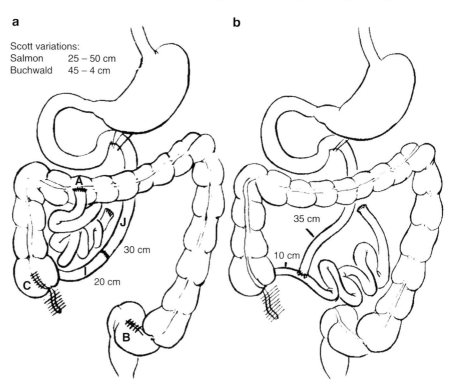

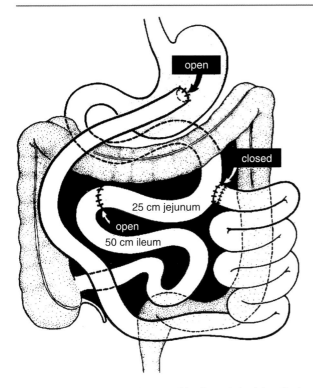

Fig. 1.3 Ileogastrostomy is a modification of the jejunoileal bypass; the bypassed segment is drained into the upper part of the stomach. Lower pressure here was supposed to prevent blind loop syndrome

This led to a reduction of stomach size and a mild malabsorption. Later Alden introduced the stapler to bariatric surgery by closing off the proximal part of the stomach with staples instead of cutting into it (Fig. 1.4b) [21].

These sutures were often instable, but the era of the stapler in bariatric surgery had begun.

In Mason's gastric bypass the segment was under tension often, but on the other hand there was no Braun's anastomosis to perform. If leakage occurred at the gastrojejunal anastomosis, secretions from the stomach, the duodenum, the gall bladder and the pancreas discharged a highly lethal complication.

For this reason Griffen developed the Roux-en-Y gastric bypass [22] which reduced the tension around the gastrojejunostomy (Fig. 1.4c).

In case of a leakage, mostly saliva would escape and most of the patients survived. The Roux segment also prevented a bile-induced gastritis in the pouch. Torres modified the Roux-en-Y gastric bypass by creating the restrictive gastric pouch vertically at the lesser curvature [23], where there are three layers of muscle tissue

and the tendency to dilate is less pronounced. Later Torres moved the afferent biliopancreatic anastomosis further distally, which created a shorter common channel and thus added a significant malabsorptive component (Fig. 1.4d) [24, 25].

Leakage, ulcers [26] around the anastomoses, dumping syndrome [27], iron- and vitamin B12 deficiency, and bowel obstruction are possible complications of the Roux-en-Y gastric bypass. Sometimes calcium deficiency leads to osteoporosis in the long run. A postoperative substitution therapy with iron, vitamin B 12 and other minerals and vitamins is therefore necessary [28].

The Roux-en-Y gastric bypass has been modified several times [29] and is considered an effective surgical method for weight loss in the United States and many other countries [30, 31]. The laparoscopic approach has become increasingly popular within the last 10 years [32, 34].

The "mini gastric bypass" is a vertical pouch at the lesser curvature, connected to the small intestine about 200 cm distal of Treitz's arch; the outcome is satisfying as well (Fig. 1.5) [35].

Treating type II diabetes as a major component of the metabolic syndrome has become an interesting topic recently. Several intestinal hormones that stimulate insulin secretion from the pancreas (so called incretins) have been identified; GLP-1 (glucagon like peptide 1) has been investigated the most extensively so far [36]. This hormone is secreted by the L-cells in the rectum. In surgical procedures that lead to a faster passage of food into the intestine, its secretion is enhanced. Another hormone, ghrelin, is secreted especially from the gastric fundus and produces hunger. Bariatric surgical procedures that include a resection of the stomach reduce hunger [37].

Biliopancreatic Diversion and Duodenal Switch

Because of the problems caused by the blind loop syndrome after jejunoileal bypass, Scopinaro developed the biliopancreatic diversion procedure in the mid-1970s in Genua, which leaves no blind loop (Fig. 1.6) [38].

Digestion and absorption of starch and fat take place in the last 50 cm of the ileum. This procedure has the best long-term results in terms of weight

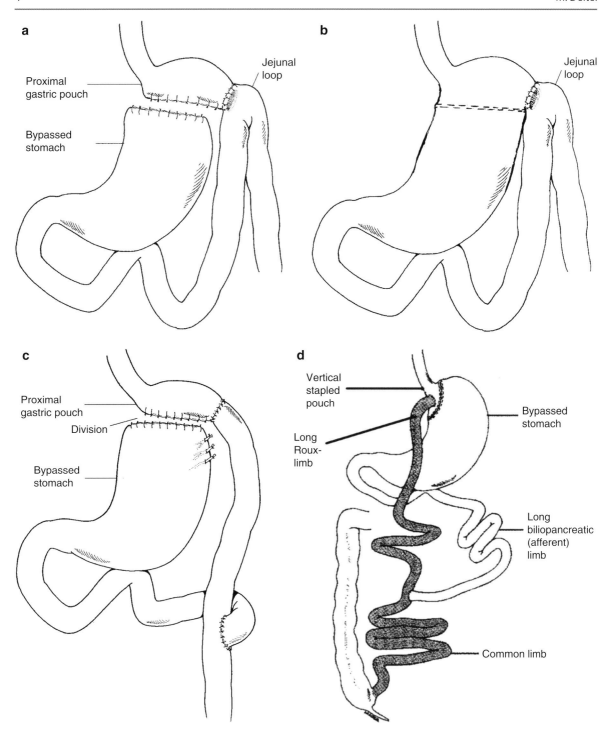

Fig. 1.4 (**a**) Loop-gastric bypass [19]. The proximally divided stomach was connected to a jejunal segment. (**b**) Alden [20] modified the loop-gastric bypass by closing the stomach with a stapler. These sutures broke often, even if a second line was added. (**c**) Griffen et al. [21] developed the Roux-en-Y gastric bypass, with which biliary reflux gastritis was prevented – the archetype of the modern gastric bypass. (**d**) Torres et al. [22] created the gastric pouch close to the lesser curvature, where the stomach wall has more muscle tissue and better blood supply. Later he prolonged the biliopancreatic and the Roux limb and shortened the common channel in order to facilitate weight loss through the addition of mild malabsorption

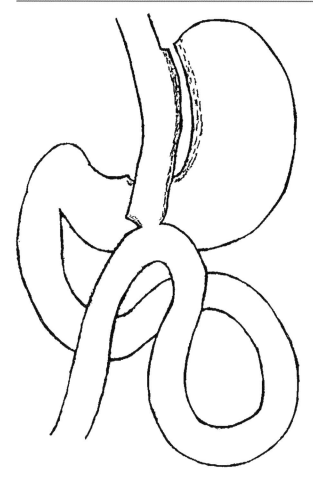

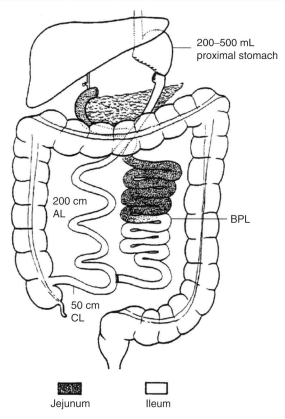

Fig. 1.5 Mini gastric bypass. The stomach is cut vertically along a 28 fr tube, beginning at the crow's foot. Gastroenterostoma is about 100 cm distal to Treitz's arch

Fig. 1.6 Biliopancreatic diversion. A distal gastrectomy is performed. The small intestine is cut 250 cm proximal to the ileocecal valve and connected to the rest of the stomach. The biliopancreatic loop (BPL) is connected to the side of the distal segment, 50 cm proximal to the ileocecal valve to create a Roux limb (200 cm), and a common loop (50 cm). The proximal stomach pouch restricts food intake, bypassed small intestine continues with reduced absorption. Cholecystectomy is performed as a prophylactic measure to prevent the formation of gall stones due to biliar stasis and rapid weight loss

loss and reduction of obesity-related diseases of all bariatric surgical procedures [39]. But close long-term monitoring of a sufficient absorption of proteins, minerals, and vitamins and supplementation is mandatory [28].

The biliopancreatic diversion was modified by Marceau and Hess through the duodenal switch [40, 41] A gastric sleeve is created along the lesser curvature and the first part of the duodenum is cut below the pylorus. The ileum is cut 250 cm proximal to the ileocecal valve; the proximal end of the duodenum is connected to the distal end of the ileum (Fig. 1.7). The long biliopancreatic section is connected to the ileum at about 75–100 cm proximal to the ileocecal valve. Leaving the pylorus unharmed prevents a dumping syndrome and duodenal ulcers.

Both the biliopancreatic diversion and the duodenal switch lead to a restriction of the stomach size initially; weight loss is maintained through the malabsorptive component.

Laparoscopic Sleeve Gastrectomy

A vertical sleeve gastrectomy as an independent procedure is usually performed with a narrower gastric sleeve than the duodenal switch (Fig. 1.8). It is performed as a first step in high risk or extremely obese patients [42, 43], who might need a duodenal switch or a Roux-en-Y gastric bypass in case of recurrent weight gain

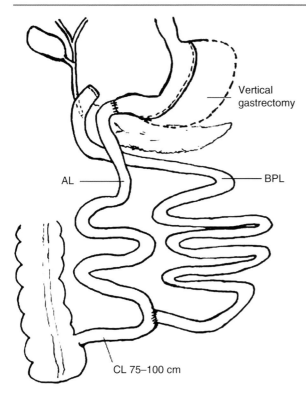

Fig. 1.7 Biliopancreatic diversion with duodenal switch. The greater curvature of the stomach is removed to limit the size. Then the ileum is cut and the alimentary loop (AL) is connected to the proximal duodenum. The biliopancreatic loop (BPL) is connected to the alimentary loop about 75–100 cm away from the ileocecal valve, thereby producing the common channel

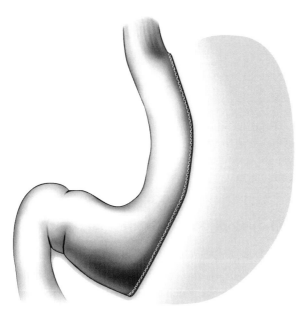

Fig. 1.8 Laparoscopic sleeve gastrectomy, as performed by many surgeons today

later. Many surgeons perform a sleeve gastrectomy in all morbidly obese patients. This restrictive technique leads to a quick emptying of the stomach [44].

Stomach Restriction

In the 1980s the search for more simple procedures led to restrictive procedures by Pace [45] and Carey [46] (Fig. 1.9a) and Gomez [47] (Fig. 1.9b) to limit the amount of food tolerated. The small horizontal proximal pouch and also the exit dilated, however. Gomez reinforced the pouch exit, but some patients suffered an obstruction of the stoma initially and then an excessive enlargement of the pouch. Mason introduced gastroplasty with a vertical band. He created a vertical pouch along the small curvature, where the muscle layers are thicker and therefore do not dilatate easily and stabilized the exit of the pouch with a non-elastic band (Fig. 1.10) [48].

The vertical gastric band and its various adaptations found widespread acceptance soon; it was later also implanted laparoscopic [49]. It later lost its popularity, however, due to recurrent weight gain in the long term.

In the early 1980s Molina in Houston developed the procedure in which the band is implanted high up around the stomach, creating only a small pouch [50]. This technique was adopted by many surgeons, also by Kuzmak in New Jersey, who perfected it. Later Forsell and Hallberg in Sweden [51] and Kuzmak [52] independently from each other developed inflatable bands. They were connected to a subcutaneously implanted reservoir via a tube. The exit of the pouch was adjusted by adding or removing saline to the band (Fig. 1.11).

The gastric band is implanted worldwide today. Weight loss is not as marked as after biliopancreatic diversion, duodenal switch or Roux-en-Y gastric bypass, but is nevertheless considered satisfactory. The gastric band has its own complications [53, 54], such as slippage or band erosion. There are also problems related to the port chamber and the tube, but surgical techniques have been developed to solve them. The perigastric pathway was used first (dissection close the stomach wall and crossing the proximal part of the omental bursa). Later the pars-flaccida-approach (high, avascular pathway, dissection of the right crus of diaphragm and the angle of His) gained more popularity, because it eliminates complications such as anterior or posterior gastric prolapse (slippage) [55, 56].

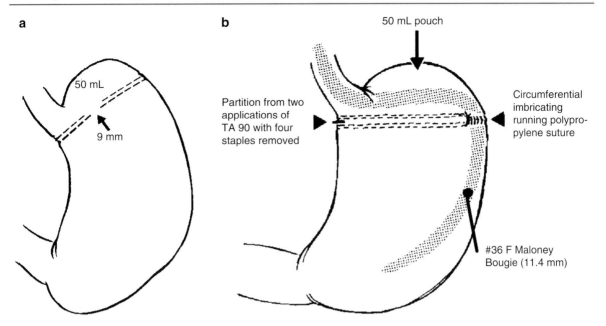

Fig. 1.9 (**a**) Cutting the stomach with a single stapler suture. (**b**) Cutting the stomach and reinforcing the exit at the greater curvature with a circular overlapping suture (Gomez 1979)

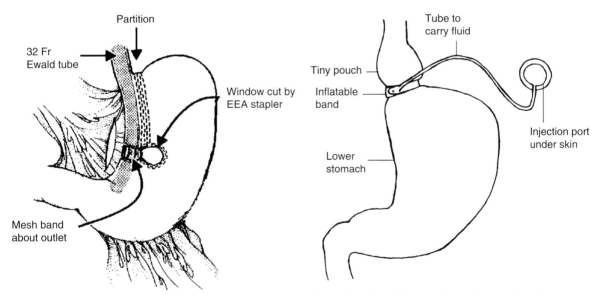

Fig. 1.10 Vertical gastroplasty [47]. A window is created in the antrum with a circular stapler and the stomach is cut vertically with the stapler; this way a small pouch is created. The exit of the pouch is reinforced with a silicone band to prevent dilatation

Fig. 1.11 Adjustable gastric band with a small proximal pouch. The port chamber is fastened to the fascia and connected to the band with a tube. Injection or removal of saline tightens or loosens the band

As with all restrictive procedures, the gastric band requires small meals, careful chewing, and slow eating to avoid vomiting. The gastric band leads to a sense of fullness early, but nutrition needs to be monitored closely. Gastric band are especially suitable for laparoscopic implantation; the procedure is reversible.

Other Procedures

Gastric pacers have been tested lately [57]. Two electrodes are implanted into the anterior gastric wall and connected to a subcutaneously implanted electric generator. This pacemaker produces regular stomach contractions that produce a sense of fullness. Weight loss success has been variable so far.

Other procedures are studies in clinical trials at the time. Large balloons are inserted inside the stomach, especially in high risk super obese patients to induce preoperative weight loss [58].

Conclusions

Morbid obesity has turned into an international health problem with severe comorbidities [59, 60]. The only successful way to lose weight is a surgical procedure. Various techniques reflect the creativity of bariatric surgeons [61]. The patient must receive help and therapy from other specialties, such as diet counseling, nursing care, psychotherapy, psychiatry, internal medicine, endocrinology, anaesthesiology, pneumology, aesthetic surgery and above all treatment in specialized hospitals.

References

1. Deitel M (2006) The obesity epidemic (ed.). Obes Surg 16:377–379
2. Wooley SC, Garner DM (1991) Obesity treatment: the high cost of false hope. J Am Diet Assoc 91:1248–1251
3. Van Itallie TB (1980) Morbid obesity: a hazardous disorder that resists conservative treatment. Am J Clin Nutr. 33:358–363
4. Deitel M, Shahi B (1992) Morbid obesity: selection of patients for surgery. J Am Coll Nutr. 11:457–466
5. National Institutes of Health Consensus Development Conference Draft Statement (1991) Gastrointestinal surgery for severe obesity. Obes Surg. 1:257–265
6. Henrikson V (1952) [Kan tunnfarmsresektion forsvaras som terapi mot fettsot? Nordisk Medicin. 47:77–44]. Can small bowel resection be defended for therapy for obesity? (translated into English in Obes Surg 1994;4:54–5)
7. Payne JH, DeWind LT, Commons RR (1963) Metabolic observations in patients with jejunocolic shunts. Am J Surg. 106:273–289
8. Lewis LA, Turnbull RB Jr, Page H (1966) Effects of jejuno-colic shunt on obesity, serum lipoproteins, lipids and electrolytes. Arch Intern Med. 117:4–16
9. Kremen AJ, Linner JH, Nelson CH (1954) An experimental evaluation of the nutritional importance of proximal and distal small intestine. Ann Surg. 140:439–444
10. Scott HW Jr, Dean RH, Shull HJ et al (1977) Results of jejunoileal bypass in 200 patients with morbid obesity. Surg Gynecol Obstet. 145:661–663
11. Salmon PA (1971) The results of small intestine bypass operations for the treatment of obesity. Surg Gynecol Obstet. 132:965–979
12. Buchwald H, Schwartz MZ, Varco RL. Surgical treatment of obesity. Adv Surg. 1973;7:235-55. Review
13. DeWind LT, Payne JH (1976) Intestinal bypass surgery for morbid obesity: long-term results. JAMA. 236:2298–2301
14. Wands JR, LaMont JT, Mann E et al. Arthritis associated with intestinal-bypass procedure for morbid obesity. N Engl J Med 1976; 294:121–4
15. Clayman RV, Williams RD (1979) Oxalate urolithiasis following jejunoileal bypass. Surg Clin North Am. 59:1071–1077
16. Deitel M, Shahi B, Anand PK et al (1993) Long-term outcome in a series of jejunoileal bypass patients. Obes Surg. 3:247–252
17. Sylvan A, Sjölund B, Januger KG (1995) Favorable long-term results with end-to-side jejunoileal bypass. Obes Surg. 5:357–363
18. Cleator IGM, Birmingham CL, Kovacevic S et al (2006) Long-term effect of ileogastrostomy surgery for morbid obesity on diabetes mellitus and sleep apnea. Obes Surg. 16:1337–1341
19. Eriksson F (1981) Bilio-intestinal bypass. Int J Obes. 5:437–447
20. Mason EE, Ito I (1967) Gastric bypass in obesity. Surg Clin North Am. 47:1345–1351
21. Alden JF (1977) Gastric and jejunoileal bypass: a comparison in the treatment of morbid obesity. Arch Surg. 112:799–806
22. Griffen WO, Young VL, Stevenson CC (1977) A prospective comparison of gastric and jejunoileal bypass procedures for morbid obesity. Ann Surg. 186:500–509
23. Torres JC, Oca CF, Garrison RN (1983) Gastric bypass Roux-en-Y gastrojejunostomy from the lesser curvature. South Med J. 76:1217–1221
24. Miller DK, Goodman GN (1989) Gastric bypass procedures. In: Deitel M (ed) Surgery for the morbidly obese patient. FD-Communications Inc., Toronto, pp 124–127
25. Brolin RE, Kenler HA, Gorman JH et al (1992) Long-limb gastric bypass in the superobese. A prospective randomized study. Ann Surg. 215:387–395
26. Capella JF, Capella RF (1999) Gastro-gastric fistulas and marginal ulcers in gastric bypass procedures for weight reduction. Obes Surg. 9:22–27
27. Deitel M (2008) The change in the dumping syndrome concept. Obes Surg. 18(12):1622–1624
28. Bloomberg RD, Fleishman A, Nalle JE et al (2005) Nutritional deficiencies following bariatric surgery: what have we learned? Obes Surg. 15:145–154
29. Fobi MAL, Lee H, Felahy B et al (2005) Choosing an operation for weight control, and the transected banded gastric bypass. Obes Surg. 15:114–121
30. Dhabuwala A, Cannan RJ, Stubbs RS (2000) Improvement in co-morbidities following weight loss from gastric bypass surgery. Obes Surg. 10:428–435
31. White S, Brooks E, Jurikova et al (2005) Long-term outcomes after gastric bypass. Obes Surg. 15:155–163
32. Wittgove AC, Clark GW (2000) Laparoscopic gastric bypass, Roux en-Y – 500 patients: technique and results, with 3–60 month follow-up. Obes Surg. 10:233–239.
33. Higa KD, Boone KB, Ho T (2000) Complications of the laparoscopic Roux-en-Y gastric bypass: 1,040 patients – What have we learned? Obes Surg. 10:509–513

34. Rosenthal RJ, Szomstein S, Kennedy CI et al (2006) Laparoscopic surgery for morbid obesity: 1,001 consecutive bariatric operations performed at the bariatric institute, Cleveland Clinic Florida. Obes Surg. 16:119–124

35. Chakhtoura G, Zinzindohoué F, Ghanem et al. (2008) Primary results of laparoscopic mini-gastric bypass in a French obesity-surgery specialized university hospital. Obes Surg. 18:1130–1133

36. Lamounier RN, Pareja JC, Tambascia MA et al (2007) Incretins: clinical physiology and bariatric surgery – correlating the entero-endocrine system and a potentially anti-dysmetabolic procedure. Obes Surg. 17:569–576

37. Frühbeck G, Diez-Caballero A, Gil MJ et al (2004) The decrease in plasma ghrelin concentrations following bariatric surgery depends on the functional integrity of the fundus. Obes Surg. 14:606–612

38. Scopinaro N, Gianetta E, Civalleri D et al (1979) Biliopancreatic bypass for obesity: II Initial experience in man. Br J Surg. 66:618–620

39. Scopinaro N, Adami GF, Marinari GM et al (1998) Biliopancreatic diversion. World J Surg. 22:936–946

40. Lagace M, Marceau P, Marceau S et al (1995) Biliopancreatic diversion with a new type of gastrectomy: some previous conclusions revisited. Obes Surg. 5:411–418

41. Hess DS, Hess DW (1998) Biliopancreatic diversion with a duodenal switch. Obes Surg. 8:267–282

42. Baltasar A, Serra C, Perez N et al (2005) Laparoscopic sleeve gastrectomy: a multi-purpose bariatric operation. Obes Surg. 15:1124–1128

43. Deitel M, Crosby RD, Gagner M (2008) The First International Consensus Summit for Sleeve Gastrectomy (SG), New York City, October 25–27, 2007. Obes Surg. 18: 487–496

44. Melissas J, Daskalakis M, Koukouraki S et al (2008) Sleeve gastrectomy a "food limiting" operation. Obes Surg. 18: 1251–1256

45. Pace WG, Martin EW Jr, Tetirick T et al (1979) Ann Surg. 190:392–400

46. Carey LC, Martin EW Jr (1981) Treatment of morbid obesity by gastric partitioning. World J Surg. 5:829–831

47. Gomez CA (1980) Gastroplasty in the surgical treatment of morbid obesity. Am J Clin Nutr. 33:406–415

48. Mason EE (1982) Vertical banded gastroplasty. Arch Surg. 117:701–706

49. Melissas J, Choretsantis G, Grammatikakis J et al (2003) Technical modification of laparoscopic vertical banded gastroplasty. Obes Surg. 13:132–135

50. Oria HE (2003) Marcel Molina. The loss of a pioneer. Obes Surg. 13:806–807

51. Forsell P, Hallberg D, Hellers G (1993) A gastric band with adjustable inner diameter for obesity surgery. Obes Surg. 3:303–306

52. Kuzmak LI (1992) Stoma adjustable silicone gastric banding. Probl Gen Surg. 9:298–303

53. Chevallier J-M, Zinzindohoue F, Douard R et al (2004) Complications after laparoscopic adjustable gastric banding for morbid obesity: experience with 1,000 patients over 7 years. Obes Surg. 14:407–414

54. Mittermair RP, Aigner F, Nehoda H (2004) Results and complications after laparoscopic adjustable gastric banding in super-obese patients, using the Swedish band. Obes Surg. 14:1327–1330

55. O'Brien PE, Dixon JB, Laurie C et al (2005) A prospective randomized trial of placement of the laparoscopic adjustable band: comparison of the perigastric and pars flaccida pathways. Obes Surg. 15:820–826

56. Dargent J (2003) Pouch dilatation and slippage after adjustable gastric banding: is it still an issue? Obes Surg. 13:111–115

57. Shikora SA (2004) Implantable gastric stimulation for the treatment of severe obesity. Obes Surg. 14:545–548

58. Sallet JA, Marchesini JB, Paiva DS et al (2004) Brazilian multicenter study of the intragastric balloon. Obes Surg. 14:991–998

59. Deitel M (1996) The development of general surgical operations, and weight-loss operations. Obes Surg. 6:206–212

60. Herrera MF, Deitel M (1991) Cardiac function in massively obese patients and the effect of weight loss. Can J Surg. 34:431–434

61. Sjostrom CD, Lissner L, Wedel H et al (1999) Reduction in incidence of diabetes, hypertension and lipid disturbance after intentional weight loss induced by bariatric surgery: the SOS intervention study. Obes Res. 7:477–484

Adjustable Gastric Banding

Michael Korenkov, Wendy A. Brown,
Andrew I. Smith, Leonid Lantsberg,
Thomas Manger, Rishi Singhal, and Paul Super

Introduction

Gastric banding is one of the so-called restrictive procedures in bariatric surgery. The aim is to limit the size of the stomach to a small pouch, which is created by tightening the gastric band (Figs. 2.1 and 2.2).

At first the idea of restricting the size of the stomach was carried out by performing gastroplasty. This procedure however was irreversible and the laparoscopic procedure faced major technical difficulties. Also the band was not adjustable, which is why this procedure is hardly performed anymore and has been replaced by adjustable gastric banding.

M. Korenkov (✉)
Abteilung für Allgemein- und Visceralchirurgie,
Klinikum Werra-Meissner, Akademisches
Lehrkrankenhaus der Universität Göttingen,
Elsa-Brendström-Straße 1, 37269 Eschwege, Germany
e-mail: michael.korenkov@klinikum-wm.de

W.A. Brown
Australian Centre for Obesity Research and Education,
Monash University Clinical School, The Alfred Hospital,
Commercial Road, Prahran, Vic, 3181, Australia
e-mail: wendy.brown@med.monash.edu.au

A.I. Smith
Australian Centre for Obesity Research and Education.
Monash University Clinical School, The Alfred Hospital,
Commercial Road, Prahran, Vic, 3181, Australia

L. Lantsberg
Surgical Unit, Chairman of Israeli Endoscopic Surgical Society,
Soroka University Hospital, Beer-Sheva, 84100, Israel
e-mail: leolant@bgu.ac.il

T. Manger
Department of General, Abdominal and Paediatric Surgery,
SRH Hospital Wald-Klinikum Gera GmbH, (Teaching Hospital
of the Friedrich-Schiller-Universität at Jena), Germany

R. Singhal • P. Super
Upper GI and Minimally Invasive Unit, Birmingham
Heartlands Hospital, Bordesley Geen East, Birmingham,
B5 9SS, Great Britain
e-mail: singhal_rishi@rediffmail.com;
paul.super@heartofengland.nhs.uk

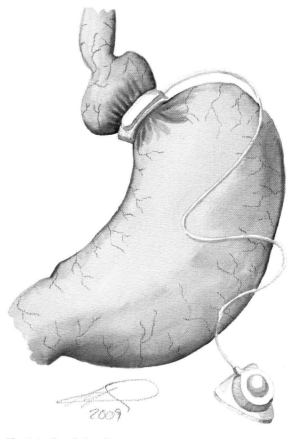

Fig. 2.1 Gastric banding

M. Korenkov (ed.), *Bariatric Surgery*,
DOI 10.1007/978-3-642-16245-9_2, © Springer-Verlag Berlin Heidelberg 2012

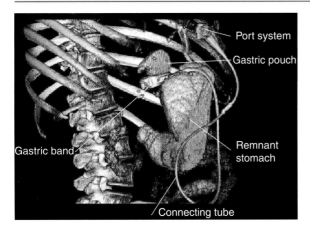

Fig. 2.2 CT-reconstruction of a gastric band (courtesy of Dr. Ingrid Harth, Radiologisches Institut, Kreiskrankenhaus Eschwege)

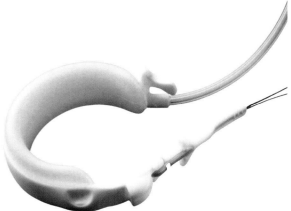

Fig. 2.4 SAGB (courtesy of Ethicon)

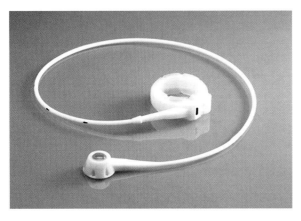

Fig. 2.3 Lap-band (courtesy of Allergan)

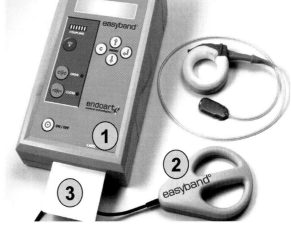

Fig. 2.5 Remote adjustable Gastric band (courtesy of Allergan). (1) A control unit sends energy and information telemetrically to the easyband through magnetic induction. (2) Antenna: magnetic induction is sent to the antenna, which is connected to the easyband. (3) A microchip saves the adjustments of the easyband

Today inflatable adjustable bands are usually chosen. A silicone ring with a soft inflatable balloon inside is connected to an access port just under the skin via a small tube. The band is then adjusted by injecting saline through the port. The most popular bands are the Lap-Band (Allergan) and the SAGB (Ethicon) (Figs. 2.3 and 2.4).

Frequent problems occur concerning the port (port rotation, leakage, difficult injections, pain around the port, exposure to radiation etc.) which is why better ports are developed today or alternatively remote adjustable gastric bands, which are tested in clinical trials at the time (Fig. 2.5).

Even though the laparascopic placement of an adjustable gastric band is considered to be one of the simpler bariatric procedures, there still are several technical difficulties and pitfalls.

The first to place an adjustable gastric band was Belachew (1983). His technique is referred to as the perigastric pathway. A higher rate of intraoperative complications (i.e., stomach perforation) and band-related complications (i.e., slippage or band migration) was observed, however. The method was therefore abandoned in favor of the pars-flaccida approach. There are only a few occasions when the perigastric pathway may be preferable.

Fig. 2.6 Positioning of the patient for laparoscopic gastric banding

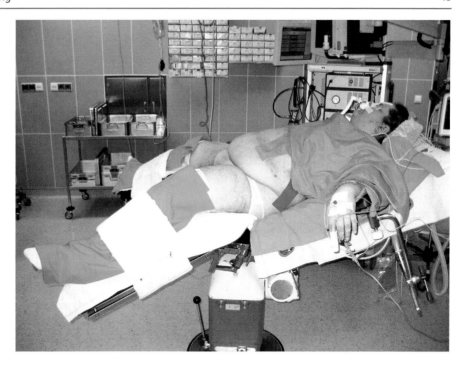

Preparation

Setting, Positioning, and the Surgical Team

- The monitor is placed on the patient's right side, either above or below the outstretched right arm. An additional monitor can be placed on the left side (Fig. 2.6 and 2.7).
- As in every laparoscopic procedure, gastric banding also begins with positioning the obese patient correctly. He is positioned in the lithotomy position, with the upper body tilted upward in a 45° angle (reversed Trendelenburg position). Adequate measures to prevent slipping are mandatory.
- The surgical team consists of the surgeon, an assistant holding the camera, a second assistant, and the scrub nurse. A post to secure the liver retractor can be used instead of a second assistant.
- The surgeon stands between the patients legs. If there is one assistant, he will stand on the patient's left side, work the camera with his left hand and a grasper with his right hand. If there are three surgeons on the team, the first assistant can stand on either side.
- The scrub nurse stands next to the patient's left leg. If the operating surgeon is left-handed, she can also stand on the right side.

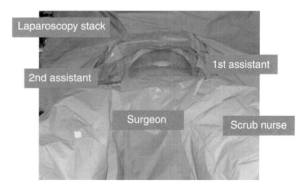

Fig. 2.7   Set up of the surgical team and the laparascopy stack

Installation of the Pneumoperitoneum

Many bariatric surgeons use the well-established approach with the extra-long Veress needle (Fig. 2.8).

Some surgeons prefer optical trocars that allow visual control of the access to the peritoneum and the creation of the pneumoperitoneum, thereby requiring only a minimal depth of puncture for entering the peritoneum and gas insufflation. They provide a good alternative to the Veress needle. We use the fiber optic equipped safety needles for the creation of the pneumoperitoneum more often now, but they are more expensive than the Veress needle (Fig. 2.9).

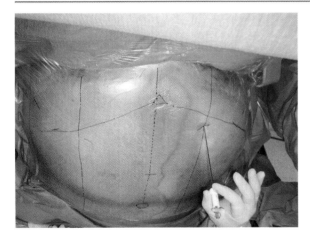

Fig. 2.8 Insertion of the Veress needle into the left upper abdomen under the costal margin

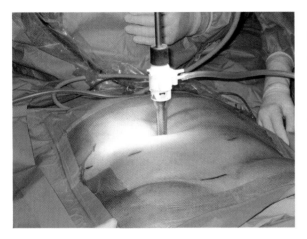

Fig. 2.9 Insertion of an optical trocar under visual control

In some rare occasions an "open" approach is chosen. The incisions are placed either supraumbilically or on the left upper abdomen, where some larger incisions for the port placement will be performed toward the end of the procedure anyway. These approaches are not suitable for severely obese patients with a BMI over 50, because a comparatively large cut will be necessary. A complete insulation is also difficult to achieve, which may lead to continuous gas leakage during the procedure.

- Place the needle in the left upper abdomen just under the left costal margin on the medioclavicular line. Another possibility is the supraumbilical approach via the incision for the camera.

We prefer the approach through the left upper abdomen, because the abdominal wall is thinner here than around the umbilicus and therefore the puncture path for the needle is shorter. This close to the costal margin the abdominal wall is also more "taut" which facilitates the insertion of the needle.

- The puncture site in the left upper abdomen will be widened after removing of Veress needle and used for the working trocar.

In obese patients with a long distance between the skin and peritoneum, one can lose the "feel" for the Veress needle during placement. In these cases we prefer the so-called double-click technique; after the second "click" the needle is not inserted any further.

- Install a maximum intraabdominal pressure of 14 mmHg.

In patients with a BMI over 50, this pressure is sometimes not high enough to lift the heavy abdominal wall sufficiently. In this case, we begin with a pressure of 20 mmHg and reduce to 14 mmHg after positioning the optic.

Positioning the Trocars

Lifting the abdominal wall for the closed approach is difficult and sometimes impossible. The abdominal wall is stretched and decompressed in the process, which elongates the distance between the skin and the peritoneum. In some cases the peritoneum cannot be reached, not even with the extra-long trocars. For these reasons we do not lift the abdominal wall from the outside, but take care to lift it by establishment of a pneumoperitoneum.

Attention: The trocar sites are indicated as seen from the patient's view and not from the surgeon's; the left working trocar is therefore inserted left to the patient's middle line (Fig. 2.10).

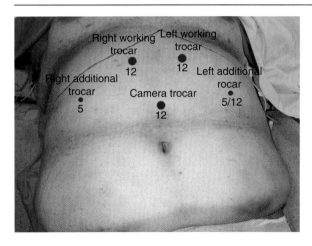

Fig. 2.10 Position of the trocars in relation to the patient

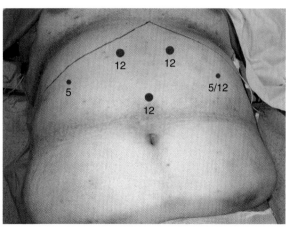

Fig. 2.11 High position of the working trocars

• Insert the first trocar in the middle line above the umbilicus.

> We suggest to insert the optical trocar slightly left of the middle line to avoid having to go through a thick ligamentum teres hepatis. In patients with a BMI under 50 we insert the first trocar a short distance left of the line between the xiphoid and the umbilicus, about one third of the distance above the umbilicus. In patients with a BMI over 50, we place the first trocar a short distance left of the middle between xiphoid and the umbilicus to avoid the optic being "too short."

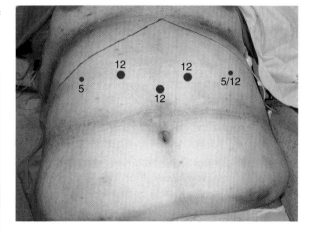

Fig. 2.12 Low position of the working trocars

• Some surgeons prefer five trocars, other use four. They are placed above the umbilicus in the upper abdomen, the exact positioning varying from surgeon to surgeon. Basically a high position is distinguished from a low position.
• For the high position place the working trocars (both 12 mm) left and right of the middle line below the xiphoid (Fig. 2.11). For the low position the trocars are placed much further laterally and lower on the medioclavicular line just under the costal margin (Fig. 2.12). The additional trocars (5 or 12 mm, depending on the graspers and the liver retractor in use) are positioned in the upper abdomen lateral to the medioclavicular line.

> Some surgeons prefer a so called *compact-pyramidal position of the trocars*. The additional trocars are placed, similar to the working trocars in the high position, left and right to the middle line, just below the xiphoid. The working trocars are placed much further down (slightly below the optical trocar) medial to the medioclavicular line (Fig. 2.13).

Surgical Technique: Pars-Flaccida Pathway

After placing the trocars and exploring the abdominal cavity with either an angled or a straight laparoscopic camera the left hepatic lobe is lifted upward

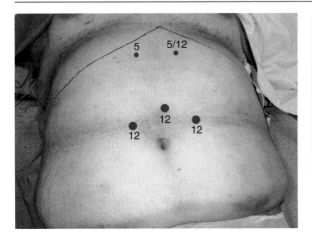

Fig. 2.13 Compact-pyramidal positioning of the trocars in laparascopic gastric banding

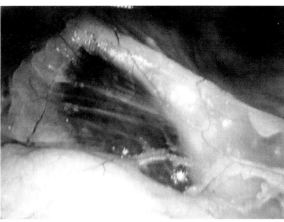

Fig. 2.14 Pars flaccida

and to the right with a liver retractor. The stomach is grasped close to the lesser curvature below the cardia and streched to the left. Now the dissection can be performed.

There are basically three different pathways:
- Pars-flaccida pathway
- Perigastric pathway
- Combined approach (perigastric/pars-flaccida).

Today the pars-flaccida approach is usually chosen. This pathway was developed by Rudolf Weiner (1997) as an alternative to the perigastric pathway and its high rate of complications (stomach perforation, slippage).

Step 1 – Dissection of the Pars Flaccida

- Place the trocars in your preferred position. Grasp the stomach through the left additional trocar with a Babcock forceps just below the cardia close to the lesser curvature and pull it to the left. The pars flaccida (the transparent section of the lesser omentum) is now visible.

Step 2 – Opening the Pars Flaccida

- Cut into the pars flaccida with a cautery hook through the left working trocar (Fig. 2.14). Grasp the perigastric fat tissue through the opened pars flaccida, using the Babcock forceps through the left additional trocar and again pull to the left.

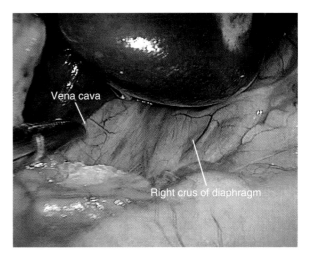

Fig. 2.15 Dissection of the right crus of diaphragm and the vena cava

Take care not to grasp the blood vessels of the lesser curvature!

Step 3 – Dissection of the Right Crus of Diaphragm

- The right crus of diaphragm is now visible.

Not to be confused with the vena cava! (Fig. 2.15).

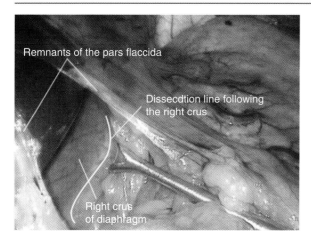

Fig. 2.16   Cutting along the right crus of diaphragm

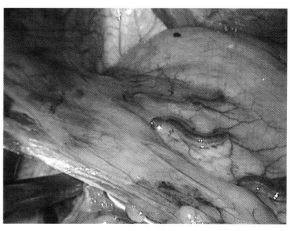

Fig. 2.17   Blunt retrogastric dissection toward the angle of His

Step 4 – Splitting the Peritoneum Along the Medial Edge of the Right Crus of Diaphragm

- Now open the peritoneum with a cautery hook close by and along the right crus of diaphragm, going caudally. To tense the peritoneum, pull the right crus of diaphragm in the opposite direction with an atraumatic grasper through the right working trocar (Fig. 2.16).

Step 5 – Preparation of a Retrogastric Channel

After opening the retroperitoneal space continue the preparation toward the angle of His. You are now between the left crus of diaphragm and the backside of the stomach.

> Do not enter the posterior mediastinal cavity behind the left crus of diaphragm.

- For the blunt dissection use the grasper (right working trocar) and the dissection probe (coagulation suction tube, left working trocar) (Fig. 2.17). To avoid sliding behind the left crus of diaphragm and thereby producing a false tunnel in the posterior mediastinal cavity, always hold the instrument in the right working trocar parallel to the stomach. We avoid producing a too broad retrogastric tunnel.
- Finish dissection in projection to the right angle of His, without cutting the tip of the instrument free

there. Dissection can take place in a practically avascular area. A slight capillary hemorrhage that might occur here will stop spontaneously.

Step 6 – Introducing the Gastric Band into the Abdomen

- After dissection the prepared gastric band is introduced into the abdomen. This can either be done through the working trocar or the working channel left after removal of the working trocar. If using the trocar, insert a guiding rod into the trocar in the left upper abdomen and remove the trocar. Use the rod to then insert a special 18-mm trocar.
- Introduce the gastric band through the "band trocar" (Fig. 2.18). Hold the band by its locking area (not by the tube) with an atraumatic grasper and introduce the stretched band into the abdomen.

> Using a 15 mm "universal" trocar from the start saves changing the trocars.

- The introduction of the band can be done in different ways. One possibility is *from the outside to the inside*: Dilate the working channel with a custom-made rod. Then push the band, held and stretched with an atraumatic grasper, into the abdomen; first the band itself, then the tube (Fig. 2.19). Another possibility is going *from the*

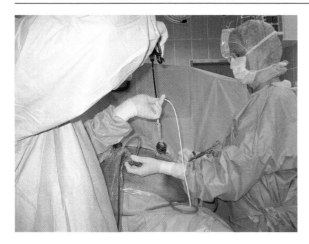

Fig. 2.18 Introduction of the gastric band through the "band trocar" into the abdomen

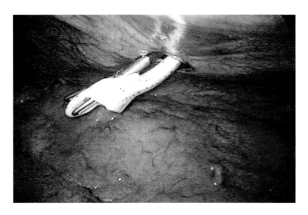

Fig. 2.19 Introduction of the gastric band through the trocar's canal into the abdomen

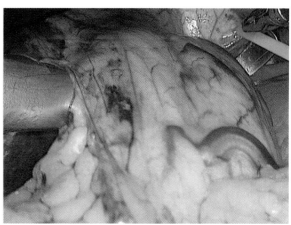

Fig. 2.20 Dissecting the tip of the flexible dissector near the angle of His

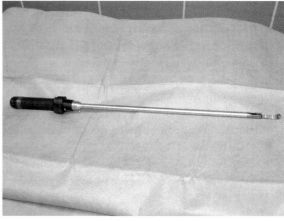

Fig. 2.21 Flexible dissector for the implantation of the lap-band

inside to the outside. Here a grasper, preferably one with a stable tip, is inserted into the abdomen through the right working trocar and out again through the left working (or the additional) trocar. This trocar is then removed, leaving the tip of the grasper showing 5 cm above skin level. Now hold the band by the locking area (not the band itself) and pull it into the abdomen. Then return the removed trocar to its place.

Step 7 – Placing the Band

- Now place the flexible dissector into the before prepared retrogastric tunnel. Dissecting the tip of the dissector near the angle of His free (Fig. 2.20). Technical details may vary at this point depending on the brand of the band.

Some surgeons prefer an atraumatic grasper or a dissector with a markedly bent tip to the flexible dissector.

Implantation of the Lap-Band

- We favor the flexible dissector for the lap-band (Fig. 2.21). The tip features a slot for the strap of the lap-band. Grasp it between the end of the strap and the beginning of the tube with a grasper and pull it into the slot from the in- or the outside.
- Then pull the strap up through the slot up to the beginning of the tube. This maneuver ensures a safe hold of the strap in the slot; it is kept from falling out while the flexible retractor is pulled back.

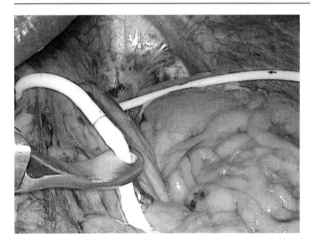

Fig. 2.22   Pulling the band around the backside of the cardia

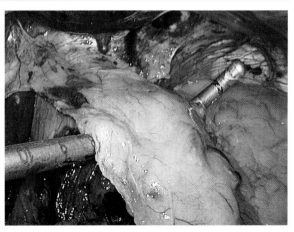

Fig. 2.24   Goldfinger for the placement of an SAGB

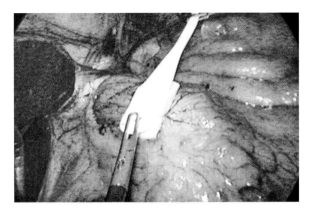

Fig. 2.23   Locking the lap-band

- Then straighten the tip of the articulating dissector and pull the end of the gastric band around the back side of the cardia. Then remove the strap from the slot with a grasper (Fig. 2.22).
- After removing the flexible retractor from the right working trocar insert a second atraumatic grasper. Close the band with the two graspers. The lap-band features a strap at the end; pull it through the loop of the locking mechanism until it is closed completely (Fig. 2.23).

> We do not use a calibration balloon for the creation of the pouch. We consider this step redundant when using the pars-flaccida pathway, because the gastric band is always located at the same place and can hardly move vertically because the preparation tunnel is very narrow.

Implantation of a SAGB

The implantation of a SAGB differs from the procedure for the lap-band in some steps.

- Retrocardiac dissection and placement of the band is performed with the so-called goldfinger instead of a flexible retractor (Fig. 2.24).
- Insert the string attached to the end of the band into the slot at the tip of the device.
- Then straighten the goldfinger and pull the band into the retrogastric tunnel.
- To close the SAGB, insert an atraumatic grasping forcep through the loop of the locking mechanism. Then grasp the other end of the band and close the band. It is not necessary to pull the entire band's tube through the loop.

Step 8 – Anterior Gastroplication

After closing the band, perform an anterior gastroplication to prevent dislocation of the band. Suture the anterior wall of the stomach to the anterior wall of the pouch with several single sutures, using nonabsorbable material. In patients with a large fat pad around the gastroesophageal junction the dissection of the serosa above the band can be difficult.

In patients with a BMI over 50 we deliberately omit anterior gastroplication, because the procedure is often difficult and may lead to serious complications, such as esophageal perforation or hemorrhage from the perigastric tissue. We believe on the other hand that the gastric band is already secured safely in the narrow preparation tunnel (pars-flaccida approach) and the massive perigastric fat tissue, especially the precardial fat pad.

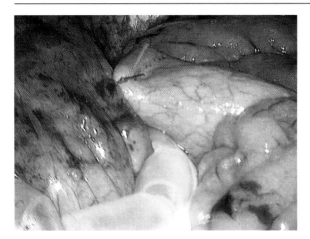

Fig. 2.25 First suture in gastroplication

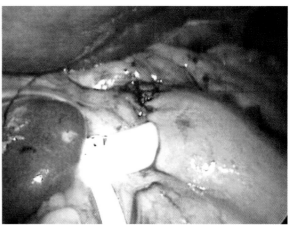

Fig. 2.26 Completed gastroplication

- For precise placement of the suture hold the gastric band with an atraumatic grasper through the left additional trocar close to the locking area. Pull the tube downward diagonally toward the right lower abdomen and hold under slight tension.
- Now grasp the anterior wall of the stomach above the band with a Babcock forceps through the right working trocar and pull cranially. This way the serosa of the stomach wall above the band can be dissected more easily.
- Place four to five single sutures (nonabsorbable).

    We consider it important to place the first suture on the left side (toward the spleen) as far laterally into the fundus as possible (Fig. 2.25).

- The sutures are directed toward the lesser curvature. This way up to five single sutures can easily be placed (Fig. 2.26). We believe that a more effective way of avoiding slippage can be thus achieved, although evident data are not available yet.
- Alternatively the gastric fundus can be sutured to the right crus of diaphragm (three sutures on average). Sometimes, however, the stomach is sutured to tightly over the band, which may lead to a persistent singultus or shoulder pain.

    Never suture the gastric fundus to the anterior wall of the esophagus. This can produce too much tension, resulting in rupture of the sutures, perforation of the esophagus, and consequent complications.

Step 9 – Implantation of the Port

The intraabdominal part of the procedure is finished after anterior gastroplication. The implantation of the port system is next. A careful execution of this part of the procedure is of great importance, as most of the late complications in gastric banding are related to the port system.

The port chamber can be placed on top of the aponeurosis of the rectus abdominis muscle in the left upper abdomen or presternally over the lower third of the sternum. In patients with a BMI under 50, we position the port in the abdominal wall; in patients with a BMI over 50, we chose the presternal location.

A port positioned in the abdominal wall in the widened insertion site of the working trocar is aesthetically more pleasing, an additional incision is not necessary. Inserting a cannula, however, is much more difficult and is usually performed under x-ray or ultrasound control. A presternally positioned port is much easier to puncture, but the port chamber is clearly visible and can cause chronic pain in women, if the elastic band of a bra runs over it.

- The tube is pulled out through one of the trocar insertion sites, depending on the chosen position. We always avoid the insertion site that will hold the port chamber. The tube might tear off due to shear forces resulting from a strong kinking of the tube. For the presternal port position, the tube is pulled out through the left working trocar, for the position in the abdominal wall through the supraumbilical trocar.
- Then the incision is enlarged to about 4–5 cm or a new horizontal incision is made presternally.

When planning a presternal position for the port in women, mark the lower edge of the bra beforehand so that the port chamber can be placed below this line. This way chronic pain which can result from pressure from the bra can be avoided.

- Insert an atraumatic grasper at the port site and move it subcutaneously over to the tube.
- Grasp the end of the tube and pull it back to the prepared pouch. Fasten a suture to the tube, with which it can be pulled back in place after the port chamber is positioned.
- Connect the tube to the port and suture the port chamber per hand or with a stapler to the fascia. Take care to fasten the port chamber straight and securely to keep it from tilting later.

Fastening the port chamber with a stapler is faster than suturing per hand, but the incision must be 1–1.5 cm larger in order to use the stapler correctly.

- After fastening the port pull the excess length of the tube back with the suture. Then remove the suture and push the excess length of the tube back into the abdomen with an atraumatic clamp.
- There are several different stapler systems commercially available, depending on the brand of the band. The implantation of the port chamber is done a little faster with a stapler than per hand, but it requires a slightly larger incision. Insert the chamber into the lower part of the stapler. Then position the stapler onto the fascia, press it down slightly, and fire. The chamber is fastened with the metal clamps in the stapler. So far there are no long-term evaluation data available comparing the fixation of the port chamber with a stapler to a suture performed by hand.

Surgical Technique: Perigastric Pathway

The perigastric pathway has almost completely been abandoned in favor of the pars-flaccida approach today, but in certain situations it can be helpful. We use this technique very rarely in revision procedures after

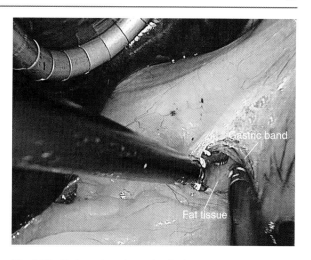

Fig. 2.27 Perigastric pathway, beginning dissection close to the lesser curvature

failed gastric banding, because the technical steps of revision procedures vary greatly, which is why we describe the perigastric pathway as a primary procedure for educational reasons.

- Dissection begins at the lesser curvature just above the first branch of the small curvatur's vessels (crow's foot). The right crus is not dissected (Fig. 2.27).

The crow's foot is not always easily found, especially not in extremely obese patients. In this case a calibration balloon can be used or the exact point of dissection is chosen by intuition.

- If a calibration balloon is used, the tube is introduced into the stomach. Make sure the tip of the tube is inside the stomach by moving it up and down slightly.
- Then fill the balloon with 25 cm^3 of saline and pull it back to the GE junction.
- The tip of the balloon marks the starting point for dissection (Fig. 2.28). When working without a calibration balloon, begin as far cranial as possible and close to the GE junction. Grasp the upper third of the stomach with the Babcock forceps (left additional trocar) and pull to the left toward the spleen.
- Grasp the densely vascularized fat tissue of the lesser curvature with the atraumatic grasper (right working trocar) and pull it toward the liver.

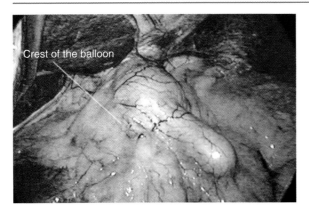

Fig. 2.28 The apex of the calibration balloon at the lesser curvature marks the starting point for dissection

- When sufficient tension is established, begin dissection in the avascular zone between stomach wall and fat tissue. Use a cautery hook or an ultrasound cutter.

  At this point a slight diffuse hemorrhage occurs usually, which stops spontaneously. Injury of a blood vessel at the lesser curvature however leads to massive bleeding, which can be quite difficult to control. The bleeding vessel must be secured tightly with ultrasound scissors or clips.

- The dissection tunnel should be narrow (only about as wide as the band itself) and run above the omental bursa at all times. After skeletonizing a small section of the lesser curvature, proceed to blunt dissection toward the angle of His, staying close to the stomach wall.

  We avoid the use of monopolar electricity or the ultrasound scissors within the retrogastric tunnel in order to protect the stomach wall from thermal injury.

- The slight diffuse hemorrhage that may occur during blunt dissection stops spontaneously. A coagulation hook is very rarely ever needed.
- After reaching the fat tissue on the opposite side, insert a flexible dissector or a "goldfinger" into the retrogastric tunnel. Dissect the tip of the instrument in the angle of His.
- Continue as above (pars-flaccida pathway).

Difficult Situations and Intraoperative Complications

Troublesome intraoperative situations during gastric banding can result from hemorrhage, anatomic abnormalities, injury of organs, or difficulties during dissection.

> There is a direct correlation between the patient's BMI and the difficulty of the procedure.

Hemorrhage

Hemorrhage occurs mostly through an injury of the left hepatic lobe with the liver retractor. Patients with a massive fatty liver (BMI over 50, long standing morbid obesity) are especially at risk. A fatty liver is easily injured by simply positioning the liver retractor or through the retracting force, but the enlarged hepatic lobe makes it difficult to get an overview of the surgical field. In an effort to see better, the hepatic lobe is pulled to the right with great force, which can result in deep tears of the liver tissue with massive hemorrhage. It can be stopped using a coagulatory hook or argon plasma coagulation without having to switch to an open conventional surgical approach. These hematostatic measures however prolong the procedure substantially.

To avoid this situation, the liver retractor should always be positioned under visual control. The retracting force of the instrument should always be distributed evenly over the backside of the liver. The retractor should always be held parallel to the bottom surface of the liver. Avoid applying high pressure to the edges of the liver during traction.

Anatomic Particularities and Difficulties During Dissection

The correct dissection of the surgical field can be difficult in patients with a high BMI. This is the result of a massively enlarged left hepatic lobe and marked perigastric fat tissue. Some bariatric surgeons do not perform gastric banding in patients with very massive obesity. Surgeons who do not fix any limits of BMI are confronted with this problem time and again.

A massively enlarged liver lobe is always in the way. A second liver retractor can be helpful here. One is introduced through the trocar in the right upper abdomen, another through a trocar in the epigastrium. An additional assistant will be necessary.

An experienced camera guide is of great importance. A very large left hepatic lobe simply cannot be retracted to the right sufficiently. To show a surgical field, the camera must be inserted under the liver. The camera guiding assistant must be able to produce a more or less sufficient image of a small operation field and keep the camera from fogging at the same time.

In rare cases, massive perigastric fat tissue prohibits the identification of the pars flaccida and the right crus of diaphragm altogether. The perigastric approach can be chosen here, but this option comes with a higher risk of intraoperative complications, such as hemorrhage from the perigastric tissue and perforation of the stomach wall. Before choosing the perigastric pathway, every option to perform the pars-flaccida technique should be explored.

- Assign an additional assistant. Place one or two additional working trocars in the left middle and upper abdomen.
- Pull the stomach toward the spleen with a grasper (left additional working trocar), holding it proximally close to the lesser curvature.
- Insert another grasper through the other additional working trocar and pull the lesser omentum also toward the spleen.
- Push the lateral parts of the lesser omentum toward the liver with the third grasper (right working trocar) and cut it with a cautery hook through the left working trocar.
- Now grasp the perigastric fat tissue (grasper through the left additional working trocar) and pull it toward the spleen.
- Then the right crus must be identified. If successful, use the pars-flaccida pathway, and implant an extra long gastric band.

If the right crus cannot be identified and the pars-flaccida pathway cannot be used, the perigastric approach is chosen as the very last option.

Early Postoperative Complications After Gastric Banding

Injuries of the backside of the stomach can occur with the perigastric approach. The number of stomach perforations has been reduced drastically by following the pars-flaccida pathway.

A *perforation of the esophagus* can occur with either technique. It is often discovered only postoperatively, with grave consequences for the patient. We believe this to be the result of a gastroesophageal instead of a gastrogastral suture during anterior gastroplication. In patients with a massive fat pad the anterior stomach wall cannot always be dissected. Some surgeons then suture the anterior stomach wall below the band to the anterior wall of the esophagus above the band. If the resulting tension is too high, this suture might break and lead to esophagus perforation. We strictly avoid gastroesophageal sutures. If the anterior wall of the stomach above the band cannot be identified, we do not perform an anterior gastroplication at all. We do not recommend suturing the stomach wall to the diaphragm, because of the danger of accidentally injuring the phrenic nerve, which can lead to persistent singultus and shoulder pain.

Therapy of a ruptured esophagus varies depending on the symptoms and extent of the damage. A conservative therapy (esophageal stent and thoracic drain) may be considered; in other cases a surgical procedure, either laparoscopic or conventional, needs to be performed.

Revision Procedures

Intraoperative complications are very rare in gastric banding, but revision procedures for late complications are necessary more often and remain a so far unsolved problem for this procedure. The procedures are performed either as emergency- or urgent operations (in complications such as slippage or band migration) or planned in cases of a malfunction of the band or inadequate weight loss.

A Water-Soluble Contrast Swallow, Performed Because of Dysphagia Even After Complete Opening of the Band, Reveals Slippage of the Band

Predisposing factors: Slippage of the band is a typical complication after gastric banding, which was very common with the perigastric approach. Weiner defines three different types of slippage: anterior, posterior, or combined. The number of cases has been reduced drastically since the introduction of the pars-flaccida pathway and the character of the slippage,

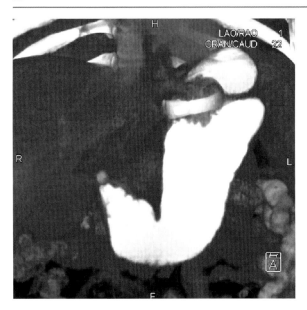

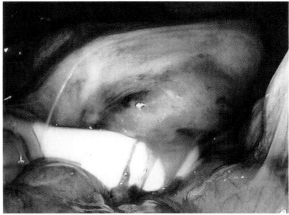

Fig. 2.30 Intraoperative picture of slippage after gastric banding

Fig. 2.29 X-ray showing anterior slippage after gastric banding (pars-flaccida approach)(Courtesy of Dr. Ingrid Harth, Radiologisches Institut, Kreiskrankenhaus Eschwege)

too, has changed. The anterior type is seen in these cases, with a part of the fundus or the anterior wall of the stomach gliding upward through the band. Depending on the clinical situation and the result of the water-soluble contrast swallow, a complete or incomplete slippage is diagnosed. With complete slippage, patients tolerate neither solids nor liquids, everything is regurgitated immediately. The water-soluble contrast swallow shows a complete stop above the band with no entrance of contrast into the rest of the stomach. In an incomplete slippage, a small amount of liquid may pass. The enlarged pouch will often be tilted to the front; the passage of contrast through the rest of the stomach will be slowed (Figs. 2.29 and 2.30).

Prevention: The introduction of the pars-flaccida technique has reduced the rate of slippages dramatically, but the problem is not completely solved. Many authors suggest various tricks and ruses to avoid slippage. Some of them are described in the following chapter. Tried and tested techniques to avoid slippage are:
• A narrow retrogastric tunnel (not wider than the band)
• At least five sutures for gastroplication (if possible)

Management: If slippage of the band is diagnosed, an emergency procedure must be performed because of the danger of ischemia and necrosis of the pouch. In case of an incomplete slippage, the procedure is to be performed urgently, because an incomplete slippage can turn into a complete slippage any time.

In *slippage after using the perigastric pathway* we remove the band and produce completely new tunnel with the pars-flaccida approach. If the band is still in working order, it is reused; if not, a new band should be implanted.

In *slippage after using the pars-flaccida pathway* we perform an endoscopic reposition of the stomach. Position of the patient, creation of the pneumoperitoneum, and placing of the trocars are done as usual. Preferably the old scars are used for placement of the trocars. If the port chamber was placed in the left upper abdomen, take care to not damage the tube while placing the trocars.

Step 1 – Transection Adhesions Between the Liver and the Lesser Curvature
• After placing the trocars identify the tube and follow it from the abdominal wall to the band.
• Then cut the scar tissue between the left hepatic lobe and the lesser curvature. The amount of tissue ranges from small transparent adhesions to thick layers of connective tissue. Several different techniques can be applied to transect the adhesions. We use an atraumatic grasper and scissors for dissection and cutting and a coagulation hook.

Step 2 – Opening the Gastric Band Tunnel and Dissection of the Lock

- After removing the adhesions dissect the locking mechanism of the band. If the procedure was performed correctly before, the lock is close to the lesser curvature.

> The operation protocol of the original procedure should be studied carefully before a revision procedure. It is important to know which kind of band was implanted in order to plan the following steps.

- The band and part of the tube close to it are foreign bodies and therefore covered with a fibrous capsule. If the band is to be reused, take care not to damage it irreversibly while transection of a fibrous capsule.
- Cut the outer layers of the fibrous capsule with scissors.
- Then open the fibrous tissue with an endodissector, until a part of the band is visible.
- Now open the capsule completely under visual control and dissect the locking mechanism.

Step 3 – Dissolving the Anterior Gastroplication

- After opening the gastric band tunnel and dissecting the locking mechanism dissolve the anterior gastroplication. There are several ways of doing so: Some surgeons cut close to the suture line with scissors. If the band has been in place for several years, it can be difficult to identify the suture line; cutting will open the stomach or produce a massive hemorrhage. We open the anterior gastroplication with a linear cutter (Endo-GIA, blue cartridge).

Step 4 – Reposition of the Dislocated Portions of the Stomach

After dissolving the anterior gastroplication reposition the dislocated parts of the stomach.
- Grasp the tube close to the band with an atraumatic grasper (right working trocar) and lift the band.
- Insert the other grasper (or preferably a Babcock forceps) (left working trocar) between the stomach wall and the band, moving upward. Grasp the protruding parts of the stomach and push them back under the band. This maneuver is, however, rarely

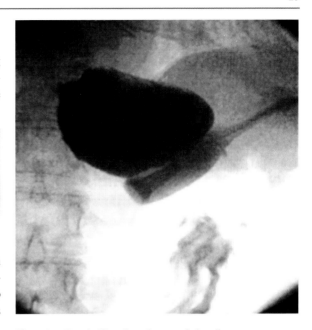

Fig. 2.31 Pouch dilatation after gastric banding

successful, which is why you should rather open the band and close it again after reposition.

Step 5 – Regastroplication

- After repositioning the stomach, perform a regastroplication. The gastro-gastric sutures are easy to place, because the stomach wall is stretched after slippage. After reposition and closure of the band, parts of the stomach can easily be pulled up over the band and sutured to wall of the pouch.
- After performing the anterior gastroplication the procedure is completed.

Dysphagia: A Water-Soluble Contrast Swallow Reveals Marked Pouch Dilatation

Predisposing factors: Inappropriate eating habits (binge-eating, compulsive eating), insufficient aftercare, and a too tight band. These factors are often combined and result in dilatation of the pouch.

Prevention: The best prophylaxis of pouch enlargement is regular follow-up examinations and timely reaction to signs of inadequate function of the band.

Diagnostic measures: If a pouch enlargement is suspected, perform a water-soluble contrast swallow. An enlargement of the pouch (without anterior tilt of the stomach) with slow passage of the contrast is usually seen in these cases (Fig. 2.31).

Management: Pouch dilatation is at first treated conservatively. The band must be opened completely and adjusted after 6 weeks. Patients should be put on a liquid diet to avoid massive weight gain during this period. After 6 weeks the band is refilled and the patient is followed-up closely. If the pouch dilates again, a surgical revision procedure is indicated (conversion into a gastric bypass or duodenal switch, gastric sleeve resection with or without removing the band or removal of the band without other procedures).

Large Amounts of Food Are Tolerated, Although the Band Is Filled and Has Been Readjusted, Intermittent "Black" Stool, Gastroscopy Reveals Intraluminal Position of a Part of the Band

Predisposing factors: The perigastric pathway definitely is a predisposing factor for these complications. Band erosions belong to the past since the introduction of the pars-flaccida pathway. The importance of other factors, such as "band too tight," "unconventional" band, port infection etc., is not scientifically proven.

Prevention: These complications can be avoided by choosing the pars-flaccida approach and "established" band brands, such as the Lap-band or the SAGB.

Management: After diagnosing band migration, the band must be removed. This is followed by another bariatric procedure to avoid excessive weight gain. If this is to be done in one operation, there are in our opinion two possibilities: a distal gastric bypass and the duodenal switch, because the operation field is far away from the migration site. We favor the distal gastric bypass, because the procedure is much easier done laparoscopic than an endoscopic duodenal switch. If the bariatric procedure is performed later, other techniques, such as the classic (proximal) gastric bypass or a sleeve gastrectomy can be performed.

If the original band was implanted through the perigastric pathway, it can easily be rebanded using the pars-flaccida approach.

Technically the removal of the migrated band is similar to band removal in case of a slippage:

- After dissection of the fibrous capsule around the band, open it to show a part of the band.

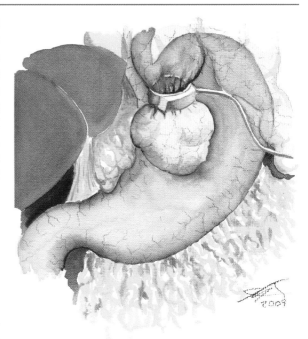

Fig. 2.32 Gastric band in a "pregastral" position

- Cut the band and remove it from the tunnel, which is by now sealed with fibrous tissue; nothing else has to be done here.

Some surgeons insist on suturing the band tunnel and the opening in the stomach wall. We believe this to be impossible and also unnecessary. The "classic" damage through band migration is situated at the back of the stomach deep inside the band tunnel and cannot be reached without major dissection work. The damage also does not reach the open abdominal cavity, but opens only into the usually rather thick fibrous tissue around the band.

- We do not position a drain tube after removal of the gastric band.

Band Cannot Be Tightened, a Water-Soluble Contrast Swallow Reveals "Pregastric" Position of the Band

Predisposing factors: This situation can occur after using the pars-flaccida-technique (Fig. 2.32). Predisposing factors are a high BMI and massive perigastric fat tissue. In very obese patients, the flexible dissector or the goldfinger can accidentally be positioned between the anterior stomach wall and the perigastric fat tissue. The tip of the retractor is dissected in the angle of His; the band is positioned and closed around perigastric fat tissue.

Prevention: This complication happens to the unexperienced bariatric surgeon. Difficulties of the procedure due to extreme obesity, such as excessive perigastric fat tissue, a large left hepatic lobe or a "too short" optic lead to a complicated and confusing situation. The surgeon must be very sure to insert the flexible dissector or the goldfinger behind the GE junction toward the angle of His. A calibration tube, inserted into the stomach during the procedure, can be helpful. The wall of the esophagus can be identified during the insertion; the instrument can then be guided around the GE junction.

Management: A faultily placed band does not have a restricting effect and needs to be removed or repositioned. An undamaged band can be reused.

A Water-Soluble Contrast Swallow Reveals Excessive Esophageal Dilatation

Predisposing factors: In some patients with normal band position and adequate adjustment of the band, an esophageal dilatation after gastric banding is seen; a late stage of the so-called gastric band-induced pseudo-achalasia. The main reason is inadequate eating habits; the patient eats much more than can fit through the adequately tightened band and then has to regurgitate due to esophageal congestion.

Prevention: This complication arises when an unsuitable patient receives a gastric band. There are, however, no reliable criteria by which to decide which patient is "suitable." The only way to reduce the incidence of this complication is consequent and close lifelong monitoring.

If a patient complains about daily nausea and vomiting, he is to be considered at risk for esophageal dilatation and must be monitored closely. If everything (band adjustment, counseling, behavior therapy) has been tried and nausea still persists, the band must be opened for a longer period of time or removed altogether.

Management: If the above mentioned conservative measures do not help, a revision procedure is indicated, which can be anything from a simple removal of the band up to conversion procedures for a gastric bypass or a duodenal switch.

Inadequate Weight Loss or "Band Intolerance"

Predisposing factors: Inadequate weight loss and the so-called band intolerance are the most frequent reasons for late revision procedures after gastric banding. Two groups of patients can be distinguished: In the first group band position and band function (ease of adjustment) are normal. Patients with band malfunction belong to the second group (difficult port puncture, frequent need of adjustment, no lasting tightening possible without leakage, or disconnection of the tube), as well as those with unwanted anatomical changes, such as beginning slippage and beginning pouch or esophageal dilatation. The two groups are described separately in the following.

Management: The following revision procedures are possible in cases of inadequate weight loss or "band intolerance":

- Removal of the gastric band
- Repositioning of the gastric band
- Addition of another bariatric procedure, such as "banded" gastric bypass or a "banded" sleeve gastrectomy
- Removal of the band and performance of another bariatric procedure, such as a gastric bypass or a duodenal switch

Weight Gain, a Water-Soluble Contrast Swallow Confirms Correct Band Position and Adjustment Without Leakage

Predisposing factors: The role of a patient history of clinical depression, binge eating, or sweet eating is discussed controversially.

Prevention: This situation is obviously due to the patient's inadequate eating habits. There are so far no valid criteria available to identify potential "failures" beforehand.

Management: If a revision procedure is indicated, either an addition of another bariatric procedure (such as "banded" gastric bypass or "banded" sleeve gastrectomy) can be considered or the removal of the band and the performance of another bariatric procedure, such as a gastric bypass or a duodenal switch.

Frequent Nausea, Tolerance for Liquids Only, Tight Band, Rapid Weight Gain After Band Adjustment; Repeated Tightening Leads to More Frequent Nausea Again, No Improvement After Several Repetitions; a Water-Soluble Contrast Swallow Reveals a Beginning Pouch Enlargement

Predisposing factors: These complaints are called "band intolerance." The factors leading to this condition are so far unknown.

Prevention: We use the rule "under 40, under 50," meaning that patients aged under 40 and with a BMI under 50 have a better outcome after gastric banding than older patients with a higher BMI. There is not much scientific evidence for this theory; it should be tested in a controlled prospective study.

Management: If a revision procedure is indicated, a band removal with or without the performance of another bariatric procedure (gastric bypass or duodenal switch) can be considered.

Pain and Redness Around the Port Chamber with Clinical Signs of an Infection

Predisposing factors: The development of an infection of the port chamber early after the implantation is usually due to faulty implantation technique without strict consideration of the rules of hygiene or it is due to a postoperatively infected hematoma around the port chamber. If the infection occurs later, the reason can either be a contamination of the port chamber during adjustment or an ascending infection after band erosion.

Prevention: The implantation of the port chamber is a very important part of gastric banding, considering that up to 25% of all patients who receive a gastric band need revision procedures because of port-related problems. But it is probably quite customary for the surgeon to leave after the intraabdominal part of the procedure and let the assistant perform the implantation of the port chamber. We recommend to have the implantation of the port chamber done by an experienced bariatric surgeon. Careful intraoperative hemostasis, strictly aseptic conditions, and the mandatory application of subcutaneous sutures on top of the fastened port chamber help reduce the number of early postoperative port infections.

Management: Port infection is a serious complication that requires the complete removal of the gastric band in many cases (Fig. 2.33). If the infection occurs late and is due to band erosion, removal of the band is

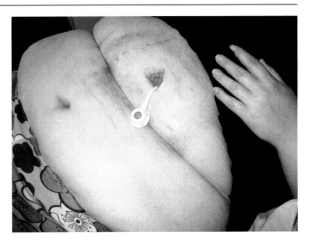

Fig. 2.33 Loose port chamber after persistent infection of the port chamber. This patient refused to have a revision procedure for a long time and continued using the port, fastened to the skin with surgical dressing

the only choice (see therapy band erosion). If the infection occurs early after the procedure, there is a chance to save the band. We recommend to remove the infected port chamber, close the end of the tube with a suture and push it into the abdomen. These patients must be monitored closely. When there are no signs of an infection any more or signs of a band erosion, a new port chamber is implanted. The end of the tube is pulled out of the abdomen in a minilaparoscopic procedure and connected to the new port chamber. If the end of the tube cannot be found, perform a laparoscopy to identify the tube.

Port Puncture Impossible: An X-Ray Reveals a Flipped Chamber

Predisposing factors: The port chamber tilts or flips over the most often if fastened to the aponeurosis of the rectus abdominis muscle in the left upper abdomen. Other predisposing factors are fastening the chamber onto fat tissue instead of onto the aponeurosis or using less than four sutures. So far there are no long-term data available regarding the influence of stapler systems on the rate of flipped over port chambers.

Prevention: We recommend positioning the port chamber presternally in patients with a BMI over 45. Less subcutaneous fat tissue and a more "taut" skin help secure the chamber tightly within the surrounding tissue. The thinner subcutaneous fat layer also facilitates the even placement of the sutures within the fascia. We recommend placing all four sutures within the planned pouch first, positioning the port chamber next and tying the knots afterward.

Management: If the port chamber is flipped over, it must be turned back into the correct position in a revision procedure. If it flips again, it should be repositioned from the left upper abdomen to a presternal position.

2.1 Surgical Technique by Wendy A. Brown and Andrew I. Smith (Australia)

Wendy A. Brown and Andrew I. Smith

Preparation

Setting, Positioning, and the Surgical Team

- The patient is positioned in the lithotomy position. We use a table with either a buttock support or an adjustable seat as the patient will ultimately be tilted head-up to around 45°.
- The legs are supported in stirrups with the knees angled toward the opposite shoulder. The legs must be kept relatively low so that when the operator is between the legs their arms and instruments do not clash with the legs.
- The surgeon will stand between the patient's legs. The assistant surgeon will stand on the patient's left and the scrub nurse will be between the assistant and the surgeon on the patient's left.
- The screen and the laparoscopic stack are at the top of the bed on the patient's right, with diathermy also on that side. The leads for the camera and the insufflator are secured at the top end of the operative field; the lead for the laparoscopic diathermy comes across to be placed in a sheath on the patient's right hip.

> We pin the hand-held diathermy on the top drape separate to the camera leads so that it will be retained at the end of the case when other equipment is passed off.

- The post for securing the liver retractor should be positioned at the level of the costal margin on the patient's right.
- Betadine is used to prepare the skin.

> We prepare the skin widely from the level of the nipple line down to the pubis in case an open procedure is required.

- The operative field is square draped from the nipple line to below the umbilicus.

> We do not use "booties" for the leg as we find these impossible to place in a clean manor in the obese. Instead, we use a large drape over each leg and then a drape across the pelvic region.

- We do not routinely use suction; however, we have it available in the theatre.
- We prefer to have a Mayo table behind the surgeon so that we may take the graspers we require. We also have a warmer for the laparoscope to be easily accessible for the assistant surgeon.
- Our patients will generally have their blood pressure monitored with a non-invasive cuff on the upper arm. Only rarely is an arterial line inserted. Intravenous access is via a peripheral line.
- DVT prophylaxis consists of subcutaneous low molecular weight heparin on induction and all patients wear compression stockings. Sequential calf compression devices are used only for high risk patients.

> We choose antibiotics to cover skin and bowel organisms. Most commonly this is flucloxacillin and ceftriaxone as a single dose on induction.

- A patient warming device is placed above the nipple line.
- The anesthetist passes a calibration tube orally that will be used to check the position of the band during the operation.

Trocar Placement and Pneumoperitoneum

- We make a 5-mm incision just below the left costal margin at a 45° angle from the umbilicus. Further port positions are as shown in the diagram below (Fig. 2.34).
- We will generally make these incisions prior to insufflation. If, however, the patient has a deep waist crease or if we are unable to palpate their

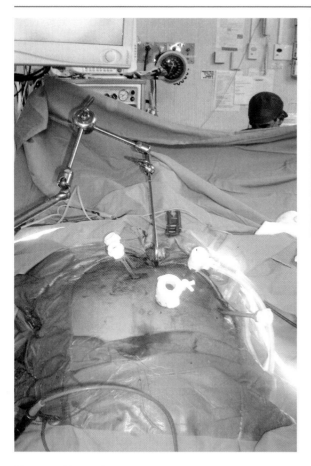

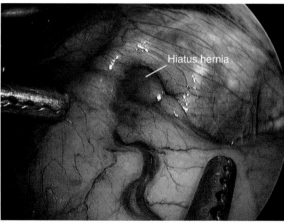

Fig. 2.35 Hiatus hernia

- The Nathanson retractor is then passed with the arm facing toward the patient's left. After the stem is inserted, it is rotated into place and the liver gently retracted toward the patient's right shoulder.
- After the liver is retracted, three further 5-mm ports and a 15-mm port are introduced. All are long ports, and are angled toward the hiatus.

Surgical Technique with Hiatoplasty

- The camera is placed in port 1. Atraumatic graspers are placed in ports 3 and 6.
- The hiatus is assessed and if a hiatus hernia is known, or if laxity is found intraoperatively, then the hiatus is explored. If no hernia is seen, then the hiatus is not explored and I would proceed to simply opening the angle of His.
- In this case, the patient was known to have a hiatus hernia. In Fig. 2.35 it can be seen that there is a clear hiatus hernia.
- To dissect out the hiatus, the angle of His is displayed by retracting the fundus with the retractor in trocar 6, and esophago-gastric fat pad with the retractor in trocar 3.
- Using the hook diathermy, dissection starts at the point where the peritoneal reflection of the esophago-gastric fat pad is clearly at the level of the spleen, above the first short gastric artery. The peritoneum is divided along the line of the left crus.
- The left crus is then completely cleared using blunt dissection, and the dissection is continued on to the

Fig. 2.34 Trocar placement

ribs, we do not site the subsequent ports until insufflation is achieved as we find that we can place them more appropriately once a pneumoperitoneum is in place.

- We currently use a 5-mm optical separating device to enter the peritoneal cavity in the left upper quadrant. This requires a 0° telescope.
- Insufflation with CO_2 is commenced at low flow (3 l/min) after confirming the catheter is in the peritoneal cavity. If the patient tolerates low flow, high flow (20 l/min) is used for the rest of the case to a maximal intraabdominal pressure of 15 mmHg.
- The patient is then tilted to a head-up position.
- The 0° laparoscope is changed to a 30° angled laparoscope which has been warming in hot water.
- The next instrument placed is the Nathanson liver retractor. Using the epigastric incision, a 5-mm trocar is used to make a pathway. This should enter the patient at a 90° angle to the skin and should be at the level of the liver edge.

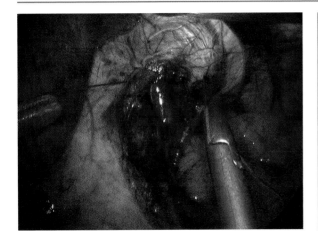

Fig. 2.36 An anterior crural repair is performed using 2/0 Ethibond in a U-shaped stitch

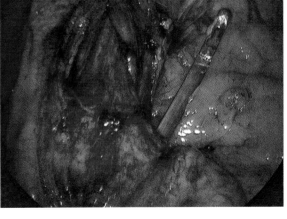

Fig. 2.37 The tip of the placer is seen in the angle of His. If less than 2.5 cm of the end of the placer is visible then a larger band size is selected

right crus. Once the crura are cleared, the esophagus is readily displayed.

- An anterior crural repair is performed using 2/0 Ethibond in a figure of 8 stitch (Fig. 2.36).
- The pars flaccida is then opened using the hook diathermy and a point just anterior to the right crus is chosen to start the dissection behind the esophagus. This is usually at the level of a line of fat crossing the base of the right crus.
- With an atraumatic grasper, retract the lesser curve fat from trocar 6.
- A blunt-nosed retractor is passed through trocar 3 and is gently advanced in front of the right crus from this point. It should pass easily.
- A lap-band placer is then passed through the same pathway via trocar 4. It is a curved instrument with a blunt end and an eye at the tip. At the beginning of the passage the convexity should face caudally. As it is gently advanced, it is rotated clockwise, so that the convexity faces cephalad.
- The tip of the placer is seen in the angle of His. It is essential that the placer comes out accurately at this point.
- The placer is then pushed through (Fig. 2.37). If less than 2.5 cm of the end of the placer is visible then a larger band size is selected.
- The band is primed with normal saline and the end of the tubing is cut at an oblique angle before introducing it into the abdomen through the 15-mm port. The tubing is then threaded through the eye of the placer.

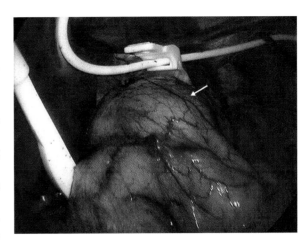

Fig. 2.38 Balloon at the end of the calibration tube, filled with 20 cm³ of air

- The placer is pulled back through to the lesser curve side. The tubing is therefore delivered through a pathway behind the esophago-gastric junction, above the lesser sac. By pulling the tubing through along this pathway, the band is placed correctly.
- Prior to closing the band the position is confirmed by passing an orogastric calibration tube. The end of this tube has a balloon on it. This is inflated with 20 cm³ of air after the tube is seen to pass through the esophago-gastric junction and into the stomach. The whole catheter is then gently pulled back until the balloon lodges at the esophago-gastric junction. The band should be seen to be lying at the equator of this balloon. This also allows us to check for hiatus herniae that may have previously been missed (Fig. 2.38).

- After confirming the position, the oro-gastric calibration tubing is removed and the band is closed.
We pull the tubing out of the body through trocar 4
and secure it to the drapes with an artery forceps so
that the buckle rotates out of the way for suturing.
We cover the exposed tubing with a betadine soaked
gauze.
- The fundus is then secured around the band by a
series of interrupted gastro-gastric sutures. We usually use 2/0 Ethibond on an atraumatic needle. We
use trocar 6 for the needle holder, and use a blunt
nosed instrument through trocar 3 as the other suturing tool. I place an atraumatic grasper through trocar 5 and use this to retract the fundus so that we
can clearly see the most lateral point on the fundus.
This is where I start my suture line
- The suture is completed into gastric tissue above
the band. If the gastric wall cannot be clearly seen,
it is important to retract or remove the esophago-
gastric fat pad so that it is well displayed. Otherwise
there is a danger that the suture will secure the band
across the esophagus and no gastric pouch will be
created.
- Generally three gastro-gastric sutures are used to
secure the fundus around the band. Take care to not
have these sutures under tension, and the sutures
should not impinge on the buckle devise of the
band, as these factors are thought to contribute to
band erosion.
- One suture is placed below the band. This gastro-
gastric suture apposes the tissue from the medial
edge of the folded fundus to the lesser curve – the
band tubing is reintroduced into the abdomen and
the buckle is rotated to sit in front of the lesser
curve. If the band is left rotated, revisional surgery
is much more difficult. The band tubing is then
passed out through trocar 5 (Fig. 2.39).
- The laparoscopic equipment is now passed off and
the trocars removed.
- The port is primed with normal saline. It is connected to the band tubing.
- The skin incision at trocar 5 is extended, and the
anterior rectus sheath is displayed by blunt dissection. Often Scarpa's fascia is very dense at this
point, so care must be taken to ensure that the correct layer is displayed. An area inferior to the exit
point of the tubing is cleared. It is important that the
tubing gently drops into the abdomen. If the angle
of entry into the abdomen is too acute the tubing is

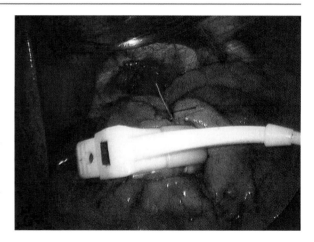

Fig. 2.39 Completed placement of a gastric band

in danger of cracking. The port is secured to the
anterior rectus sheath with either 2/0 Prolene sutures
or with one of the commercially available stapling
devices.
- Deep tissues are closed with vicryl and the skin is
closed with subcuticular monocryl. If the patient
has a particularly heavy apron, then we will generally reinforce the port incision with interrupted
prolene sutures.

2.2 Surgical Technique by Leonid Lantsberg (Israel)

Leonid Lantsberg

Introduction

Keep it simple and stupid (KISS). As long as you
follow the simple principles and rules and avoid doing
stupid mistakes, the chances of getting into trouble
with this surgical procedure are very little. My preferred technique is the pars-flaccida approach, which
is used to overcome the problems associated with the
perigastric technique.

Preparation

Setting, Positioning, and the Surgical Team

Instrument requirements:
- One "Goldfinger"
- Two atraumatic graspers

- Two needle holders
- A 45° scope

Suction and electrocautery are needed in rare cases and should be requested only if necessary during the procedure.

- The patient lies on the operating table in the "French position" (surgeon standing between the patient's legs), head up 20°–30°, and tilted to the right (left shoulder up) 10°–15°.
- A five trocar approach is used (three 10 mm and two 5 mm) to obtain pars flaccida retrogastric blunt dissection to create a tunnel for the band.

> If the patient has a big left liver lobe (mainly males) introd uce a sixth trocar in advance and ask for a second assistant.

- Have a constant contact with the anesthetist; if the patient shows bradycardia, hypotension, or desaturation (due to ventilation difficulties) reduce or deflate the abdomen completely until the problem is resolved.
- Good abdominal wall muscle relaxation is mandatory for achieving a free intraabdominal maneuver environment. In a patient with a "heavy abdominal wall" (highly resistant to insufflations) increase the insufflation pressure up to 18 mmHg.

Trocar Placement

A Veress needle is usually inserted in the left upper quadrant, but if the patient has a scar from previous surgery, keep away from it as far as possible.

Insert the first trocar for the camera high enough so you can reach the appropriate structures (such as GE junction, crus of diaphragm etc.) usually around 20–25 cm below the xiphoid.

> Use the length of your palm as a measure for the distance below the xiphoid to the point of the trocar insertion.

- A 10-mm trocar will be inserted next in the left upper quadrant in anterior axillary line below 10th rib. This trocar is used for stomach fundus retraction and its inlet is used for band introduction into the abdominal cavity in later stages of the operation.

- Two 5-mm working trocars are inserted approximately at the crossing of the midclavicular and hypogastric lines on each side.
- The last 10-mm trocar is inserted through a transverse subxiphoidal incision and is used for retraction of the left hepatic lobe by a single grasper and for subcutaneous presternal pocket creation for the port positioning at the end of the procedure.

Surgical Technique: Pars-Flaccida Approach (SABG)

- Identification of the left crus is achieved by disruption of the gastrophrenic ligament through a small 1–1.5 cm dissection created by a "goldfinger."

> The size of the dissection is crucial since a preserved gastrophrenic ligament is used as a band-anchor, in an attempt to minimize the incidence of slippage.

- Now open the pars flaccida just anterior to the caudate lobe of liver followed by the identification of the right crus.
- Create a retrogastric tunnel under direct vision by using a "goldfinger" and a needle holder and gently progress toward retro/supragastric fat which is recognized by the typical yellow color.
- Only when reaching the fat pad the surgeon will bend the "goldfinger" (the right side assistant should simultaneously grip and pull the fundus downward using atraumatic forceps). The tip of the "goldfinger" should appear superior and posterior to the fundus without any additional tissue on it.

Rules for the creation of the retrogastric tunnel
- Gentle, cautious, and powerless smooth motions toward the GE junction behind the posterior gastric wall will prevent gastric wall perforation.
- The tunnel should be created high enough, just above the lesser sac, in order to prevent the possibility of posterior slippage (no need for a gastrostenometer once experience in the procedure has been gained).

Intrabdominal Band Introduction

- Opening the gastric band kit only after the completion of the retrogastric tunnel will prevent wasting bands which will not be inserted for different uncommon intraoperative situations (such as inability to create the tunnel, bleeding, perforations etc.) and will also minimize band exposure, thus decreasing the risk of infection. Preparation of the band on the bedside table before insertion should include examination of band's integrity (water filling or vacuum tests), the addition of a thread loop when necessary (for specific modules in which this is not built in) and creation of a notch at the distal edge of the connecting tube in order to preserve the band vacuum in a flattened position for the whole procedure.
- Remove the 10 mm left upper sided trocar.
- The flattened band should be mounted on a needle holder and inserted intraabdominally through the same inlet.

Positioning of the Band

- Anchor the thread loop on the "goldfinger" groove and pull the "goldfinger" under direct vision from the exit site.

> Be sure that no excessive tissue exists between the band and the gastric wall at the point of exit.
>
> The use of excessive force or lack of visualization during this maneuver may lead to a tear of the thread loop or the band and in worse cases induce gastric wall damage.
>
> If the band does not progress smoothly through the tunnel, stop pulling! Extract the band from the tunnel and recreate the tunnel using the "goldfinger."

Band Closure

- Band closure should be accomplished by using its mechanism followed by a visual and manual confirmation of a good seal Buckles should be directed toward the liver.

> In my experience, no gastro-gastric or gastro-phrenic sutures are required for band fixation. It does not seem to reduce the anterior slippage rate and further more even increases the risk of intragastric band migration.

- After locking the band, be sure it is positioned in a loose and appropriate manner so that no additional structures are incarcerated between the band and the stomach. If the band is too large (VANGUARD or AP-LARGE for example), 2–3 cc of saline should be injected into the band in order to prevent acute gastric incarceration due to band slippage which will require emergency reoperation.

> If at any stage of the procedure a loss of vacuum or injected fluids is detected, the band has a puncture and should be replaced by a new one. For this reason and others, always have a spare band at hand.

Connection of the Band to the Port

- Retrieve the connecting tube through the epigastric port using grasping forceps.
- Deflate the abdomen and create a subcutaneous presternal pocket by hand.
- Clamp the connecting tube and cut the notch before connecting the tube to the port. A good positioning of the port in the pocket will not require additional sutures for fixation.

> Be sure there are no twisting forces on the port that may cause future port rotation and use a gentle traction maneuver to confirm the port-tube connection.

Revision Procedures

Band Slippage

The rear (dorsal slipping) or front (anterior slipping) stomach wall shifts upward through the band are called band slippage. This is the most common complication (6–12%), mainly caused by operational circumstances. Upon introducing a contrast medium, the pouch will look eccentric on x-rays. Due to the enlargement of the pouch, a valve-like mechanism occurs, in which passage to the main stomach is progressively obstructed by parts of the stomach wall (partial to complete stoma occlusion). As the pouch increases in size, a part of the stomach wall can cause a shift of the gastrostoma which progressively obstructs the passage. Inflammatory changes can also lead to an obstruction.

This is reflected in intolerance toward solid food and then to liquids until obstruction is complete:

- Chronic: Increasing passage disorders for solid foods; repeated vomiting after meals; regurgitation (back-flow of food remains, indigestion, also at night). Progressively increasing capacity limitations even for liquids; drinking is only possible in little sips; solid food is not tolerated anymore at all, excessive weight-loss, reflux symptoms (pain or heartburn), general complaints like tiredness and deficient nutrition. Left untreated, any chronic form can escalate into an acute form.
- Acute: Complete halt of food passage. Consequences of untreated total food intolerance, dehydration, electrolyte imbalance, prerenal failure (caused by dehydration), extremely heightened risk of aspiration mostly at night (breathing reflux stomach contents into the airways causing a risk of pneumonia). I use the term "wet pillow syndrome" which describes the patients as they wake up in the morning with a puddle of saliva on their pillow.
- Conservative management:
  - Complete opening the stomach band
  - Insertion of a naso-gastric tube to relieve the pouch and to avoid aspiration
  - Immediate intravenous rehydration and balancing electrolytes
  - Start administration of an antacid (e.g., Omeprazole) to protect against or treat mucosal changes within the pouch and add substitutive therapy (iron, vitamins, etc.)

Laparoscopic band reposition without exchanging the band is usually possible by creating a new path (Fig. 2.40).

Band Migration

An erosion of the stomach or penetration of the stomach wall by the band occurs very rarely (<2%). It usually occurs more than 2 years after the original surgery. The causes of this are still being discussed but may include:

- Primary undiscovered stomach wall injuries
- Pressure-related stomach wall necrosis caused by strong filling of the band
- A secondary infection along the band system

There may be a complete lack of symptoms or the only sign may be regaining of weight – or there may be pain complaints related to an infection of the upper abdomen. Diagnosis is made after decongesting the band by a gastroscopy, which enables viewing of the

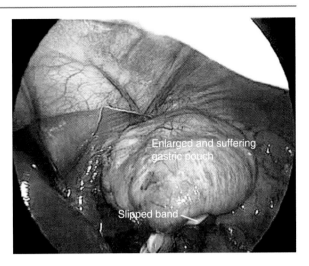

Fig. 2.40 Acute anterior slippage

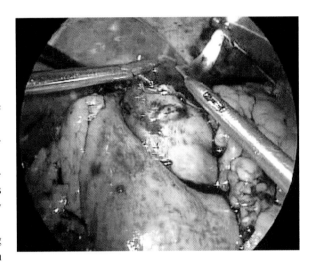

Fig. 2.41 Removal of the migrated band

whole band and not only the constricted part at the stomach entrance and by X-ray contrast swallow revealing an inability to adjust the band. Treatment consists of removal of the band (Fig. 2.41) and securely closing the stomach wall.

If the stomach wall was penetrated completely, the band may be removed endoscopically after severing the catheter. Three to six months later most patients will regain weight and an additional bariatric procedure will be required. According to my experience, rebanding these patients 4–5 months later is the preferable strategy due to the fact that this procedure remains to be the one with the least number of complications.

Esophageal Dilatation

Severe deviations in function (dysfunctional movement, motility) and anatomy of the esophagus after using gastric bands have been reported. How often and how long after surgery they appear, under optimal conditions and operative techniques, is unclear so far. Esophageal dysfunction is usually indicated by discomfort. It may either result from continuing increased pressure on the esophagus, or from the effects of exposure to stomach acids with the corresponding inflammatory reactions of the mucous membrane. Should these dysfunctions manifest themselves, they may be visualized radiologically, endoscopically, and by corresponding pressure and acid measurements. This allows for diagnostic differentiation and determination of further treatments.

If the esophageal diseases cannot be controlled by adjusting the band or eating habits, removal of the gastric band or laparoscopic band unlocking must be considered. In later stages, patient may regain weight, thus, performing rebanding (my preference) or an alternative procedure (sleeve resection, Roux-en-Y gastric bypass) may become necessary.

Gastric Pouch Dilatation

There are several different forms; namely early and late stage and acute and chronic pouch enlargements. An early dilatation may occur a few weeks after surgery; this is usually caused by an incorrectly positioned band. The main effect of this is a creation of a pouch that is too large. The late-stage form manifests itself after weeks, often even after a year, and is usually caused by abnormal eating habits like meal sizes that are too large (possibly even pre-operative binge-eating), or a gastrostoma that is too constricted. This may also include a sliding hiatal hernia (diaphragmatic hernias with an upward-shifting stomach entrance) in front of an otherwise well-positioned band. Radiological visualization will show a concentric pouch. If left untreated (complete deflation, laparoscopic band reposition), the dilatation may progress into real "slipping," including upward-shifting of the stomach wall above the band.

Stoma Occlusion

Unchewed chunks of food may cause a shifting gastrostoma with subsequent complete halt of food and liquid passage. Thus, it is of utmost importance to chew very consciously. Certain foods may have to

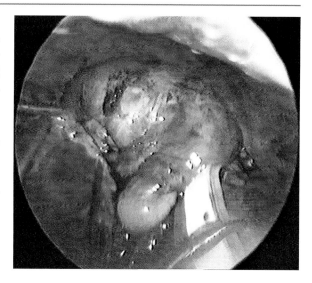

Fig. 2.42 Gastric pouch necrosis

be avoided completely under certain circumstances, especially with repeated vomiting (long-grained vegetables, legumes, coarse-grained meats, pasta). Initially an attempt is made to remove the congestion by opening the band and drinking fluids. If this is unsuccessful, a gastroscopy is almost always sufficient. If congested for more than 6 h the band should remain open for approx. 1 week, and acid reducing treatment should be implemented to treat inflammation and swelling of the mucous membrane. If the time needed to restore passage through the band exceeds 6 h, then there is a risk of acute pouch extension with stomach rupture. In this case, emergency intervention with partial gastrectomy may be necessary (Fig. 2.42).

2.3   Surgical Technique by Thomas Manger (Germany)

Thomas Manger

Introduction

The treatment of morbid obesity with gastric banding was begun in 1983 by Kuzmak. Today this technique is performed almost worldwide in about 25% of all bariatric procedures. In Europe gastric banding is the most widespread procedure (more than 70%) [1]. The prospective multicenter study on quality standards in bariatric surgery in Germany we conducted shows that gastric banding was the most frequently performed procedure until 2006. From 2007 on, combined malabsorptive procedures have been performed more often, so gastric banding moved back to second place behind the Roux-en-Y gastric bypass [4].

Gastric banding is a little invasive technique with low morbidity and mortality. A great advantage is that it can be performed laparoscopic (in 98.4%) and that the procedure is reversible. Conversion rates are low (0.7%). The pars-flaccida approach for band implantation has established itself in 98% of all procedures. About 73% of all surgeons calibrate the pouch, only 9% do not cover the band with stomach serosa.

Long-term results are mostly affected by band-related problems, such as complications with the port (0.4–6.8%), pouch dilatation/slippage (1.4–21%) and band migration (0.3–11%). This results in a revision rate of up to 4% per year [2–4].

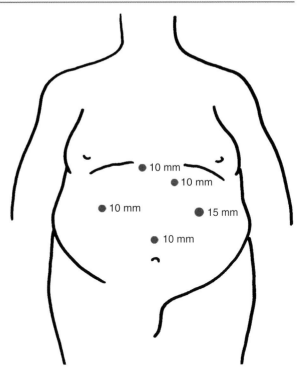

Fig. 2.43 Placement of the trocars

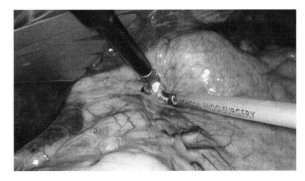

Fig. 2.44 Calibration of the pouch with 25 mL of saline by carefully pulling it toward the GE junction; dissection begins at the equatorial plane at the lesser curvature

Preparation

Setting, Positioning, and the Surgical Team
- The patient is positioned half sitting (15–30° anti-Trendelenburg position) with spread legs in general anesthesia on a 2.5 cm gel mat. Cardia and stomach are exposed this way; gravity lowers other internal organs out of the way.
- You as the surgeon stand between the patient's legs.
- The monitor and the first assistant are positioned on the patient's right side.
- After a single shot antibiotic prophylaxis the pneumoperitoneum is created with 15 mmHg pressure.
- This first trocar is inserted 25 cm below the xiphoid through a 10 cm cut into the fascia between two Kocher's forceps.
- The other four working trocars (11–15 mm) are inserted according to Fig. 2.43.

Surgical Technique

Calibration of the Gastric Pouch
- Determine the position of the band with a calibration tube. It is inserted into the stomach by the anesthetist and filled with 25 mL of saline. Then it is carefully pulled back up unto the GE junction (Fig. 2.44).

- Mark the equatorial plane of the balloon by ticking the serosa with an electrical device at the lesser and the greater curvature.
- Empty the balloon and remove it.

Creation of the Retrogastric Channel, Pars-Flaccida Approach
- Begin dissection of the hepatogastric ligament close to the lesser curvature in an avascular area, taking care to spare the hepatic branch of the vagus nerve.

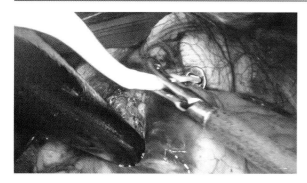

Fig. 2.45 Flexible retractor with retrogastric tunnel, connection to the gastric band

- Continue up to the right crus of diaphragm, dissecting the backside of the stomach under visual control. The medial border of the right crus can now be seen next to the loose connective tissue between the left and the right crus.
- Now pull the greater curvature in mediocaudal direction with a large grasper and open the peritoneum at the marked spot proximal to gastric blood vessels near the angle of His; the cut is about 10-mm long.
- Dissect and mobilize the stomach wall alongside the greater curvature up to the left crus of diaphragm, using a 30° angled camera.

Retrogastric Tunnel
- Passage through the retrogastric tunnel is possible with an atraumatic angled blunt dissector. We prefer the flexible retractor; the flat and approximately finger-wide tip can be angled and allows safe dissection.
- Insert the dissector through the paraxiphoid trocar No 3 alongside the lesser curvature up to the right crus of diaphragm.
- Form a 90° angle with the instrument and insert it with gentle pressure into the retrogastric tunnel. Push it through the prepared channel behind the stomach to the greater curvature. If done correctly, the tip of the angled dissector will appear in the angle of His at the greater curvature (Fig. 2.45).

Inserting the Band
- We use the Lap-band (INAMED Health, Santa Barbara, USA) or the Swedisch Gastric Band (SAGB/Obtech, Ethicon-Endo-Surgery).
- Insert the band into the abdomen through the 15-mm trocar.

- Place the strap of the band into the slot of the flexible retractor and pull the band back through the retrogastric channel.
- Now you can position the band around the cardia in the equatorial plane and lock it with or without a special instrument.

Covering the Band
- Position the lock of the gastric band medially, dorsal to the left hepatic lobe.
- Cover the band completely with serosa beginning far dorsally at the greater curvature. Place 3–4 seromuscular single sutures with absorbable monofilament material.
- Pull the tube of the gastric band out of the abdomen through trocar No 4.
- Remove the instruments under visual control and desufflate the pneumoperitoneum.

Positioning the Port Chamber
- Fasten the port chamber on the fascia of the rectus sheath in the middle upper abdomen with four nonabsorbable single sutures. Widen the skin incision for trocar No 1 for this step and guide the silicone tube to trocar No 4 subcutaneously.

> Take great care to prevent kinking of the tube close to the port chamber.

- After connecting the port chamber with the tube, check the function of the band by injecting 2 mL of saline in the chamber (huber needle). Remove the saline completely afterward.
- Close fascia and skin of all trocar incisions.

Aftercare

Let patients drink immediately after surgery. Reaffirm the correct position of the band radiologically before the patient is released from hospital. An emergency health card informs other doctors about the procedure. Tightening of the band is performed no earlier than 6–8 weeks after the procedure on an outpatient basis, depending on the individual patient's situation. The first filling is usually performed when weight loss stagnates. Lifelong aftercare is mandatory.

2.4   Surgical Technique by Karl Miller, (Austria)

Karl Miller

Introduction

Minimal invasive or laparoscopic techniques have found their way into almost all surgical disciplines and have been performed much more frequently since the early 1990s due to constant technical improvements. Vertical banded gastroplasty, gastric bypass, and even biliopancreatic diversions are performed laparoscopic [1–3]. The least invasive laparoscopic procedure is the implantation of the adjustable gastric band.

In bariatric surgery, the surgical procedure is not the final point, but the beginning of the treatment.

Regular aftercare and cooperation of the patient are crucial for success.

Indication for Surgery

Indication for surgery is defined in evidence-based guidelines. A BMI over 40 defines severe obesity that needs to be treated. Surgical therapy is justified if it is the patient's wish and the surgeon believes it to be indicated, too. A BMI over 40 is about 45 kg excess weight over ideal body weight in a person with average height. Patients with a BMI between 35 and 40 should be considered for surgery if they suffer from comorbidities that can be improved substantially through weight loss.

The patient must be able to take care of himself or otherwise have somebody at hand to secure aftercare. High motivation on the side of the patient and interdisciplinary treatment are much more important for success than strict exclusion criteria that are changed yearly anyway.

Adjustment of the band, psychological care, and dietary advice constitute a major part of therapy with the adjustable gastric band. If aftercare cannot be guaranteed, absolutely refrain from performing the procedure.

Follow the guidelines of the American Society for Bariatric and Metabolic Surgery (ASMBS) and the International Federation for the Surgery of Obesity (IFSO) requiring a hospital to have sufficient experience in both open and laparoscopic abdominal surgery. It must also offer qualified nutritionists, psychologists, a motivated nursing staff, and if possible a support group. Special examination couches, operating tables, beds, and instruments in case of the need to switch to conventional surgery must be provided as well as facilities for perioperative monitoring. The necessity of well trained and experienced surgeons is obvious.

Information of the patient, especially the first counseling interview, is time-consuming and of great importance. There is almost no other surgical procedure in which success or failure is so dependent on the patient's cooperation. Patients must learn about obesity as a disease, current surgical procedures, laparoscopic band implantation, possible complications, warning symptoms, and aftercare. Patients with extreme morbid obesity (triple obesity, BMI over 60), severe eating disorders such as binge eating or insulin-dependent type II diabetes should rather be treated with complex procedures, such as a gastric bypass or biliopancreatic diversion.

Preoperative Proceedings

- Apart from taking the medical history and a physical examination, endocrinological diseases must be treated sufficiently. An internal medical examination, an abdominal ultrasound scan and spirometry are recommendable.
- Existing gallstones should be removed during the same procedure, as massive weight loss often leads to gallstone-related complications.
- The patient is introduced to the anesthetist several days before the procedure with the examination results. Dietary advice and a psychological examination are mandatory.
- It makes sense to have compression stockings custom made before admittance to the hospital. Patients bring a cost acceptance declaration from their health insurance company (Table 2.1).
- In our department we conduct the educational talks not on the day of the procedure, but some time earlier.

Perioperative Care

- We recommend perioperative antibiotic prophylaxis (cephalosporin single shot) and low molecular weight heparin (medium to high risk).
- The patient may drink small amounts of tea immediately after the procedure. A water-soluble contrast swallow is performed the next day, and then the step-by-step return to the recommended diet begins.

Table 2.1 Checklist for perioperative measures and diagnostics

Information of the patient, medical history, physical examination

Internal preoperative examination

Blood tests preoperatively

Spirometry

Abdominal ultrasound scan

Gastroscopy if indicated

Functional diagnostics of the upper gastrointestinal tract if indicated

Tests on metabolism if indicated

Dietary advice

Psychological tests

Fitting of compression stockings

Application for cost acceptance declaration from the health insurance company

Schedule appointment for procedure (not in first interview)

Table 2.2 Postoperative measures

Time after surgery	Measure
Day 1	Water-soluble contrast swallow
Day 7/8	Removal of the stitches
Weeks 4–6	Dietary advice, band adjustment, (water-soluble contrast swallow)
Month 3	Clinical examination, band adjustment if necessary
Months 6–9	Clinical examination, band adjustment if necessary
From then on once a year	Ultrasound scan, medical history, quality control, physical examination, water-soluble contrast swallow

Optional and according to demand: psychological care, dietary advice, and support groups anytime

- More dietary counseling should take place before the band is tightened for the first time.
- Further control examinations depend on the procedure and individual needs of the patient (Table 2.2)

Preparation

Setting, Positioning, and the Surgical Team
- The patient is positioned overstreched slightly with spread legs.
- The pneumoperitoneum (12 mmHg) is created from the left middle upper abdomen. The patient is brought into an anti-Trendelenburg position only after the trocars are placed to avoid an injury of the liver.

Positioning the Trocars

There are many different suggestions for positioning the trocars. Their placement depends on the patient's habitus and is the key to success in extreme obesity. In contrast to normal abdominal walls the trocars cannot be tilted within obese abdominal walls. Preoperative assessment of the size of the left hepatic lobe with an ultrasound scan can be very useful.

- The first incision for the optic trocar is placed about a hand width below the xiphoid a little left to the middle line and should be performed under visual control to avoid injury of the liver.
- The liver retractor is inserted in the right middle/upper abdomen or in the epigastrium.
- Through a puncture with a long needle in the epigastrium right to the middle line the best position for a dissector and later the closing instrument is determined.
- The trocar for the dissector and for the insertion of the band is placed in the left middle/upper abdomen. The 15-mm trocar for the insertion of the band can be placed here.
- Insertion of another 5-mm trocar next to the left costal arch is optional; it can be used to tense the stomach wall or to retract the greater omentum.

Surgical Technique

After placing the trocars lift the left hepatic lobe far enough to display the diaphragm. The band must always be placed around the upper part of the stomach and not the esophagus. There are three different techniques for band implantation. Perigastric placement after creation of a retrogastric channel has been abandoned in the last years in favor of the so-called pars-flaccida approach. A combined procedure (pars-flaccida to perigastric) needs to be performed especially in patients with massive fat tissue around the cardia.

Perigastric Approach
- Insert the gastric tube that comes with the band into the stomach, fill the balloon at the tip with 15–20 m³ of air and pull it back to the GE junction.
- Dissect a 0.5 cm opening at the equatorial plane at the lesser curvature. Continue dissecting along the stomach wall on the backside up to the angle of His, but take care not to open the omental bursa.
- At the greater curvature dissect the left crus of diaphragm and the GE junction in the angle of His. Do

not cut the gastrophrenic ligament; the band will be positioned within it.

- Insert the dissector (we prefer the "goldfinger") through the opening up the lesser curvature and place it into the angle of His inside the gastrophrenic ligament by bending the tip.
- The band can only be inserted into the abdomen through 15 or 18 mm trocar. You can also position the band around the GE junction with an angled atraumatic grasper.
- Before locking the band, fill the balloon at the tip of the gastric tube with 15 mL of air. The band will lock below this pouch; no further sutures are necessary to secure it.
- To avoid slippage of the band, add 3–4 seromuscular single sutures to the front side of the stomach.
- Pull the end of the tube out through the 15 or 18 mm trocar and connect it to the port.
- Fasten the port with four nonabsorbable sutures (upon or under the front fascia of the rectus sheath) near the incision for the 15 or 18 mm trocar. You could also use a port stapler (Fig. 2.46a and b).

Pars-Flaccida Approach

- After reaching the operative site, open the pars flaccida of the lesser omentum to display the right crus of diaphragm.
- Create a channel in the avascular part of the gastrophrenic ligament by dissecting in the angle between the crus of diaphragm and the GE junction.
- The band is prepared for implantation by rinsing it with saline and testing for tightness.
- Insert the band system into the abdomen through the 15 or 18 mm trocar.
- Above the omental bursa, dissection is performed with an atraumatic forceps, the retrogastric channel is created with the atraumatic flexible "goldfinger." Fat tissue around the lesser curvature and the ventral vagus nerve are included within the band system in this technique. A 2-0 Ethibond suture at the end of the band system connects it to the "goldfinger."

We recommend fastening the fundus to the left crus of diaphragm to keep the fundus from slipping proximally (Fig 2.47).

- Three to four nonabsorbable sutures are placed onto the front wall of the stomach to avoid slippage of the band.

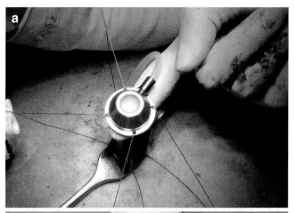

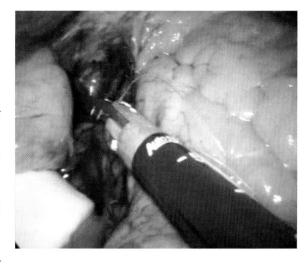

Fig. 2.46 (**a**) Fastening the port with four nonabsorbable sutures. The sutures are placed first, then the port is positioned onto the fascia, then the knots are tied. (**b**) Fastening the port chamber with a port stapler

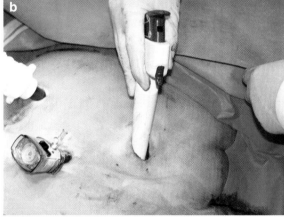

Fig. 2.47 The fundus is sutured to the left crus of diaphragm to prevent proximal slippage

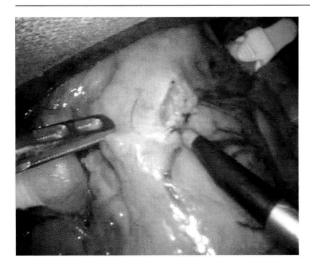

Fig. 2.48 In patients with massive fat pads the band might be too small. Dissect a channel between the stomach and the fat pad before locking the band

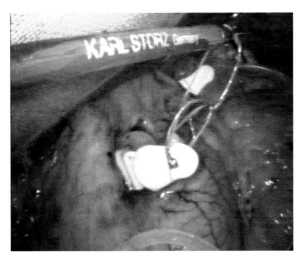

Fig. 2.49 The left part of the band is pulled between the stomach and the fat pad with a "goldfinger" or the flexible dissector and then locked

Combined Technique

The band might be too short in patients with massive fat tissue around the cardia.

Before locking the band, it is first positioned following the pars-flaccida approach, and then a channel is created between the stomach wall and the surrounding fat tissue (Fig. 2.48). Then the band is pulled through with the "goldfinger" or a dissector and finally is locked close to the stomach wall (Fig. 2.49).

Latest developments in surgical technique can be summarized as following:

Table 2.3 Complications after placement of an adjustable gastric band [4–26]

Complication	Incidence (%)
Perioperative complications	
Lethality	0–2.1
Injury of the gastric wall	0–3.5
Pneumothorax	0–0.2
Hemorrhage	0.5–2.0
Late complications	
Pouch dilatation with/without slippage	0–13.4
Banderosion	0–4.6
Complications concerning the port and the band system	0.5–10.4
Wound infection	0–7.7
Motility disorders (clinically apparent)	0–1.5

- Reduction of the pouch to 15 cm^3
- Placement of the band above the omental bursa
- Pars-flaccida approach
- The band should be within the gastrophrenic ligament
- Band is secured tightly with sutures at the front wall of the stomach
- If the omental bursa is opened, the band is placed so far away from the GE junction that additional stay sutures need to be placed on the back of the stomach.
- The band should not be filled in the first weeks after surgery to avoid vomiting. This could lead to a breakdown of the stay sutures and slippage of the band.
- If the band is too tight, the combined technique is chosen.

Difficult Situations and Intraoperative Complications

Complications can arise early or later (Table 2.3). Preventing complications altogether is first priority. Thorough training and an interdisciplinary treatment concept have been mentioned before. The incidence of surgical complications such as slippage or band erosion has been lowered significantly by following the pars-flaccida approach [4].

Perioperative Complications
Mortality

Perioperative deaths have been reported after perforation or necrosis of the stomach wall, cardiogenic shock, and pulmonary embolism. Large centers figure mortality of adjustable gastric band surgery to be about 0–0.1% [5–8].

Injury of the Stomach Wall

The stomach wall can be injured fairly easy in confusing situations. During the "learning curve," the first 50 procedures, usually one or two stomach perforations occur [8–11]. The incidence of this complication is about 0–3.5% [9].

If the perforation is located distally of the band, the latter can be implanted after suturing the injury. This complication can be avoided by working carefully and using suitable atraumatic instruments.

We recommend injecting 5 mL methylene blue with 15 mL saline through the gastric tube before positioning the gastric band, if the procedure is difficult or the site confusing.

Other Perioperative Complications

Other complications, such as hemorrhage or pneumothorax, can also occur, just as in conventional abdominal surgery. Literature reviews confirm that complication rates are lower in laparoscopic procedures than in conventional surgery. Always have an effective hemostyptic, such as FloSeal (Baxter), at hand.

Late Complications

Pouch Dilatation with Slippage of the Band

Many authors report pouch dilatation at the backside of the stomach near the omental bursa [9–12]. The frequency of this complication was lowered significantly by placing stay sutures to the backside of the stomach or by positioning the band above the omental bursa and within the gastrophrenic ligament [4–13]. O'Brien conducted an impressive study with 350 patients; he reduced the incidence of pouch dilatations and band slippage from 30% to 2.5% by placing sutures on the backside of the stomach [14]. Pouch dilatations usually occur about 8 months post surgery [13].

Pouch Dilatation Without Slippage of the Band

This rarely reported complication [15] is probably due to a pouch that was created too large from the beginning [13]. Desaive published a study comparing revision rates after two different pouch sizes: 25 cm³: 33%, 15 cm³: 5.1% [16]. The size of the pouch can be measured perioperatively with the calibration balloon that comes with the system (BioEnterics Corporation) or a gastric tube with an excentric balloon fastened to the tip (Ethicon). The size of the pouch should not exceed 15 cm³.

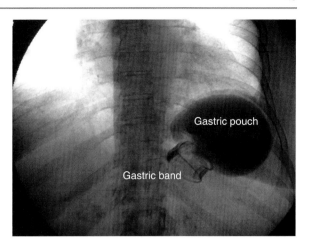

Fig. 2.50 Complete slippage after gastric banding. Contrast cannot pass into the remnant stomach, the pouch is dilated

Pouch dilatation is marked by early impaired food ingestion. Possible causes are eating beyond satiety, eating too fast, induced vomiting, or consuming large amounts of carbonated drinks. Chelala showed that repeated vomiting can lead to pouch dilatation [17]. An adjustment of the band should therefore be performed a few weeks after the implantation.

Therapy of Pouch Dilatation and Band Slippage

This complication can be avoided by correct positioning of the band (above the omental bursa) and intraoperative measurement of the pouch. Diagnosis is made with an X-ray showing an asymmetrical pouch. Extreme dilatations lead to complete obstruction ("internal herniation"; Fig. 2.50); an emergency procedure is required.

If the problem is recognized early, the band can be adjusted by removing saline to widen the exit. Sometimes the pouch dilatation can thus be reversed. Alvarez-Cordero succeeded in doing so in three out of eight cases [18]. If the procedure is not successful, the band needs to be repositioned.

One can either reposition the old band or remove it and position a new band correctly. This procedure can well be performed laparoscopic [19].

Band Erosion

Migration of the band into the stomach is usually treated by removal of the system (Fig. 2.51). Dargent has treated 500 patients; 3 of whom experienced band erosion 17, 18, and 21 months after surgery. One patient needed a 2/3 gastrectomy, in the other two cases the band was removed laparoscopic [4].

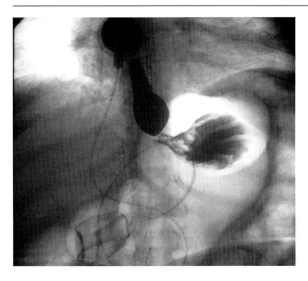

Fig. 2.51 Band erosion X-ray. The band has migrated through the stomach wall completely and is now inside the distal stomach

Band erosion is usually diagnosed because of symptom-free weight gain or heartburn and upper abdominal pain. In an analysis of 3,800 patients wearing the Lap-Band an erosion rate of 0.6% was found. Reasons might be increased pressure within the band (overfilling), injury of the stomach wall during dissection or sutures and clips. No definite cause however has been verified. The gastric band can be removed gastroscopically with a band cutter (AMI, Austria) or with a laparoscopy.

Complications of the Port System and the Tube

Use nonabsorbable sutures to prevent the *port chamber from flipping over*. The port should be positioned a few centimeters away from the point at which the tube exits the abdomen to prevent kinking.

Port inflammation can be caused by band erosion; colonization of the port chamber by germs comes through the stomach. Always perform gastroscopy in case of port inflammation for this reason. Insufficient hygiene while puncturing the port is also discussed.

Leakage of the band usually results in symptom-free weight gain. Leakage can be proved by injecting Jopamiro or Uromiro. Very small leaks can take hours to days before they show symptoms, i.e., days later the patient can suddenly eat much more. In this case a thallium-201-szintigraphy can show the miniature leak

[22]. If the diagnosis is made, either the port or the complete system are exchanged.

Management of port inflammation without erosion includes removal of the port, filling of the band with the before used amount of saline, closure of the tube, and placement of the tube into the peritoneum. If inflammation persists, the complete system will have to be removed. A new port or band system can be implanted laparoscopic 6–8-weeks later [23].

Esophageal Dysmotility

Greenstein postulates that preexisting esophageal hernia and/or esophageal dysmotility predispose to revision procedures [24]. In this study, patients with esophageal dysmotility have revision rates of 33%, so do patients with hiatus hernia. But he had an allover revision rate of 18%; all of these were among his first 30 patients. We found no such correlation for our patients [25]. Morbidly obese patients have symptom-free esophageal dysmotility in up to 60%. If dysmotility becomes symptomatic after surgery (achalasia – like signs in radiological and manometrical examinations), we recommend removing the saline from the band completely or removing the entire band system laparoscopic and performing a different bariatric procedure, such as a gastric bypass.

Adjuvant Pharmaceutical Therapy

If the band system is dysfunctional, patients can receive Orlistat 3×120 mg to avoid weight gain while waiting for the revision procedure. Our pilot study proved that patients continued to lose weight with Orlistat even if the band was dysfunctional or removed [26].

Summary

Obesity and morbid obesity are a chronic multifactorial disease in need of treatment. We believe that the laparoscopic implantation of an adjustable gastric band is an efficient treatment for most of the morbidly obese patients. Stomach or intestine do not have to be opened, anatomy and physiology of the gastrointestinal tract are left intact. Late metabolic complications are not to be expected. Weight loss and food intake can be adjusted individually according to the patient's needs. Eighty percent can expect to lose 50–60% of their excess weight.

Removal of the band and restoration of the original situation is much easier than after other procedures.

Surgical technique is difficult in the beginning, but easy later on and bears comparatively little risk as long as the safety recommendations are followed.

In bariatric surgery, the surgical procedure is not the final point, but the beginning of the treatment.

Regular aftercare and cooperation of the patient are crucial for success.

2.5   Surgical Technique by Rishi Singhal and Paul Super (Great Britain)

Rishi Singhal and Paul Super

Preparation

Setting, Positioning, and the Surgical Team
- Patients are positioned in reverse Trendelenburg position either with legs straight or in leg supports.

Trocar Placement
Five laparoscopic ports are used (15 mm, 10 mm, and 3×5 mm). Essentially these are placed as high as possible on the abdomen as long as they are not above the left lobe of liver. Where the liver is large, they must be placed in a correspondingly lower position so that the instruments clear under the liver.
- The 5-mm liver retractor (Snowden Pencer Inc.) is placed via the mid-clavicular LUQ port site.
- The surgeon's left hand working port (5 mm) is just to the right of the midline.
- The 30° camera port (10 mm) is medial to the left mid-clavicular line.
- The surgeon's right hand working port (15 mm) is lateral to the mid-claviciular line. It is used for introduction of the band and for suturing.

> Bleeding from the epigastric artery is minimized by always being lateral to the mid-clavicular point.

- A final 5-mm port is placed in the anterior axillary line and used for assistant retraction, usually on the stomach but also on the band during fixation suturing.

In order to enable smooth instrument control and manipulation all ports should be directed through the abdominal wall in the direction of the hiatus. This ensures that instruments pass through the ports smoothly with little drag on the port edges. This is most important in BMI greater than 50 where the thicker abdominal walls make pivoting of the port to change direction in the abdomen very difficult if not impossible. The greater the abdominal wall thickness, the greater the requirement to have all ports inserted in the direction of the cardia. The exception is that for the liver retractor which is inserted in the direction of the left iliac fossa.

Surgical Technique: Pars-Flaccida Approach, SAGB

> All dissection in our practice is carried out with simple hook diathermy.

- Surgery starts with the creation of a window in the lesser omentum. Usually a large cruciate incision is all that is required and this is made in the avascular portion below the hepatic branches of vagus and vessel bundle which run transversely from the left lobe of liver to the cardia.
- Fat pads attached to the cardia can be retracted by the assistant to the left to reveal the right crus.
- A 2-cm vertical incision is made in the myomesium over the medial border of the right crus to reveal the muscle surface.
- Gentle retraction of the fascia to the left and the crural bundle to the right allows a grasper to probe the path of least resistance and to pass between the cardia and the aorta and at the same time to pass in front of the left crus which at this stage can usually be seen behind the cardia in the lower BMI patients.
- Next attention is drawn to the angle of His and to display the left crus.
- The peritoneal reflection of the angle of His is taken down. The assistant retracts the fundus close to the cardia downward, and the surgeon retracts the fat pad over the cardia to the right. This maneuver usually reveals the left crus.

- The crus is followed downward in a caudal direction and a similar 2 cm vertical incision is made in the myomesium over the left crus using the hook diathermy. This mirrors the incision in the myomesium made over the right crus.

  Occasionally a sliding hiatus hernia is encountered and if less than 3 cm, usually band insertion alone is all that is required. The band reduces the hernia and subsequently will produce fibrosis of the band tunnel and prevent prolapse of the stomach and band above the hiatus. If the hiatus hernia is greater than 4 cm we always carry out a 2-suture posterior crural repair (nonabsorbable sutures) from the right side of the cardia which is fairly straightforward given the dissection over the right crus which we have already undertaken as part of our insertion technique. In this case we incise the myomesium over the medial border of the right crus over a 5-cm length and the assistant retracts the cardia to the patients left to display both crura.

Delivery of the Band

- A blunt retrogastric dissector is passed from the opening in the myomesium over the right crus, behind the cardia to the opening in the myomesium over the left crus where it exits into the abdomen.

  Many types are available and we favor the Goldfinger (Snowden Pencer Inc).

- The band is usually prepared by priming with normal Saline and almost fully aspirating.
- A 2/0 vicryl loop is secured to the band and this usually fits snugly into the groove on the retro-gastric dissector.
- The band is delivered into the abdomen via the 15-mm port. The band is fastened below the perigastric fat pad which we never resect.

  If the fat pad is bulky we favor the use of a larger size gastric band and pull the fat pad cranially above the band.

Gastric Fixation (Tunnellating) Sutures

We have developed the "Birmingham Stitch" which incorporates a plication suture to gather up the redundant superior fundus which is fixed high up on the left crus. We believe this significantly reduces the risk of slippage.

- This is started high on the fundus approximately 5 cm lateral and parallel to the band and plicates up the fundus in a line toward the angle of His (Figs. 2.52 and 2.53).
- Next two gastro-gastric sutures are inserted, the first from the anterior fundus and the second from the fundus close to the lesser curve, each suture again plicating the fundus in a line parallel to the band and approximately 5 cm lateral to it. These sutures are nonabsorbable and extra-corporeal suturing is used which allows multiple (up to 10) points of suture fixation to be drawn together as the suture loop closes securely.

  If there has been any minor bleeding from the sutures or dissection then this can be controlled using a small swab inserted via the 15-mm port. Formal irrigation is seldom necessary.

- The band tubing is delivered into the abdominal wall via the 10-mm camera port site.
- We always place the adjustment port over the xiphisternum and so we enlarge the 5-mm incision closest to the site. Using the hook diathermy, we then clear a 2 cm area of muscle fascia over the linea alba as high up as possible.

  We feel that the subcutaneaous fat layer is thinnest here and patients prefer the port not to be near the left costal margin where some surgeons place the port. This area is relatively avascular with less risk of hematomas (and infection). Besides this, the port in this position is more easily palpable for subsequent port adjustments.

- Three or four nonabsorbable sutures are placed in the linea alba and a tunnel is made from this port wound to the 10-mm tubing exit wound. It is important that

Fig. 2.52 Diagram of the Birmingham stitch

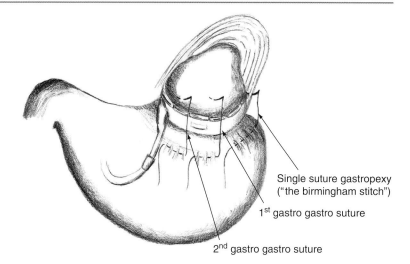

Single suture gastropexy
("the birmingham stitch")

1st gastro gastro suture

2nd gastro gastro suture

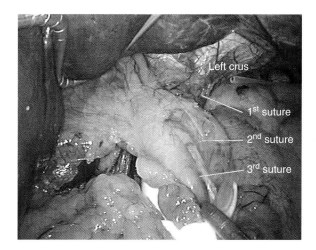

Left crus

1st suture

2nd suture

3rd suture

Fig. 2.53 Positions of gastropexia and gastrogastric sutures

this subcutaneous tunnel for the tubing is in contact with the fascia and that the tubing is exiting a 10-mm port wound. This facilitates easy replacement of the tubing into the abdomen without any further requirement for laparoscopy.

• When the adjustment port is attached to the tubing it is extremely important to remove any axial twist in the tubing so that there are no axial forces on the port which we believe are the most common reason for subsequent port rotation.

Wound Closure

• We never try to suture the fascial or muscle layer in any of our port sites. A fine absorbable suture is used to close the superficial fascia over the port and all wounds are closed with tissue glue.

If there is a persistent ooze from the 10 mm or 15 mm port sites then a large surgicel pack (Johnson and Johnson) is inserted beneath the fascial layer to compress any bleeding. If the bleeding is brisk then the facia should be sutured directly to secure hemostasis.

Band Adjustments

• We favor radiological adjustments at 3 monthly intervals which always ensures an appropriate and optimal band fill and patient satiety. In addition, inappropriate band fills are largely avoided if radiology detects esophageal dilatation and if pouch enlargements are the reasons for lack of satiety.

Difficult Situations and Intraoperative Complications

Early Postoperative Dysphagia

This is usually because too much residual fluid was left in the band system at the end of surgery. If this persists after 24 h and the patient cannot tolerate sips, we remove all residual band fluid by deflation.

If dysphagia to liquids persists, a trial of a short course of Hydrocortisone 100 mg twice daily for 2 days usually improves swallowing.

If not, a repeat laparoscopy should be performed and a larger size of band inserted, usually by suturing the new band to the opened end of the band being removed. This means that one band replaces the other without disturbing the tunnel sutures covering the band.

Early Postoperative Pain and Sepsis

At the end of the procedure we always perform a local anesthetic block of each of the wounds using 0.5% bupivicaine or equivalent. This is introduced into the rectus sheath taking care not to damage the band tubing in those port sites close to the adjustment port.

In nearly all cases Diclofenac 100 mg and paracetamol 1.0 g are given rectally at the end of the procedure which gives gradual pain control over the first few postoperative hours. Postoperative opiates are avoided since this impedes early resumption of oral intake and early mobilization (important factors in the prevention thrombo-embolism and in the promotion of same day discharge).

It is uncommon to have *severe postoperative pain* following gastric banding although shoulder pain may persist for several days if there has been any accumulation of hematoma in the subphrenic area or if any gastric fixation sutures have been inserted into the right hemi-diaphragm (suturing into the left crus does not cause shoulder pain).

If patients develop severe pain in the postoperative period which is constant and associated with sepsis then this must be investigated by contrast swallow looking specifically for evidence of leak secondary to gastric trauma at the time of insertion. This pain may be upper abdominal or epigastric but usually chest pain. Even if the contrast study is normal and pain and sepsis persist we would advocate early laparoscopy and direct inspection of the band with methylene blue testing of the gastric pouch as such a complication remains a possibility.

If evidence of a *gastric perforation* exists then this should be treated by band removal and drainage of the area. Usually any perforation is tiny, usually affecting the posterior cardia and will heal spontaneously without any requirement for suture repair.

Early Postoperative Bleeding

This is usually port-site bleeding and usually from the port in the left upper quadrant which is the largest. Normally the bleeding is greatest after administration of anti-coagulation in which case the bleeding should stop spontaneously and surgical control of the bleeding will not be necessary. If signs of bleeding persist then the patient should be returned to the theatre for repeat laparoscopy, washout, and suture of the bleeding point.

Port Site Infection

This may be a simple superficial problem but may also be a feature of a true band infection. We advocate laparoscopy in all cases in order to inspect the tubing. If the band tubing is clearly visible and free of omental adhesions then the band is unlikely to be infected. In this circumstance we would cut the tubing and remove the port at the end of the operation with subsequent re-laparoscopy and replacement of a new port 3 months later. Antibiotic cover for *Staphylococcus aureus* should be given. If at the initial laparoscopy the band tubing is covered in omental adhesions and not directly visible then usually there is a band infection. We favor immediate band removal (without taking down fixation sutures) and subsequent band replacement 6 months later when inflammation and fibrosis will have almost fully resolved.

Punctured Band Balloon

This usually is only a feature with bands which have thin balloons which are not pre-formed such as the old type Swedish band (Ethicon). The puncture is usually seen using contrast radiology as the leaks are due to material failure. A fracture line allows contrast to escape from the balloon into the tissues following contrast injection into the port. In this case we laparoscope the patient and exchange one band for another using a lower profile band. This is usually done without taking down the fixation sutures as the replacement band can be attached to the old band using a single suture. As one band is removed, the new band replaces it in the same retro-gastric tunnel.

Esophageal and Pouch Dilatation

These radiological findings are secondary to high pressures in the stomach and esophagus and develop gradually and chronically due to overeating. In some cases they will always appear if the band has been tightened inappropriately beyond optimum and are an inevitable consequence of a normal fluid and soft food intake. In the first instance the band should be partially deflated and the patient given further dietary advice regarding optimal meal consistency and volume. If there is a large pouch dilation then this usually behaves like a partial slippage and the patient may well obstruct again even with a partially deflated band. The key here is to have a lower threshold for radiological evaluation if there is a past history of these complications developing.

Partial Band Slippage – Responds Clinically to Band Deflation

A partial slippage usually will respond to full deflation of the band. This means that patients who had obstructive symptoms to fluids will now be able to drink. The band cannot be inflated fully without first being replaced higher around the cardia. This only makes sense if the patient has had successful weight loss whilst the band was in a good position before the slippage developed. If the patient demonstrated no success with the lap-band system the slippage of the band should be considered a reason for band removal and subsequent conversion to another type of bariatric surgery.

Full Slippage – No Clinical Response to Band Deflation

This is a surgical emergency, the consequences of which could result in gastric necrosis, leak, and death of the patient. Immediate laparoscopy once fluid resuscitation has taken place should be performed with band removal. The fundus may have been strangulated above the band and exhibit signs of necrosis. Once decompressed by band removal one usually finds a loose and redundant fundus which is amenable to excision if there is any suggestion of gastric necrosis. Excision is facilitated by laparoscopic stapling with articulated stapling device which cuts and seals the resected tissues.

Band Erosion or Migration into the Gastric Lumen

This is a rare complication in some units and common in others. This suggests that surgical techniques and band fill protocols in some way influence this complication. It is the experience of the authors of this chapter that erosion is always preceded by partial slippage which perhaps results in stretching and pressure necrosis of the gastric wall over the top edge of the band which results in erosion developing. Once erosion has occurred the band can be cut endoscopically using a band cutting device. The band is then pulled into the stomach lumen and removed endoscopically. If this is

not possible or not available then removal for erosion can be carried out laparoscopic but the band may only be accessible via a gastrotomy made high on the fundus. The band should be grasped, cut with scissors, and pulled into the abdominal cavity followed by closure of the gastrotomy.

References

2.3 Surgical technique

1. Buchwald H, Avidor Y, Braunwald E, Jensen MD, Pories W, Fahrbach K, Schoelles K (2004) Bariatric surgery. A systematic review and meta-analysis. YAMA 292:1724–1737
2. Stroh C, Hohmann U, Schramm H, Manger T (2005) Langzeitergebnisse nach Gastric Banding. Zentralbl Chir 130: 410–418
3. Stroh C, Hohmann U, Will U et al (2008) Experiences of two centers of bariatric surgery in the treatment of intragastrale band migration after gastric banding – the importance of the German multicenter observational study for quality assurance in obesity surgery 2005–2006. Int J Colorectal Dis 23(9):901–908
4. Stroh C, Birk D, Flade-Kuthe R et al (2009) A nationwide survey on bariatric surgery in Germany-results 2005–2007. Obes Surg 19(1):105–112

2.4 Surgical technique

1. Chua Ty, Mendiola RM (1995) Laparoscopic vertical banded gastroplasty: the Milwaukee experience. Obes Surg 5:77–80
2. Wittgrove AC, Clark GW, Schubert KR (1996) Laparoscopic gastric bypass, Roux-en-Y: technique and results in 75 patients with 3–30 months follow-up. Obes Surg 6:500–504
3. Cleator IGM, Litwin D, Phang PT, Brosseuk DT, Rae AJ (1994) Laparoscopic ileogastrostomy for morbid obesity. Obes Surg 4:358–360
4. Fried M, Miller K, Kormanova K (2004) Literature review of comparative studies of complications with Swedish band and Lap-Band®. Obes Surg 14:256–260
5. Dargent J (1999) Laparoscopic adjustable gastric banding: lessons from the first 500 patients in a Sinle Institution. Obes Surg 9:446–452
6. Favretti F, Cadiere GB, Segato G, De Marchi F et al (1999) Lap-band for the treatment of morbid obesity. A 6-year experience of 509 patients. Obes Surg 9:327
7. Klaiber Ch, Metzger A, Forsell P (2000) Laparoskopisches gastric banding. Chirurg 71:146–151
8. Miller K, Pump A, Hell E (2007) Vertical banded gastroplasty versus adjustable gastric banding: prospective long-term follow-up study.Surg Obes Relat Dis 3(1):84–90
9. Belva PH, Takieddine M, Lefebvre JC, Vaneukem P (1998) Laparoscopic LAP-BAND gastroplasty: European results. Obes Surg 8:364

10. De Jong JR, van Ramshorst B (1998) Re-interventions after laparoscopic gastric banding. Obes Surg 8:386

11. Elmore U, Restuccia A, Perrotta N, Polito D, De Leo A, Silecchia G, Basso N (1998) Laparoscopic Adjustable Silicon Gastric Banding (LASGB): analyses of 64 consecutive patients. Obes Surg 8:399

12. Angrisani L, Lorenzo M, Santoro T, Nicodemi O, Da Prato D, Ciannella M, Persico G, Tesauro B (1998) Follow-up of LAP-BAND Complications. Obes Surg 8:384

13. Chapman AE, Kiroff G, Game P et al (2004) Laparoscopic adjustable gastric banding in the treatment of obesity: a systematic literature review. Surgery 135:326–351

14. O'Brian P, Brown W, Smith A, Chapman L, Kotzander A, Dixon J, Stephens M (1998) The LAP-BAND provides effective control of morbid obesity – a prospective study of 350 patients followed for up to 4 years, Obes Surg 8:398

15. Mizrahi S, Avinoah E (2007) Technical tips for laparoscopic gastric banding: 6 years' experience in 2800 procedures by a single surgical team. Am J Surg 193:160–165

16. Desaive C (1995) Influence of the initial volume of the gastric pouch on the rate of complication after adjustable silicone gastric banding. Obes Surg 5:247

17. Chelala E, Cadiére GB, Favretti F, Himpens J, Vertruyen M, Bruyns J, Maroquin L, Lise M (1997) Conversions and complications in 185 laparoscopic adjustable silicone gastric banding cases. Surg Endosc 11:268–271

18. Alvarez-Cordero R, Ramirez-Wiella G, Aragon-Viruette E, Toledo-Delgado A (1998) Laparoscopic gastric banding: initial two year experience. Obes Surg 8:360

19. Miller K, Hell E (1999) Laparoscopic adjustable gastric banding: a prospective 4-year follow-up study. Obes Surg 9:183–187

20. Forsel P, Hellers G, Hell E (1998) The Swedish adjustable gastric banding (SAGB) for morbid obesity – weight loss, complications, pouch volume, and stoma diameter in a four-year follow up. Acta Chir Austriaca 30:161–165

21. Silecchia G, Polito D, De Leo A, Trentino P, Restuccia A, Basso N (1997) Major complications following laparoscopic adjustable silicone gastric banding (LAGB): a proposal for a minimally invasive treatment. Obes Surg 7:304

22. Miller K, Rettenbacher L, Hell E (1996) Adjustments and leak detection of the adjustable silicone gastric band (ASGB) and Lap-band TM adjustable gastric (LAGB) band system. Obes Surg 6:406–411

23. Miller K., Hell E (1999) Laparoscopic treatment of complications after adjustable gastric banding. Obes Surg 9:352–353

24. Greenstein RJ, Nissan A, Jaffin B (1998) Esophageal anatomy and function in laparoscopic gastric restrictive bariatric surgery: implications for patient selection. Obes Surg 8:199–206

25. Miller K, Amerhauser A, Rettenbacher L, Hell E (1999) Esophageal motility after vertical banded gastroplasty and laparoscopic adjustable gastric banding. Eur J Coelio-Surg 29:61

26. Miller K, Hell E (1999) Orlistat treatment after failure of the adjustable gastric band system. Obes Surg 4:333

Further Reading

2 Adjustable Gastic Banding

Cunneen SA (2008) Review of meta-analytic comparisons of bariatric surgery with a focus on laparoscopic adjustable gastric banding. Surg Obes Relat Dis 4(3 Suppl): 47–55

Dapri G, Cadiere GB, Himpens J (2009) Feasibility and technique of laparoscopic conversion of adjustable gastric banding to sleeve gastrectomy. Surg Obes Relat Dis 5(1): 72–76

Dargent J (2008) Isolated food intolerance after adjustable gastric banding: a major cause of long-term band removal. Obes Surg 18(7):829–832

Gagner M, Milone L, Yung E, Broseus A, Gumbs AA (2008) Causes of early mortality after laparoscopic adjustable gastric banding. Obes Surg 206(4):664–649

Iannelli A, Negri C, Piche T, Becaud A, Gugenheim J (2008) Iatrogenic injury of the intrathoracic esophagus sustained during a gastric banding procedure. Obes Surg 18(6): 742–744

Hudson SM, Dixon JB, O'Brien PE (2002) Sweet eating is not a predictor of outcome after Lap-Band placement. Can we finally bury the myth? Obes Surg 12(6): 789–794

Korenkov M, Sauerland S, Yuucel N, Köhler L, Goh P, Schierholz J, Troidl H (2003) Port function after laparoscopic adjustable gastric banding for morbid obesity. Surg Endosc 17(7):1068–10671

Korenkov M, Kneist W, Heintz A, Junginger Th (2004) Technical alternatives in laparoscopic placement of an adjustable gastric band: experience of two German university hospitals. Obes Surg 14:806–810

Miller KA, Miller KA (2008) Evolution of gastric band implantation and port fixation techniques. Surg Obes Relat Dis 4(3 Suppl):22–30

Prosch H, Tscherney R, Kriwanek S, Tscholakoff D (2008) Radiographical imaging of the normal anatomy and complications after gastric banding. Br J Radiol 81:753–757

Snyder B, Nguen A, Scarbourough T, Yu S, Wilson E (2009) Comparison of those who succeed in losing significant excessive weight after bariatric surgery and those who fail. Surg Endosc 23(10):2302–2306. Epub 2009 Jan 30

Stroh C, Birk D, Flade-Kuthe R, Frenken M, Herbig B, Höhne S, Köhler H, Lange V, Ludwig K, Matkowitz R, Meyer G, Pick P, Horbach T, Krause S, Schäfer L, Schlensak M, Shang E, Sonnenberg T, Susewind M, Voigt H, Weiner R, Wolff S, Lippert H, Wolf AM, Schmidt U, Manger T (2009) Bariatric Surgery Working Group: A nationwide survey on bariatric surgery in Germany – results 2005-2007. Obes Surg 19:105–112

Wölnerhanssen BK, Peters T, Kern B, Schötzau A, Ackermann C, von Füe M, Peterli R (2008) Predictors of outcome in treatment of morbid obesity by laparoscopic adjustable gastric banding: results of a prospective study of 380 patients. Surg Obes Relat Dis 4(4):500–506

2.1   Surgical technique

Dixon JB, O'Brien PE (2002) Neck circumference a good predictor of raised insulin and free androgen index in obese premenopausal women: changes with weight loss. Clin Endocrinol (Oxf) 57(6):769–778

Colles SL et al (2006) Preoperative weight loss with a very-low-energy diet: quantitation of changes in liver and abdominal fat by serial imaging. Am J Clin Nutr 84(2):304–311

2.4   Surgical technique

Council on Scientific Affairs (1988) Treatment of obesity in adults. JAMA 260:2547–2551

Segal L, Carter R, Zimmet P (1994) The cost of obesity, the Australian perspective. PharmacoEconomics 5(suppl. 1): 45–52

Martin LF, Hunter S, Lauve R, O'Leary JP. Severe obesity: expensive to society, frustrating to treat, but important to confront. South Med J 1995, 88, 9, 895–902.

National Institute of Health Consensus Statement. (1991) Gastrointestinal surgery for severe obesity. Obes Surg 1: 243–256

Finigan KM, Martin LF, Robinson AF, Roth N (1997) Improvement in quality of life one year after gastric Lap-Band®. Obes Surg 7:281

Miller K, Mayer E, Pichler M, Hell E (1997) Quality-of-life outcomes of patients with the LAP-BAND® versus non-operative treatment of obesity. Preliminary results of an ongoing long-term follow-up study. Obes Surg. 7:280

Pories WJ, Swanson MS, MacDonald KG et al (1995) Who would have thought it? An operation proves to be the most effective therapy for adult-onset diabetes mellitus. Ann Surg 222:339–352

Chapman AE, Kiroff G, Game P et al (2004) Laparoscopic adjustable gastric banding in the treatment of obesity: a systematic literature review. Surgery 135:326–351

Fried M, Hainer V, Basdevant A et al (2007) Clinical guidelines inter-disciplinary European guidelines on surgery of severe obesity. Int J Obes 10:1–9

Sugerman HJ, Brewer WH, Shiffman ML et al (1995) A multicenter, placebo-controlled, randomized, double-blind, prospective trial of prophylactic ursodiol for the prevention of gallstone formation following gastric-bypass-induced rapid weight loss. Am J Surg 169:91–96

Miller K, Hell E, Lang B, Lengauer E (2003) Gallstone formation prophylaxis following gastric restrictive procedures for weight loss: a randomized doubleblind placebo controlled trial. Ann Surg 238:697–702

Proximal (Classic) Gastric Bypass

3

Michael Korenkov, Guy-Bernard Cadière,
Kelvin D. Higa, Ahad Khan, Antonio Iannelli,
Gintaras Antanavicius, Sayeed Ikramuddin,
Rudolf A. Weiner, and Manuel Garcia-Caballero

M. Korenkov
Abteilung für Allgemein- und Visceralchirurgie,
Klinikum Werra-Meissner, Akademisches Lehrkrankenhaus der
Universität Göttingen, Elsa-Brendström-Straße 1, 37269
Eschwege, Germany
e-mail: michael.korenkov@klinikum-wm.de

G.-B. Cadière
CHU Saint-Pierre, Clinique de Chirurgie Digestive,
Rue Haute 322, B-1000 Bruxelles, Belgium
e-mail: guy-bernard_cadiere@stpierre-bru.be

K.D. Higa • A. Iannelli
Service de Chirurgie Digestive et Transplantation Hépatique
Hôpital Archet Nice, Cedex

Faculté de Médecine,
Université de Nice-Sophia-Antipolis Nice,

Centre Hospitalier Universitaire de Nice, Pôle Digestif Nice,
France

A. Khan (✉)
USA

G. Antanavicius • S. Ikramuddin
Department of Surgery, University of Minnesota, MMC 290,
420 Delaware St SE, Minneapolis, MN 55455, USA
e-mail: gintas444@yahoo.com; ikram001@umn.edu

R.A. Weiner
Head of the Department of Visceral- and bariatric Surgery,
Krankenhaus Sachsenhausen,
Schulstr. 31, D-60594 Frankfurt
e-mail: rweiner@khs-ffm.de

M. Garcia-Caballero
Department of Surgery, University Malaga,
Facultad de Medicina
29080-Malaga, Spain
e-mail: gcaballe@uma.es

Introduction

The intention of this procedure is a restriction of the size of the stomach by cutting it proximally and the creation of malabsorption by dividing the small intestine into an alimentary (Roux limb) and a biliopancreatic segment (Fig. 3.1). Both goals (restriction and malabsorption) are reached in one operation; it is therefore referred to as "combined procedure."

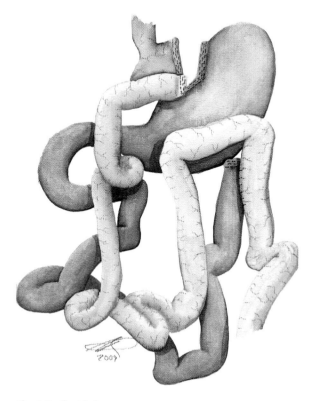

Fig. 3.1 Gastric bypass

M. Korenkov (ed.), *Bariatric Surgery*,
DOI 10.1007/978-3-642-16245-9_3, © Springer-Verlag Berlin Heidelberg 2012

The Roux-en-Y gastric bypass is a standard procedure in bariatric surgery. But there is no procedure with more technical modifications in the field; every large bariatric center has its own variation. The most significant differences are seen concerning the gastroenteral anastomosis. Among the many topics discussed among specialists are questions as whether to suture by hand or to use a stapler, to follow the retrocolic or the antecolic pathway, to use the linear or the circular stapler and if to operate completely laparoscopic or hand assisted. The jejunojejunostomy can also be performed in different ways; surgeons discuss an end-to-side or a side-to-side anastomosis, as well as completely stapler technique, combination from stapler and hand suturing or hand suturing techniques. The best length for the Roux limb and the biliopancreatic segment is also discussed.

Preparation

Setting, Positioning, and the Surgical Team
Positioning the patient is usually not a matter of discussion.

- The patient is positioned just like in gastric banding with widespread legs (lithotomy position) and the upper body is tilted upward in a 45° angle (reversed Trendelenburg position). Some surgeons position the patient lying flat on his back and then stand on the patient's left side.
- Adequate measures to prevent slipping are mandatory.
- The surgical team consists of the surgeon, an assistant holding the camera, a second assistant (not mandatory) and the scrub nurse. Mechanical retractor system can be used instead of a second assistant.
- The surgeon stands between the patient's legs. If there is one assistant, he will stand on the patient's left side, work the camera with his left hand and a grasper with his right hand.
- The pneumoperitoneum is created as in gastric banding, see page. 14).

Positioning the Trocars
The gastric bypass is performed using five or six trocars, all of which are positioned above the umbilicus. If an additional trocar is needed, it is not advisable to place it below or on the same level as the umbilicus.

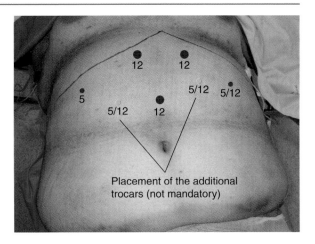

Fig. 3.2 High position of the trocars

The abdominal wall is much thicker here in morbidly obese patients; even extra long trocars might turn out to be too short. Even if the tip of the trocar reaches the abdominal cavity, the pressure of the surrounding fat tissue is very high; precise intraoperative manipulations will be very difficult to perform and the instruments may be damaged.

The position of the optical trocar is undisputed. It is inserted about 20 cm below the xiphoid a little left to the middle line.

The working trocars can be positioned "high" or "low," as in gastric banding (see page 15).

For the *high position of the trocars* the working trocars are placed high up in the epigastrium a little left and right to the middle line. The additional trocar for the liver retractor is placed below the left costal margin, the other additional trocar for the grasper is placed below the right costal margin. An eventually necessary additional working trocar can be placed in the right middle or upper abdomen (Fig. 3.2).

For the *low position of the trocars*, the optic trocar, two working trocars, and an additional trocar are all placed roughly in one line. The additional trocar for the liver retractor is placed in the epigastrium. If an additional working trocar becomes necessary, it is inserted below the right costal margin (Fig. 3.3).

Surgical Technique

After positioning the trocars, inspect the abdominal cavity to decide whether the procedure can be performed as planned. For the classic (proximal) gastric

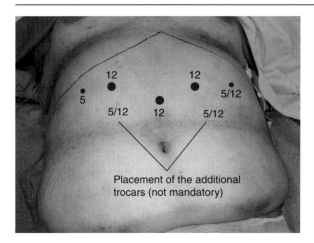

Fig. 3.3 Low position of the trocars

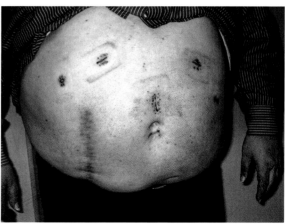

Fig. 3.4 Scars after laparotomy because of appendicitis with perforation. Laparoscopy revealed massive intraabdominal adhesions; some segments of the small intestine were stuck tightly within the lower abdomen. Instead of performing gastric bypass surgery, a sleeve gastrectomy was performed as a first step

bypass a mobilized section of the small intestine must be pulled up into the upper abdomen to create the gastrojejunostomy.

- Before cutting the stomach make sure the anatomical situation is suitable for this maneuver. Limiting factors are very short and fatty mesentery, especially in very obese male patients, as well as massive intraabdominal adhesions with segments of the small intestine stuck together (Fig. 3.4).

> To avoid the unpleasant situation of producing a gastrojejunal anastomosis under tension, we do not begin the procedure with cutting the stomach, but with measuring and preparation of the jejunal segments. This is especially recommendable in patients with a BMI over 50 or after abdominal surgery in the patient's history, such as appendectomy or surgery in the lower abdomen. In patients with a BMI under 45, little visceral fat tissue and no known complications in their history, the procedure can very well be begun by cutting the stomach. If the Roux limb cannot be pulled up tension free, change plans and perform another procedure, such as a duodenal switch, a sleeve gastrectomy, or the distal "single anastomosis gastric bypass" (see M. Garcia-Caballero, p. 103-107).

Step 1 – Measuring the Small Intestine

- Tilt the patient head down for this step (Trendelenburg position).
- Move from between the patient's legs to his left side.
- Remove the liver retractor to avoid accidental liver injury.
- In patients with a BMI below 45, begin with exposure of Treitz's arch. Hold the greater omentum with two graspers and pull it upward.
- Then identify the transverse colon, grasp it with the same instruments and pull it up also.
- Then measure the jejunum up to the intended incision spot.

> The small intestine can be measured with a tape measure or a specially marked grasper or simply estimated.

- If you use a *tape measure* (a commercially available measure or a surgical one, such as 5 mm mersilene band), grasp the first jejunal segment at Treitz's arch together with the end of the measure, preferably using a grasper with a wide end.
- Grasp the measure a bit further down with a second grasper (of the same design), stretch it and measure the jejunal segment distal to Treitz's arch.

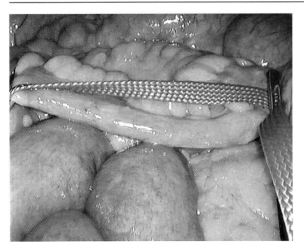

Fig. 3.5 Measuring the small intestine with a mersilene band

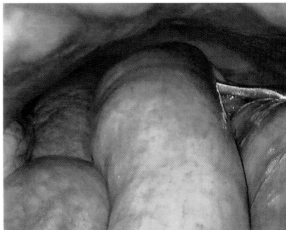

Fig. 3.6 Bringing the chosen jejunal segment up to the proximal stomach

- Then open the first grasper and take over the jejunum and the measure.
- Now open the second grasper, take the measure, stretch it and measure the next segment. We tie one end of the measure to the atraumatic grasper to speed up this step (Fig. 3.5).
- If you use *graspers with distance marks*, measuring is done much faster than with a tape measure; a distance of 5 cm is preferable.
- If you *estimate*, grasp the jejunum at Treitz's arch with a grasper. Then position another grasper about 10 cm further distal. Keep switching graspers, positioning them always the same distance from each other.

The identification of Treitz's arch and the measurement of the jejunum can be difficult in patients with a higher BMI. In these cases it is advisable to begin measuring at the ileocecal valve. Intraabdominal adhesions can cause problems. Even comparatively small procedures, such as an appendectomy or surgery in the lower abdomen can result in tight adhesions between the greater omentum and the peritoneum, so that the omentum is stuck tightly in the lower abdomen. The following steps can be extremely difficult in these cases, especially in very obese patients with heavy fat tissue in the omentum. In order to see better, the patient must be tilted even further head down. If a patient has undergone lower abdominal surgery before, install shoulder rests before the procedure to prevent the patient from slipping off the table.

Step 2 – Transecting the Jejunum

Before cutting the jejunum at the measured point, define which route the Roux limb is to take to the pouch. It can be done antecolic–antegastric, retrocolic–retrogastric, or retrocolic–antegastric. The antecolic–antegastric pathway is technically the most simple to perform and is therefore usually chosen. The other two pathways are only suitable for patients with a short and fatty mesentery, if the antecolic pathway would lead to high tension between the Roux limb and the pouch.

- Before you cut, pull the chosen jejunal segment up to the future pouch to test for tension (Fig. 3.6).

Attention: If this test shows tension, try the neighboring jejunal segment in either direction instead.

- When a tension-free situation is established, skeletonize the mesentery around the future cut with ultrasound scissors.
- The camera is then usually removed from the supraimbilical trocar and inserted into the left working trocar or the left additional trocar, depending on the intraoperative situation.
- Insert a grasper through the supraumbilical camera trocar and pull the small intestine up into the middle abdomen close to the anterior abdominal wall.
- The assistant grasps the intestine with an atraumatic grasper (right working trocar) about 10 cm away from the surgeon's grasper to tense it between the two graspers.
- Then cut a window into the mesentery.

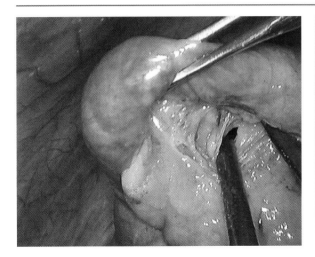

Fig. 3.7 Opening in the mesentery before cutting the jejunum

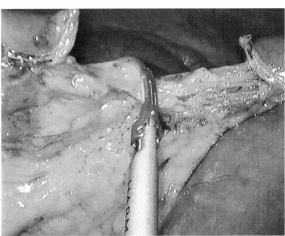

Fig. 3.9 Dissection of the mesentery with ultrasound scissors after cutting the jejunum

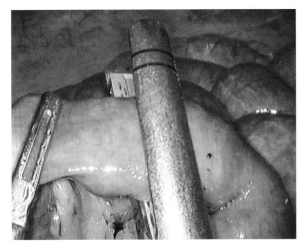

Fig. 3.8 Cutting the jejunum with a linear stapler (blue cartridge)

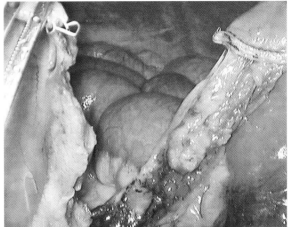

Fig. 3.10 Opening the mesentery half way down

To avoid hemorrhage from the fat tissue in the mesentery, we begin dissection with a coagulatory monopolar hook instead of the ultrasound scissors.

- After opening the upper layer of the mesentery, continue dissection with a blunt dissector or a coagulation suction tube until the backside is reached. The opening must be large enough to allow passage of the stapler (Fig. 3.7).
- Cut the jejunum with a linear stapler (blue cartridge) (Fig. 3.8).
- Then cut the mesentery with the ultrasound scissors about halfway down (Figs. 3.9 and 3.10).

If this dissection is not sufficient for a tension-free anastomosis, continue mobilizing the mesentery down to the peritoneum on the back.

If it is not possible to pull the jejunum up tension free, change plans and switch to another procedure, such as a duodenal switch, a sleeve gastrectomy, or the distal "single anastomosis gastric bypass." The patient must be told beforehand that the planned procedure might not be possible to perform and that in case of certain circumstances a different operation will have to be performed.

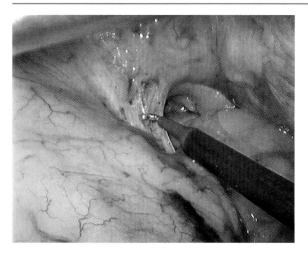

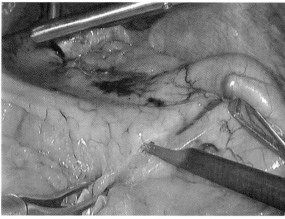

Fig. 3.12 Opening the lesser omentum with a monopolar hook

Fig. 3.11 Angle of His, beginning dissection with a monopolar hook

Step 3 – Mobilization of the Angle of His

- Insert the liver retractor back into the trocar and pull the liver upward and to the right to show the GE junction.
- Begin dissection by mobilizing the angle of His. Pull the stomach to the right toward the liver with a grasper (right working trocar), holding it by the upper end.
- Grasp the greater omentum close to the gastric fundus (left additional trocar) and pull it down. The angle of His is now visible and can be mobilized.
- Use ultrasound scissors or a monopolar hook until the left crus of diaphragm is visible (Fig. 3.11).

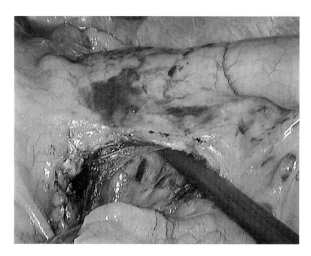

Fig. 3.13 Beginning retrogastral dissection, then opening the omental bursa

Cutting the gastrophrenic ligament between the gastric fundus and the diaphragm is usually sufficient for an adequate dissection of the angle of His. In some very rare cases the cranial short gastric arteries must be cut.

- Cut the hepatogastric ligament (lesser omentum) close to the stomach between the first and the second, or sometimes between the second and the third branch of the "crow's foot."

This step should be begun with a monopolar hook and not the ultrasound scissors because using the scissors in this area can result in hemorrhage more often (Fig. 3.12).

Step 4 – Dissection of the Retrogastric Tunnel

Many surgeons begin the procedure with this step. Open the omental bursa coming from the lesser curvature and create a retrogastric tunnel leading toward the angle of His.

- Grasp the upper part of the stomach close to the lesser curvature (left additional trocar) and pull it toward the spleen.

- After opening the lesser omentum, continue with retrogastric blunt dissection and open the omental bursa (Figs. 3.12 and 3.13).

A slight diffuse hemorrhage usually occurs during dissection; it will soon stop spontaneously.

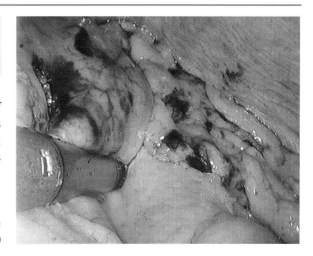

Fig. 3.14 Cutting the stomach. The first stapler is positioned horizontally

- Continue the blunt dissection toward the angle of His. There are two different possibilities for this maneuver. You can finish the retrogastric tunnel first and then cut the stomach or dissect and cut as you go along.

Step 5 – Transecting the Stomach

- After dissecting the retrogastric tunnel, cut the stomach to create a small pouch with about 15–20 cm³. Use a linear stapler for this step; we chose a 45 mm Endo-GIA with a blue cartridge and an angled tip.
- Cut the stomach bit by bit, going horizontally first (Fig. 3.14). Make sure the stomach tube has been pulled back into the esophagus before.

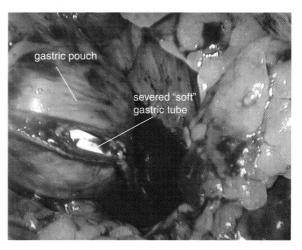

Fig. 3.15 Entrapment of the gastric tube in the stapler suture while creating the stomach pouch

Accidentally "stapling" the stomach tube can have dramatic consequences. In this situation (Fig. 3.15) the anesthesiologist was asked to pull the stomach tube back. The stomach was cut after he had answered that the tip of the tube was almost up in the mouth. When firing the second cartridge, the tube was cut. Using the stapler was normal; no difficulties indicated a possible entrapment of the tube. The sections of the suture in the pouch and the rest of the stomach were opened with scissors; the remainders of the tube were removed. The openings were then stapled close again. Creating the pouch-enteroanastomosis was difficult, however, because the pouch had become too small. It was done completely by hand; postoperative recovery was normal. Since then, we always have the stomach tube removed completely before stapling and have it replaced afterward, even although our anesthesiological colleagues object (Fig. 3.15).

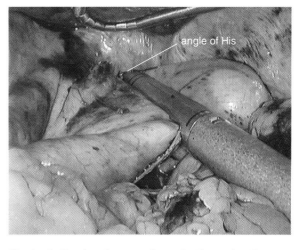

Fig. 3.16 Creating the stomach pouch. The cutting line runs parallel to the lesser curvature towards the angle of His

- Next point the stapler upward tangentially, holding it almost parallel to the lesser curvature.
- Continue going upward almost vertically until the stomach is completely cut (Fig. 3.16).

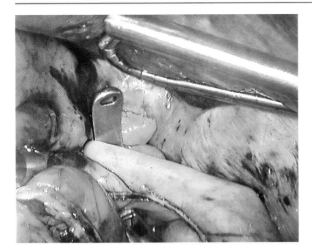

Fig. 3.17 Last "bridge" of stomach tissue. The tip of the flexible dissector is cut free in the angle of His

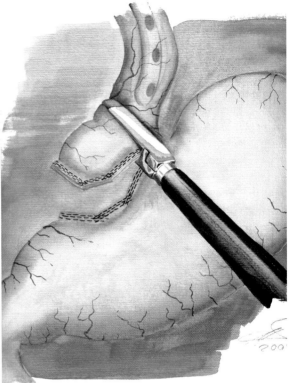

Fig. 3.18 Accidentally cutting the esophagus instead of the stomach

- A complete transsection of the stomach is mandatory. Before you proceed, make sure there is no tissue left between the pouch and the rest of the stomach (Fig. 3.17).

Keep the following in mind while cutting the stomach:

Hemorrhage from the stapler suture: It will stop without any other measure most of the times. We recommend a staple suture reinforcement to avoid hemorrhage or to add a suture on the bleeding point.

Affect the esophagus with one of the vertical cuts: A clear identification of the anatomical situation can be difficult at times, especially in very obese patients with massive fat pads around the GE junction, which can lead to this technical mistake with its fatal result (Fig. 3.18). To avoid it, insert a calibration balloon into the pouch. Also make sure to dissect the angle of His very clearly. A flexible dissector or the "goldfinger" are helpful here. If the esophagus is stapled accidentally, switch to open laparotomy immediately. If a tension-free esophagoenteral anastomosis can be created with a 21 or 25 mm circular stapler, it is a good solution for this situation. If not, the proximal remnant stomach must be connected to the esophagus as ultima ratio. To avoid a gastroesophageal reflux and to achieve the desired weight loss, per-

form a duodenal switch with a sleeve gastrectomy, either immediately or in a second procedure.

Including the fundus to the gastric pouch: To close the secretion of ghrelin off completely from the passage of food, the fundus must remain part of the remnant stomach. An incompletely detached fundus can result in inadequate weight loss due to remaining ghrelin production (hypothesis; Figs. 3.19 and 3.20).

Step 6 – Cutting the Greater Omentum (Not Mandatory)

A very fatty omentum can lead to a certain tension between the pouch and the alimentary segment. Sometimes the pars libera of the greater omentum has to be cut in order to relieve the tension on the anastomosis.

- Position the patient flat on the back or in a slight Trendelenburg position.

Fig. 3.19 Cutting lines for the creation of the stomach pouch

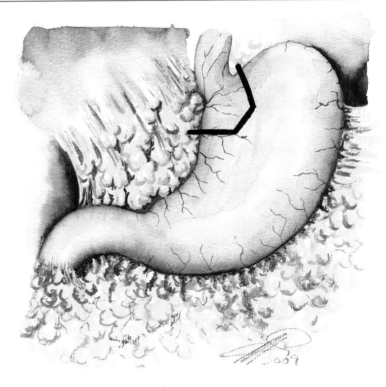

left working trocar and the right additional trocar) and fold it upward.

- Tense the greater omentum between the two instruments and cut down to the transverse colon with ultrasound scissors.

Take care to avoid thermal damage to the stomach wall or accidentally opening the intestine. In very obese patients, the wall of the colon is covered with a thick layer of fat, which can make the identification of the transverse colon difficult. We dissect the cranial segment of the greater omentum with scissors, partly cutting, partly dissecting bluntly, without electricity. Small hemorrhages can be stopped precisely with a bipolar hook.

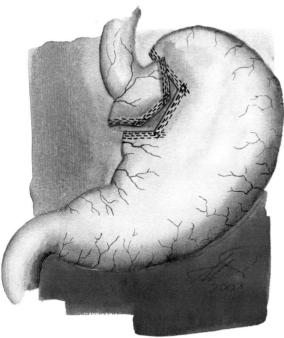

Fig. 3.20 Finished stomach pouch. The fundus must remain part of the remnant stomach completely

- Grasp the loose end of the greater omentum with two graspers (preferably babcock forceps, using the

Step 7 – Creation of the Gastroenteral Anastomosis

The next steps depend on the exact technique used. Today linear stapler sutures, circular stapler sutures, and handmade anastomoses are performed. So far no technique has proven to be superior.

Creating a Linear Stapler Anastomosis

To create the linear stapler anastomosis, the Roux limb is connected with its side to the front part of the pouch with a linear stapler suture. For the antecolic–antegastric pathway you can transect the jejunum, pull the Roux limb up to the pouch and connect them with the linear stapler. You can also connect the jejunal segment to the pouch first and then cut the segment off close to the stomach with the linear stapler.

In both methods it is very important not to confuse the two jejunal segments. In patients with less intraabdominal fat tissue, we cut the jejunum after creating the anastomosis. In patients with massive intraabdominal fat tissue, we cut the jejunum first and then pull the Roux limb upward.

For the retrocolic–retrogastric pathway, the jejunum is always cut first and pulled up afterward.

For the linear antecolic-antegastric gastroenteral anastomosis we favor the following technique:

- Fasten the side of the Roux loop to the anterior wall of the pouch with a few stay sutures.
- After fastening it, inspect the Roux limb very carefully, considering especially the following three aspects:
  - Tension between the Roux limb and the pouch
  - Blood supply of the Roux limb
  - A possible twisting of the Roux limb (this happens more often if following the retrocolic pathway)
- If the segment that is fastened to the pouch is tension-free and well-supplied with blood, cut small openings for the stapler into the pouch and the jejunum (opposite to the mesentery) with the ultrasound scissors, approximately 3 cm from the stay suture.
- Then insert the 45 mm Endo GIA into both openings (left working trocar), close it and fire. The resulting defect in the anterior side of the anastomosis is closed by hand.
- Place absorbable single sutures at the ends of the opening and tie the knots.
- Grasp the corner sutures with two graspers (endodissectors) and pull the upper one in cranial direction. The grasper can be inserted through the right additional trocar (instead of the liver retractor).

If the left hepatic lobe still needs to be held, insert an additional 5 mm trocar into the right upper or middle abdomen.

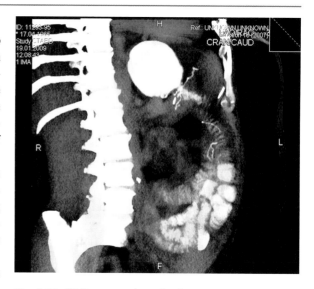

Fig. 3.21 CT-Reconstruction of a linear pouch-enteroanastomosis (courtesy of Dr. Ingrid Harth, Radiologisches Institut, Kreiskrankenhaus Eschwege)

- Then insert the stomach tube through the pouch into the Roux limb. The remaining opening is tensed between two graspers and closed with two absorbable running sutures (2-0).
- Suture going "outside-inside-inside-outside" and tie them together in the middle of the opening.
- Then close the lumen of the Roux loop below the tip of the stomach tube with an atraumatic intestinal forceps and inject about 50 mL methylene blue through the tube. If no leakage is seen, the creation of the gastroenteral anastomosis is finished (Fig. 3.21).

If the jejunal segment was not cut before the creation of the gastroenteral anastomosis, do so before testing for tightness of the anastomosis. Make sure you cut the correct segment!

Creating an Anastomosis with the Circular Stapler

For this technique there are several different ways to position the anvil. It can be inserted into the pouch from the abdominal cave or through mouth and esophagus (transorally). At first we created circular anastomoses with a circular stapler inserted transabdominally, but now we prefer the linear stapler. We have no own experience with the transoral technique and therefore refrain from describing it here (see Gagner, p. 148–153).

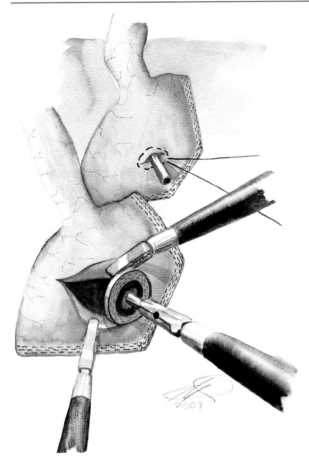

Fig. 3.22 Inserting the anvil into the pouch and creating a purse string suture

For the transabdominal technique proceed as following:

- Insert the anvil of the 25 mm circular stapler through the left working trocar into the abdominal cavity. This trocar will later be used for the circular stapler.
- Remove the 12 mm trocar and enlarge the cut in the skin to 2–2.5 cm. Dilate the trocar channel far enough to accommodate the 25 mm stapler with the anvil.
- Then open the stapler, remove the anvil from the device, and hold it with a special grasper.
- Remove the stapler and insert a 20 mm trocar or the "old" 12 mm trocar back into the channel. If you use the 12 mm trocar, insulate the opening with a gauze strip.
- There are two different ways of inserting the anvil into the stomach pouch. One method requires a small cut into the anterior wall of the stomach with an ultrasound scalpel. Then prepare a purse-string suture with a nonabsorbable monofilament suture. Now insert the anvil into the pouch and close the purse-string suture (Fig. 3.22).

- The other method is easier to perform:
- Cut a small opening into the anterior wall of the future pouch before cutting off the stomach completely.
- Now cut a 2 cm gastrotomy into the fundus of the remnant pouch close to the stapled seam.
- Insert a grasper through the cut in the pouch into the cut in the remnant stomach (right working trocar). Grasp the handle of the anvil and pull it in until the handle comes out through the gastrotomy in the pouch. This way it is secured tightly inside the pouch and does not need to be fastened otherwise. The gastrotomy in the remnant stomach is resected during the definitive creation of the remnant pouch and removed from the abdomen through a widened opening in the left upper abdomen (Fig. 3.23).
- Open the stapled suture in the jejunum segment with scissors or the ultrasound scalpel and hold it with two babcock forceps (right working trocar, left additional trocar).
- Widen the opening in the left upper abdomen and remove the working trocar. Insert the stapler inside its protective sheath into the abdomen and then into the jejunum.
- Screw the tip of the stapler through the wall of the Roux loop opposite to the mesentery. Reposition one of the babcock forceps (right working trocar) to hold the jejunal wall under tension.
- After screwing the stapler off completely, remove the babcock forceps altogether and replace with a special grasper.
- Grasp the handle of the anvil with this instrument and connect the anvil with the stapler body.
- After checking the correct position of the Roux loop (twisted?) fire the stapler.
- Remove the stapler and close the opening with the linear stapler.
- Then check for leakage, following the above mentioned instructions.

Creating the Anastomosis by Hand

There are several variations of this technique. We prefer to connect the end of the pouch to the side of the jejunum. Suture the backside of the anastomosis in a double line. We close the first line with seroserous single sutures (vicryl 2-0), tying extracorporeal knots, because it can be done faster than intracorporeal knots. We position open sutures in the corners and 3–4 between them, as in the conventional method. Then perform gastrotomy and enterotomy with ultrasound scissors. Close the back line with a 2-0 vicryl running

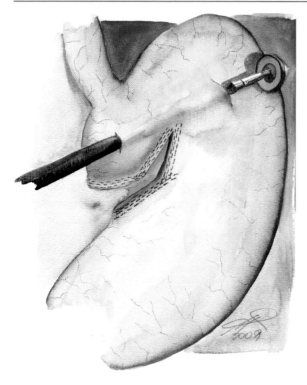

Fig. 3.23 Inserting the anvil through the remnant stomach

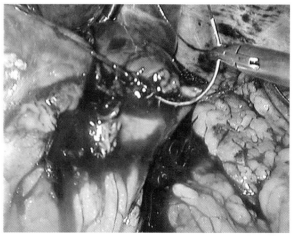

Fig. 3.24 Closing the anterior section of the gastroenteral anastomosis by hand

suture. Then insert a stomach tube through the opening into the Roux limb. The front side of the anastomosis is closed with a simple interrupted suture through all layers, using a 2-0 vicryl suture. Perform a test for leakage as described above (Fig. 3.24).

> We do not create the anastomosis by hand routinely, only in situations not suitable for the linear stapler.

Retrocolic Position of the Roux Limb

Situations requiring the retrocolic positioning of the Roux limb are rare, but not altogether avoidable. Every bariatric surgeon should therefore be familiar with this technique.

- Test the jejunum carefully for mobility before you cut. If the chosen segment cannot be pulled up far enough without tension and no other segment is available, the retrocolic approach is an option.
- Cut the greater omentum from the pars libera down to the edge of the stomach first. Cut a wide opening into the omental bursa.

- Now create an opening in the avascular zone of the transverse mesocolon. Just left to Treitz's arch there are usually the least amount of fat tissue and no blood vessels. This area is almost transparent, even in very obese male patients.

> This is not always easy, because these are patients with vast amounts of intraabdominal fat tissue. Performing diaphanoscopy to identify the avascular zone is quite laborious in laparoscopy. We use a second camera with an additional light (as used in rectoscopy). It is inserted through the left working trocar. The light connected to the camera should be held sidewise to reduce glare.

- After cutting the greater omentum and opening the omental bursa stretch the transverse colon between two babcock forceps (right working trocar and left additional trocar) and pull upward.
- Begin dissection about 3 cm above and a little to the left of the duodenal-jejunal junction. You will need an additional trocar; we place a 5 mm trocar between the working trocar and the additional trocar in the right upper abdomen. Use blunt instruments with rounded tips, such as a coagulation suction tube or a palpation probe.
- Diffuse hemorrhage is controlled with the coagulation suction tube and monopolar electricity.
- Continue dissecting in cranial – ventral direction.

In very obese patients the fat tissue in the mesentery is hard to distinguish from the pancreas; in confusing situations, injuries can occur. We recommend to move the transverse colon occasionally during dissection and to look at the omental bursa to make sure you are proceeding in the right direction.

The opening can also be closed with a linear stapler. We believe this technique to be questionable for two reasons: stenosis can occur or if, in an effort to avoid stenosis, too little tissue is grasped, leakage. To reduce the risk of these complications, some authors recommend using two stapler cartridges for the enteroenteral anastomosis: one going craniad, the other caudad.

Step 8 – Creating the Enteroenteral Anastomosis

The side-to-side anastomosis is usually created with the linear stapler. Except for differences in the closure of the enterotomy, surgical technique varies little at this step.

- After defining the Roux limb and the biliopancreatic segment at the correct length, align the two segments and connect them with a single traction suture.
- Create small openings in the two segments opposite to the mesentery with an ultrasound scalpel.
- Insert the jaws of 45 mm Endo GIA linear stapler into the openings and close the anastomosis.
- Inspect the suture. Hemorrhage is rare, but not always avoidable.

For small diffuse hemorrhage we use a coagulation suction tube with monopolar electricity. A suture is rarely necessary.

- Then close the openings with two parallel, approximately 15 cm long continuous sutures with a 2.0 vicryl suture. Place the sutures parallel to the running direction of the bowel. Begin the upper suture at the cranial end of the opening and tie a knot.
- Work continuously in and out of serosa and mucosa. The assistant must keep the suture under tension with a grasper (left working trocar). Close half of the opening.
- Begin another suture at the caudal corner and work toward the middle, using the same technique.
- Tie both ends together, making sure that both sutures are tightened sufficiently to avoid leakage.

Step 9 – Closing the Mesentery

In this last step all artificial openings in the mesentery must be closed again. The technique for this step should be chosen according to the intraoperative situation. We most often prefer single sutures with absorbable material. Many other authors prefer non-absorbable material.

This part of the procedure must be performed very carefully. Even with the relief of having finished the difficult last step successfully and the urge to finish the whole operation soon, the surgeon must take time and care for this step. All openings in the mesentery must be identified and closed.

Difficult Situations and Intraoperative Complications

Intraoperative difficulties during gastric bypass surgery are usually the result of the following problems:
- Intraoperative hemorrhage
- Impaired blood supply in the pouch ("blue pouch")
- Impaired blood supply in the Roux segment ("blue loop")

Intraoperative hemorrhage during gastric bypass surgery can arise from the stapler suture, the lesser omentum, the retrogastric cavity, or the mesentery of the small intestine.

Hemorrhage from the stapler suture can be stopped quite easily with a single suture. Hemorrhage from the mesentery is also usually unproblematic and can be controlled with a suture or coagulation. Hemorrhage from the retrogastric cavity during the creation of the pouch usually stops spontaneously and rarely causes any serious trouble.

Hemorrhage from the lesser omentum however can be quite difficult from a surgical point of view. In some cases a large hematoma can result, which can impair the blood supply of the pouch.

A Large Hematoma Has Developed in the Pouch near the Lesser Curvature

Predisposing factors: Cutting fat tissue with the ultrasound scissor without dissecting the tip of the scalpel first and thus injuring a blood vessel.

Prevention: Do not use the ultrasound scissor to create the retrogastric channel for transsection of the stomach. We recommend beginning the dissection at the lesser curvature, using a monopolar hook. A small portion of the surface of the lesser omentum is opened first, then dissection is continued bit by bit through the fat tissue. Blood vessels can be identified, dissected and, if necessary, cut under visual control.

Management: The hematoma impairs blood supply to the pouch and can cause the pouchenteral anastomosis to break. On the other hand, hemostatic measures close to the lesser curvature can also impair blood supply of the pouch. If the hematoma in the lesser omentum does not increase in size and the front and back sides of the pouch are well supplied with blood, we recommend to let it be.

However, if the hematoma does grow larger or the stomach wall turns purple in color, it needs to be treated. The peritoneum of the lesser omentum must be opened, the hematoma removed, and bleeding blood vessels must be closed with sutures, coagulation, or clips.

A Final Inspection at the End of the Procedure Reveals an Impaired Blood Supply of the Roux Segment ("Blue Loop")

Predisposing factors: An overly generous removal of the mesentery at the end of the Roux segment or a twisting of the Roux segment with consequent compression of the mesenterial blood vessels.

Prevention: Do not remove a too broad portion of the mesentery of the intestine. From a surgical point of view, this is not necessary, as the gastroenteral anastomosis is created side-by-side. Take care to avoid twisting the Roux segment while pulling it upward.

Management: Impaired blood supply of the Roux loop often does not show before the end of the procedure. At this point the surgeon tends to compromise more easily; decisions are likely to be influenced by a more negligent attitude. We recommend to undo the anastomosis, reposition the segment, and close the anastomosis again. If difficulties arise, do not hesitate to switch to a conventional surgical approach.

Revision Procedures Due To Surgical Complications

Revision procedures after gastric bypass surgery are divided into two groups, depending on their cause; procedures due to surgical complications and procedures to correct the negative effects of the anatomical changes (see below).

Postoperative complications are classified based on the anatomy of the gastric bypass:
- Complications in the pouch, the pouch-enteral anastomosis and in the blind loop
- Complications in the remnant stomach and the duodenum
- Complications around the enteroenteral anastomosis
- Complications in the remaining intestine

Based on the appearance of the problem, the complications are classified as following:
- Septic complications due to leakage or necrosis
- Hemorrhage
- Bowel obstruction/ileus
- Special cases

1. Septic Complications (Pouch Necrosis, Leak of the Gastroenteral Anastomosis, the Stapler Suture, or the Enteroenteral Anastomosis)

Relaparoscopy Because of Septic Deterioration of the General Condition Early After the Procedure Reveals a Necrotic Gastric Pouch

Predisposing factors: This complication is very rare, but not completely unknown. Blood supply for the pouch is based on blood vessels from the lesser curvature. Predisposing factors for pouch necrosis are an impairment of the blood supply due to a hematoma or because the blood vessels have been cut deliberately as a hemostatic measure.

Prevention: Avoid the formation of a hematoma around the lesser curvature.

Management: Pouch necrosis is a critical life-threatening situation. Therapy is the emergency removal of the pouch, a closure of the esophagus, and the insertion of a jejunostoma into the also closed blind Roux loop.

Another variation here is the closure of the Roux loop and the insertion of a gastrostoma into the remnant stomach. The esophagus is drained through a soft nasal tube or a salivary fistula at the neck. After the patients' general condition has improved sufficiently, a second procedure is performed. The remnant stomach is turned into a gastric sleeve and connected to the esophagus.

Other techniques, such as placing a segment of the Roux loop between the esophagus and the remnant stomach, are also possible.

Septic Deterioration of the General Condition Early After the Procedure; a Water-Soluble Contrast Swallow Reveals Leakage of the Gastroenteral Anastomosis

Predisposing factors: Leakage of the gastroenteral anastomosis is a significant complication of gastric bypass surgery with an incidence between 1% and 5%. The most important predisposing factor is little surgical experience. The significance of other factors, such as BMI, gender, age, open surgical approach, and the antecolic position of the Roux loop is discussed controversially today.

Prevention: Unfortunately there is no easy way to avoid this complication. Basic surgical guidelines must be followed strictly: a tension-free anastomosis and undisturbed blood supply of the segments are essential. Before stomach and jejunum are cut, make sure that the Roux segment can be pulled upward tension-free.

A test for leakage during the procedure with methylene blue or a gastroscopy is mandatory.

Management: Therapy of leakage of the gastroenteral anastomosis is not necessarily surgical. If the patient's condition is stable and the leakage small, a conservative approach can be tried.

The *conservative therapy* consists of complete food restriction and enteral feeding through a tube, which is placed deep into the Roux segment (endoscopically or radiologically controlled), as well as broad-spectrum antibiotics and an adequate drainage, which is either positioned during the procedure (as a prophylactic measure) or inserted later. However, emergency procedures are performed very much more often.

A *relaparoscopy* is performed first to assess the extent of the procedure and whether it can be done laparoscopic safely.

The simplest procedure is the laparoscopic closure of the broken suture. After this, a test for leakage must be performed intraoperatively. Most broken anastomoses can be treated this way successfully.

In some cases, however, the opening is too large and extensive local inflammation results in "brittle" tissue; a suture cannot solve the problem. These situations are especially difficult and require advanced surgical skills.

One possibility is *drainage from the leak* via a gastrostoma. A Foley catheter is inserted into the broken suture. Then a small balloon is inflated and the tube is pulled out through a small incision, usually situated in the left middle or upper abdomen. Try to suture the serosa of the pouch and the Roux-segment to the peritoneum close to the tube.

In very difficult cases, when the gastroenteral anastomosis and the stapler suture of the pouch are both broken, therapy is similar to that in cases of pouch necrosis.

Septic Deterioration of the General Condition After the Procedure; an Abdominal CT with a Water-Soluble Contrast Swallow Reveals a Little Free Air and a Possible Leakage Around the Enteroenteral Anastomosis

Predisposing factors: This complication is rare, but not completely unknown. Predisposing factors are technical mistakes during the creation of the anastomosis and intestinal obstruction below the entroenteral anastomosis.

Prevention: For more unexperienced bariatric surgeons we recommend creating a side-to-side anastomosis with a linear stapler and closing the enterotomy by hand. This technique is the easiest when operating laparoscopic. At the end of the procedure, the anastomosis must be inspected very carefully from all sides, especially the upper and the lower end of the enteroenteral anastomosis. The two segments must be pulled apart for this. The next step should only be performed if the anastomosis looks absolutely flawless.

Management: Therapy of a broken enteroenteral anastomosis is always surgical. If the opening is only small, an additional suture closes the broken part sufficiently. A larger opening with marked perifocal inflammation however requires the removal of the segments with the first anastomosis and the creation of a new enteroenteral anastomosis.

At the end of every procedure due to a broken enteroenteral anastomosis a complete revision of the entire small intestine must be performed to identify and remove kinks and other possible obstructions.

2. Gastrointestinal Hemorrhage (Mallory-Weiss Syndrome, Ulcers Around the Anastomosis and Hemorrhage from the Stapler Suture, a Duodenal Ulcer or the Enteroenteral Anastomosis)

Gastrointestinal hemorrhage after gastric bypass surgery happens. Early onset hemorrhage is distinguished from late post-operative hemorrhage. Depending on the anatomy of the gastric bypass, the origin of the hemorrhage can have different locations.

Very often, gastrointestinal hemorrhage after gastric bypass surgery stops spontaneously without any treatment; one or two blood transfusions usually are sufficient. In a few cases interventional or surgical measures have to be taken.

The following situations are classified depending on the origin of the hemorrhage.

Severe, Hemodynamically Relevant Hemorrhage from the Upper Gastrointestinal Tract After Gastric Bypass Surgery, Gastroscopy Reveals Mallory-Weiss Syndrome

Predisposing factors: This source is quite unusual after gastric bypass surgery, but possible. Excessive postoperative vomiting might be the cause.

Prevention: If the patient begins to feel sick early after the procedure, take anti-emetic measures in time. Patients must know the risks of excessive vomiting before they leave the hospital.

Management: Treatment of choice are endoscopic injections around the bleeding area. Hemorrhage from an ulcer around the anastomosis or the stapler suture is treated in a similar way.

Emergency Admittance to the Hospital Years After Gastric Bypass Surgery Because of Melena, Hypotension and Tachycardia, No Source of Bleeding in Emergency Gastroscopy and Coloscopy, Angio-CT Reveals a Possible Hemorrhage from the Duodenum

Predisposing factors: This kind of hemorrhage is very rare, predisposing factors are unknown.

Prevention: The incidence of bleeding duodenal ulcers after gastric bypass surgery is very low, therefore the benefit of prophylactic measures cannot be easily assessed. Some bariatric surgeons nevertheless recommend a life-long therapy with proton pump inhibitors after gastric bypass surgery.

Management: The method of choice is the angiographic embolization of the bleeding blood vessel. If the bleeding cannot be stopped, an emergency procedure must be performed, preferably a laparatomy. A duodenotomy is followed by suturing the bleeding vessel. If this vessel is not found, we recommend an intraoperative endoscopic examination through the remnant stomach (Fig. 3.25).

3. Intestinal Obstruction/Ileus (Blind-Loop Syndrome, Stenosis of the Jejunojejunostomy, Incarcerated Internal Hernia, Adhesions, Stenosis of the Roux Loop in the Mesocolon)

Severe Sickness and Dysphagia, a Water-Soluble Contrast Swallow Reveals a Massively Dilated Blind Loop with a Large Deposit of Contrast and a Very Slow Passage Through the Roux Loop

Predisposing factors: A blind-loop syndrome occurs only very rarely and is the consequence of a technically faulty gastroenteral anastomosis. Two major aspects are to be mentioned:

- The blind loop is below the Roux loop (Fig. 3.26).
- The blind loop is too long (Fig. 3.27).

Prevention: Make sure the blind loop remains above the Roux segment during the creation of the gastroenteral anastomosis, and that it is as short as possible. If the small intestine is cut after the creation of the gastroenteral anastomosis, take care to not accidentally cut the pouch and the anastomosis.

If the intestine is cut before the creation of the gastroenteral anastomosis, the blind loop must not be too long; you might need to shorten it close to the stomach.

Management: A blind-loop syndrome requires surgical therapy; the procedure includes the removal of the dilated blind loop with or without the creation of a new gastroenteral anastomosis, depending on the cause of the problem and the anatomical situation.

Fig. 3.25 Intraoperative flexible gastroscopy through the remnant stomach to identify the bleeding duodenal ulcer

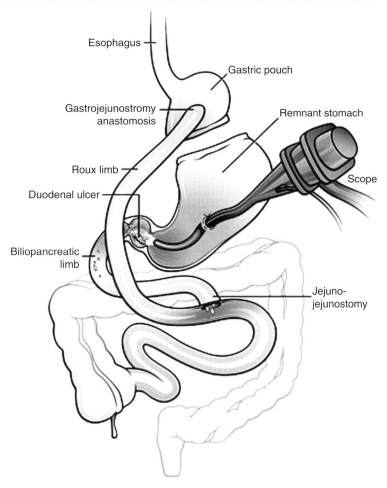

Fig. 3.25 Intraoperative flexible gastroscopy through the remnant stomach to identify the bleeding duodenal ulcer

Esophagus

Gastric pouch

Gastrojejunostromy anastomosis

Remnant stomach

Roux limb

Scope

Duodenal ulcer

Biliopancreatic limb

Jejuno-jejunostomy

Massive Nausea and Dysphagia, a Water-Soluble Contrast Swallow Reveals a Complete Bowel Obstruction Within the Roux Segment

Predisposing factors: A complete obstruction can be the result of a twisted Roux segment (very rarely) or a compression of the Roux segment in the mesenterial opening (retrocolic pathway, Fig. 3.28).

Prevention: We recommend the antecolic pathway. For especially heavy patients with a short mesocolon and marked perivisceral fat tissue we recommend the duodenal switch in two steps or the distal gastric bypass.

Management: An ileus due to a complete obstruction in the Roux segment must be treated surgically, either laparoscopically or open. Different procedures are performed, depending on the reason for the obstruction. In case of a stenosis around the mesenterial opening we recommend creating a new enteroenteral anastomosis between the segments below and above the obstruction. We prefer a side-to-side anastomosis with the linear stapler.

Massive Nausea and Dysphagia, a Water-Soluble Contrast Swallow Reveals a Complete Bowel Obstruction Around the Enteroenteral Anastomosis

Prediposing factors: An ileus with a complete obstruction due to a stenosis of the jejunojejunal anastomosis is the result of the technique used to create the anastomosis. Closing the openings created for the stapler with the stapler might be a predisposing factor, but there are no data so far available to prove this.

Prevention: The enteroenteral anastomosis is best created with two linear staplers. One stapler is directed caudally, the other one cranially. This way, the opening remains in the middle of the anastomosis, which minimizes the risk of stenosis.

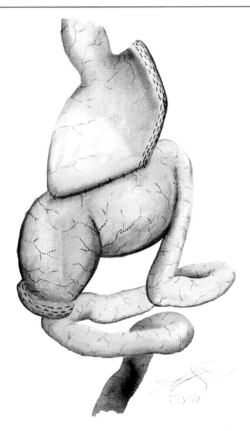

Fig. 3.26 The blind loop is situated below the alimentary (Roux) loop. Food goes there first; the resulting kinking leads to an obstructed passage and dysphagia

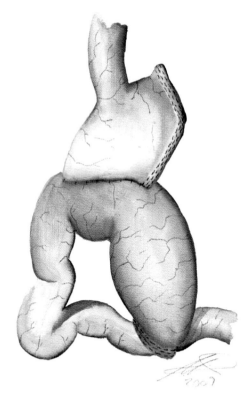

Fig. 3.27 The blind loop is too long. Food does not pass through the Roux limb, but accumulates in the blind loop

Management: An ileus due to a complete obstruction around the jejunojejunal anastomosis must be treated surgically. The extent of the procedure is determined depending on the individual patient's situation. A new enteroenteral anastomosis between the biliopancreatic segment above and the Roux segment below the stenosis is created most often in these cases.

Massive Nausea and Dysphagia; an Abdominal CT-Scan with a Water-Soluble Contrast Swallow Reveals a Complete Bowel Obstruction and a Dilated Lower Small Intestine

Predisposing factors: The most common causes for small bowel obstruction after gastric bypass surgery are an incarcerated internal hernia and intraabdominal adhesions.

Prevention: The only way to avoid internal herniation is the consistent closure of every single opening within the mesentery during the procedure. So far there is no effective measure against intraabdominal adhesions after surgical procedures.

Management: Radiologically proven complete bowel obstruction requires an immediate emergency procedure. It is justified to begin laparoscopic, but do not hesitate to switch to an open approach if any difficulties arise.

Repeated Nausea and Bilious Vomiting, a Water-Soluble Contrast Swallow Reveals a Dilated Pouch and an Obstruction of the Roux Segment near the Gastroenteral Anastomosis; Revision Shows, That the Biliopancreatic and not the Roux Segment Was Connected to the Stomach Pouch

Predisposing factors: Little experience in endoscopic bariatric surgery, difficult intraoperative conditions, and working under time pressure can lead to this complication (Fig. 3.29).

Prevention: The definite (!) identification of the Roux segment before closing the gastroenteral

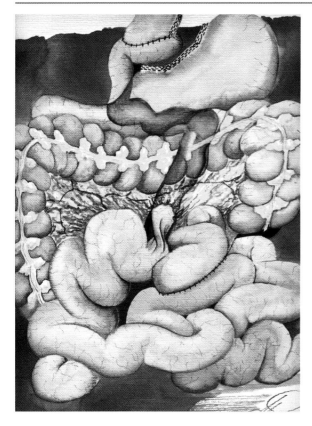

Fig. 3.28 Twisted Roux loop, retrocolic pathway

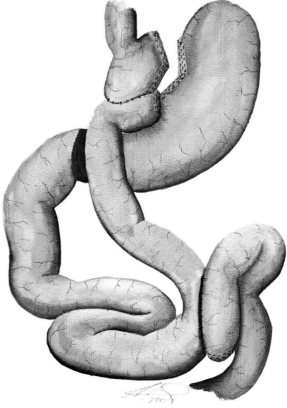

Fig. 3.29 "Wrong loop." The biliopancreatic loop was accidentally connected to the stomach pouch

anastomosis or cutting the intestine, depending on the technique, is mandatory.

Management: If this complication is suspected, surgical revision must be performed immediately. The gastroenteral anastomosis must be removed and a new anastomosis between the stomach pouch and the Roux segment must be created. The enteroenteral anastomosis can be kept or not, depending on the length of the Roux loop.

4. Special Cases (Gastrogastric Fistula)
A Water-Soluble Contrast Swallow Reveals a Thin Connection Between the Pouch and the Remnant Stomach

Predisposing factors: The gastrogastric fistula is a specific complication after gastric bypass surgery. It is caused by:

- An incompletely cut stomach
- A breakdown of the stapler suture closing the stomach pouch (Fig. 3.30)
- A penetrating ulcer around the anastomosis.

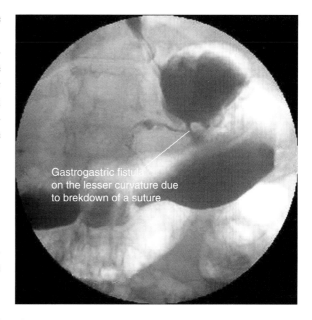

Gastrogastric fistula on the lesser curvature due to brekdown of a suture

Fig. 3.30 Gastrogastric fistula after breakdown of the stapler suture at the pouch. The fistula was removed in a revision procedure because the patient was gaining weight

Prevention: The stomach must always be cut completely. Dissect the left angle of His at the end of this step of the procedure. If an ulcer around the anastomosis is seen endoscopically, the patient must be put on proton pump inhibitors for a longer period of time.

Management: Therapy of a gastrogastric fistula varies, depending on the patient's individual condition and the anatomical situation. If no symptoms are seen, no therapy is necessary at all. If the patient however stops losing weight, reports persistent upper abdominal pain or has a refractory ulcer around the anastomosis, surgical revision must be performed.

In most cases an endoscopical closure of the fistula is possible. The extent of the procedure however depends on the individual situation. The following procedures can be performed:
- Cutting the fistula
- Complete or partial removal of the remnant stomach
- Removal and reconstruction of the pouchenteral anastomosis und cutting the fistula

A gastroscopy is performed during the procedure quite often to identify the fistula.

Revision Procedures Due To Anatomical Changes to the Gastrointestinal Tract

Typical reasons for revision procedures due to anatomical changes to the gastrointestinal tract are:
- Dumping syndrome, or respectively refractory hyperinsulinemia
- Repeated spasmodic abdominal pain
- Inadequate weight loss

Repeated Postprandial Weakness, Fits of Perspiration, and Spasmodic Abdominal Pain After Gastric Bypass Surgery

Predisposing factors: Complaints of dumping-like symptoms, more or less pronounced, are not unusual after gastric bypass surgery. The mechanism of the dumping syndrome and postprandial hypoglycemia are discussed controversially, especially theories like nesidioblastosis (hyperinsulinemia due to hypertrophy of the beta cells) or the late-dumping theory.

Prevention: Dumping-like symptoms after eating sweets are basically the desired effect of gastric bypass surgery. The mechanism of a massive refractory dumping syndrome is not sufficiently understood and therefore no surgical advice can be given as to how it can be prevented.

Management: Every case of massive dumping-like complaints must be assessed individually and interdisciplinary. Detailed endocrinological examinations are necessary in these cases. If dietary measures do not help, surgical revision might be an option in some cases. Operation procedures vary and must be discussed individually and interdisciplinary. Possibilities include a reconstruction of the gastroduodenal passage, a new gastroenteral anastomosis, or a partial resection of the pancreas.

Repeated Diffuse Abdominal Pain After Gastric Bypass Surgery Without Any Pathological Radiologic or Endoscopic Findings

Predisposing factors: Some patients develop persistent abdominal pain after gastric bypass surgery. Diagnostic measures in these cases include standard endoscopic examinations (gastroscopy, coloscopy) and radiological tests, in this case a CT-scan of the abdomen with a water-soluble contrast swallow. In many cases these tests however reveal no pathological findings. The exact cause of this repeated abdominal pain after malabsorptive and combined bariatric procedures is unknown. An increased bacterial colonization of the small intestine is discussed.

Prevention: As the cause of repeated abdominal pain is unknown, there are no special prophylactic measures known, either.

Management: Every case of repeated abdominal pain without an objectifiable cause poses a difficult therapeutic dilemma. If dietary measures, antibiotics, and other symptomatic remedies fail to improve the situation, diagnostic laparoscopy is performed in some cases. Success can be achieved by removing adhesions or a beginning internal hernia.

Weight Gain After Gastric Bypass Surgery; Water-Soluble Contrast Swallow Reveals Only a Slight Dilatation of the Pouch

Predisposing factors: About 20% of all patients do not lose weight as might be expected after gastric bypass surgery. If the procedure was performed correctly, the reason for these failures is unknown. The correct length of the Roux loop and the biliopancreatic segment are

Fig. 3.31 Positioning of surgical team and equipment

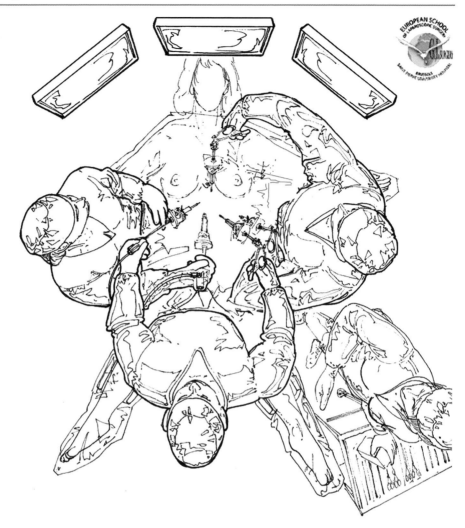

discussed, but so far there are no evidence-based data available.

Prevention: Criteria for the individual choice of the right bariatric procedure have not been assessed scientifically yet and are still discussed.

Management: If a revision procedure is indicated, the following techniques are possible:
- Implantation of an adjustable gastric band around the pouch
- Prolongation of the Roux loop
- Conversion to a biliopancreatic diversion

The exact technique for the revision procedure is determined individually. We recommend the adjustable gastric band, as its implantation is the least traumatic and it bears the smallest risk of metabolic decompensation.

3.1   Surgical Technique by Guy-Bernard Cadière (Belgium)

Guy-Bernard Cadière

Preparation

Setting, Positioning, and the Surgical Team
- The patient is positioned on his back with spread legs.
- The surgeon stands between the patient's legs, the scrub nurse on the patient's left side, the first assistant on the right side, the second assistant on the left side (Fig. 3.31).

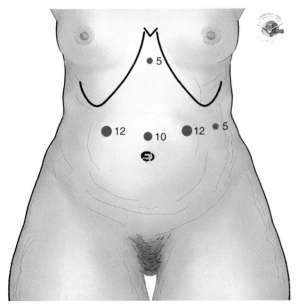

Fig. 3.32 Trocar placement

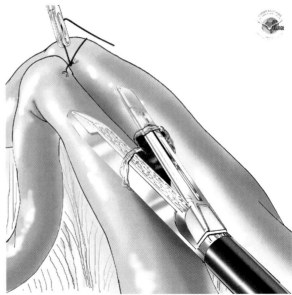

Fig. 3.33 Side-to-side enteroenteral anastomosis with a linear stapler

Creation of the Pneumoperitoneum and Placement of the Trocars

A pneumoperitoneum with 16 mmHg is created using a Veress needle in the left upper quadrant.

The trocars are placed as following (Fig. 3.32):

- T1: 10 mm trocar for the optic system (30°) close to the middle line on the left, 20 cm beneath the xiphoid
- T2: 5 mm trocar on the left anterior axillary line, 5 cm below the costal margin
- T3: 12 mm trocar in the left upper quadrant on the left midclavicular line, between the trocars T1 and T2
- T4: 12 mm trocar in the right upper quadrant on the right midclavicular line
- T5: directly distal and left of the xiphoid

Surgical Technique

Identification of the Biliodigestive Loop, Measurement of the Roux Loop, and Jejunojejunal Anastomosis

- The patient is positioned flat on his back, tilted slightly to the right.
- Lift the omentum and the transverse colon.
- After identifying Treitz's arch, follow the small intestine downward, letting the segments slide on the patient's left side as you go to avoid mesenterial twisting. The aim is to display the first segment that can be pulled up to the stomach following the antecolic pathway without tension.

- A grasper (T5) holds the intestine carefully in this position. Sometimes this can lead to injury of the serosa; then an atraumatic grasper is required. The segment on the patient's right side is the alimentary loop and marked with the cautery hook. The segment on the left is the biliopancreatic loop.
- Measure 150 cm of the alimentary loop. Fasten it to the biliopancreatic loop with a single suture.
- Pull the suture up to the upper part of the stomach with a grasper (T5).
- Open the alimentary and the biliopancreatic loop with the cautery hook.
- Insert a linear stapler (T3, white cartridge) into the openings and fire (Fig. 3.33).
- Graspers in T2 and T4 carefully hold the biliopancreatic and the alimentary loop.
- The openings are closed with two running sutures (PDS 2-0) that begin in the corners and meet in the middle where they are tied together (Fig. 3.34).

There are several ways to create the jejunojejunal anastomosis:

- Side-to-side anastomosis with a stapler (Fig. 3.35)
- End-to-side anastomosis completely by hand (Fig. 3.36)

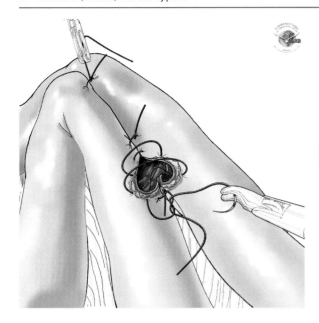

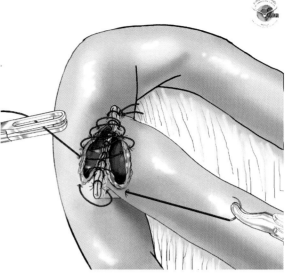

Fig. 3.36 End-to-side anastomosis done completely by hand

Fig. 3.34 Closure of the enterotomy with two running sutures (PDS2–0) that begin in the corners, run toward each other and are tied together in the middle

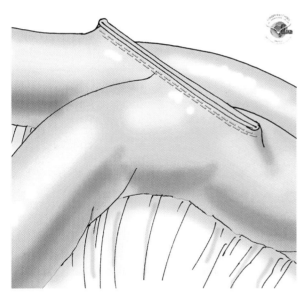

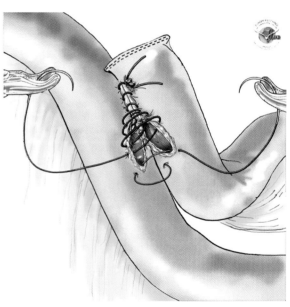

Fig. 3.37 Side-to-side anastomosis done completely by hand

Fig. 3.35 Closure of the enterotomy with a linear stapler after a completely mechanical creation of a side-to-side anastomosis

- Side-to-side anastomosis completely by hand (Fig. 3.37)

Creating the side-to-side anastomosis with a stapler requires three cartridges; this is quite expensive compared to other techniques and the lumen of the anastomosis is often too large.

If the biliopancreatic segment is wide enough, suture by hand. A side-to-side anastomosis can also be done by hand, although this is technically more demanding.

Regardless of the technique, the opening in the mesentery between the biliopancreatic and the alimentary loop must be closed with a purse-string suture (polypropylene 2-0 or 1) (Fig. 3.38). We prefer the purse-string suture to the running suture, because the anastomosis remains more flexible and a kinking of

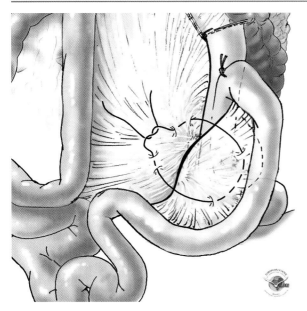

Fig. 3.38 Closure of the mesenterial opening between the alimentary and the biliopancreatic loop after jejunojejunal anastomosis with a purse string suture (polypropylene 2–0 or 1)

the intestine is prevented this way. This is a common cause for dilatation and bursting of the remnant pouch.

- For a better view, pull the suture between the biliopancreatic and the alimentary segment up with a grasper (T5). This relieves tension around the purse-string suture and facilitates closure.

Creation of the Gastric Pouch

- The patient is now tilted into an anti-Trendelenburg position.
- Tick the gastrolienal ligament with the cautery hook in the angle of His. Display the third vessel of the lesser curvature, coming from the GE junction. Dissection begins between Latarjet's nerve and the stomach serosa where the omental bursa can be reached.

> To avoid hemorrhage, begin dissection with the cautery hook and continue with the ultrasound cutter.

- The first stapler cut through the stomach is positioned horizontally with a single blue cartridge (T4).
- Further cut go vertically toward the angle of His (T3, blue cartridge).

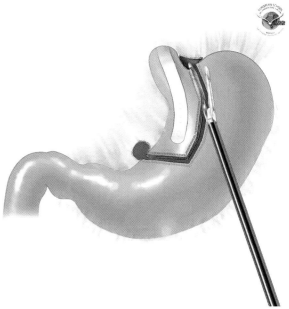

Fig. 3.39 Creation of the gastric pouch. The vertical cut must be placed as close as possible to the lesser curvature. To prevent stenosis, the anesthetist must protect the stomach by inserting a 34 Fr gastric tube

- The vertical cut must be placed as close as possible to the lesser curvature. To prevent stenosis, the anesthetist must protect the stomach by inserting a 34 Fr gastric tube (Fig. 3.39).

> A branch of the lienal artery usually goes to the backside of the stomach. It could be injured, so stay to the right of it.

Gastrojejunostoma and Closure of Petersen's Space

The gastrojejunal anastomosis can be created in different ways: circular mechanically, linear mechanically, or completely by hand.

Transabdominal Anastomosis with a Circular Stapler

- After cutting the stomach horizontally with a single cut with a linear stapler (blue cartridge), create a small incision into the stomach wall in the middle of the suture line. Insert a grasper (T4) into it, pushing it in craniolateral direction up to the fundus.
- Create another incision over the tip of the grasper to push it through slowly and carefully. The anvil of a

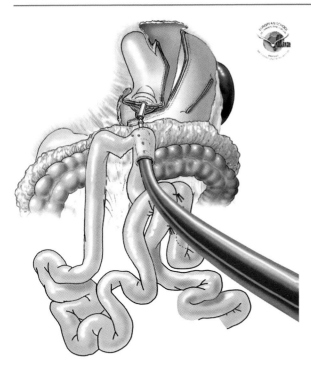

Fig. 3.40 Creating the gastroenteral anastomosis with a circular stapler

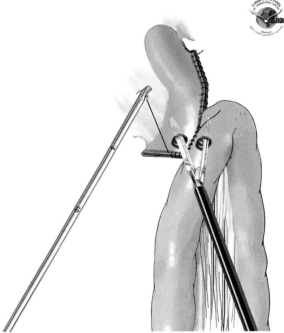

Fig. 3.41 Creating the gastroenteral anastomosis with a linear stapler

25 mm circular stapler is inserted into the abdomen with a silicone drain through the channel for T3. The T3-channel is protected by plastic covering as soon as the abdominal wall is covered, too. The silicone drain is taken by the grasper coming out of the stomach and pulled inside.

- Pull the silicone drain toward the lesser curvature until it comes out of the stomach again together with the handle of the anvil.
- Cut the desired pouch from the remnant stomach by firing a linear stapler in vertical direction (T3, blue cartridge). The 34 Fr gastric tube serves as a guide rail.
- Close the gastrostomy you used to insert the anvil with the linear stapler (blue cartridge) or a running suture.
- Insert the 25 mm circular stapler through a widened channel for T3 into the opening in the alimentary segment.
- Screw the handle through the wall of intestine and connect it to the anvil.
- Screw the instrument together, fire, and remove it afterward (Fig. 3.40).
- Place two sutures into the corners of the anastomosis for safety.

- Now close the openings needed for the stapler with the linear stapler (T3, white cartridge).
- Close the channel for T3 layer by layer.

Creating the Anastomosis with the Linear Stapler

- Begin at the gastric pouch just beneath the GE junction with a 3 cm running suture (PDS1). This suture follows the vertical part of the stapler suture at the pouch. When approaching the horizontal part, the sutures also go through the pouch itself and the alimentary segment. It is lifted carefully and held close to the stomach with a grasper (T2).
- Cut openings into the stomach and the intestine with the cautery hook, the second assistant pulls the seam in caudal direction with a grasper.

The jaws of the linear stapler (blue cartridge) are inserted only partially into the openings and then fired to keep the anastomosis short. This way the anastomosis is placed onto the anterior wall of the stomach (Fig. 3.41).

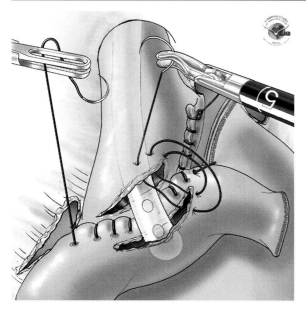

Fig. 3.42 Before closing the anterior wall of the anastomosis the 34 Fr gastric tube is pushed forwards into the alimentary segment

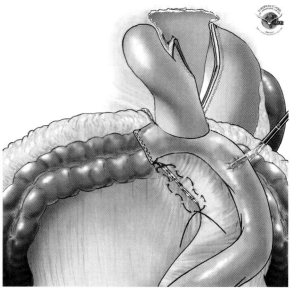

Fig. 3.43 Closing Petersen's space with a purse string suture (polypropylene 2/0 or 1)

- Close the openings with absorbable suture (PDS1).
- The last step is the transsection of the small intestine between the gastrojejunostomy and the biliodigestive segment with the linear stapler (T3, white cartridge).

Anastomosis Completely by Hand
- Cut the intestine between the biliodigestive and the beforehand marked alimentary segment with the linear stapler (T3, white cartridge).
- Begin at the gastric pouch just beneath the GE junction with a 3 cm running suture (PDS1). This suture follows the vertical part of the stapler suture at the pouch. When approaching the horizontal part, the sutures also go through the pouch itself and the alimentary segment. It is lifted carefully and held close to the stomach with a grasper (T2).
- Create a gastrotomy and an enterotomy next to the running suture, each about 2 cm long. Begin another running suture (PDS 1) in the middle of the front wall of the anastomosis that runs to the posterior wall in the middle (Fig. 3.42). Then you begin a new suture.
- The 34 Fr gastric tube is pushed forward into the alimentary segment by the anesthetist before the suture is completed. It serves as a guiding rail during the completion of the anastomosis.

- To prevent leakage at the corners of the sutures, continue the posterior suture around the angle up to the anterior wall of the anastomosis.
- Then tie the two running sutures together on the anterior stomach wall.
- Remove the redundant blind loop with the linear stapler (T3, white cartridge).

Petersen's space is a possible surgically produced defect between the alimentary segment and the mesentery of the transverse colon. It needs to be closed to prevent internal herniation, regardless of the technique chosen for the gastrojejunostomy (Fig. 3.43).
- We prefer to close the opening with a purse-string suture (PDS 2-0 or 1). The alimentary segment remains on the patient's left side due to the tilt of the operating table. Two graspers (T2 and T5) pull the mesentery of the transverse colon upward. The purse-string suture is placed next to Treitz's arch at the lowest point of the mesenterial defect.

Testing the Anastomoses for Leakage
- The gastric tube is pulled back into the pouch by the anesthetist.
- The patient is moved into the Trendelenburg position.
- Emerge the gastrojejunostomy in saline.
- Close the alimentary segment temporarily with an atraumatic forceps (T4). Then the anesthetist injects

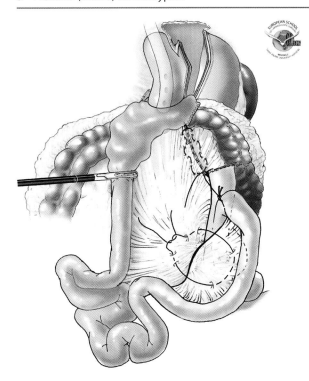

Fig. 3.44 Performing the test for leakage. The alimentary segment is closed with a grasper; air is injected through the gastric tube

air into the tube. The absence of air bubbles proves the integrity of the gastrojejunostomy (Fig. 3.44).

- Afterward, move the alimentary segment until the air has reached the jejunojejunal anastomosis. The air is still compressed and therefore tests the integrity of the enteroenteral anastomosis in the same way.
- Place a drainage tube (T2) near the gastrojejunostomy close to the upper part of the spleen as a last step.
- Close the channel for T3 with an absorbable suture (Vicryl 1), if the cut does not run obliquely. Always suture it after using the circular stapler.

3.2 Surgical Technique by Kelvin Higa (USA)

Kelvin Higa and Ahad Khan

Introduction

Gastric bypass was introduced by Mason in 1966 and has survived through various modifications to become one of the most common, yet demanding laparoscopic

bariatric procedures [1, 2]. The history of the gastric bypass has taught us the importance of pouch orientation and size, even more appropriate with the advent of minimally invasive techniques [3].

Although the laparoscopic gastric bypass is technically challenging and is associated with a long-learning curve, the outcomes greatly favor this approach over the open procedure [4, 5]. Many techniques have been described relating to the method of gastrojejunal anastomosis: trans-oral or trans-gastric circular stapler, linear cutter, or hand-sewn [6–9]. Few authors have reported on limb lengths and routing of the Roux limb, retro-colic or ante-colic, retro-gastric or ante-gastric [10–12].

It is our opinion, however, that safety and performance are not optimized by a single step; it is the evolution of the procedure by systematic analysis and deliberate actions that will limit complications. What follows is a description, not only of how we perform the laparoscopic gastric bypass, but why. We caution the reader that opinion is not fact, but that experience derived from a case series can be as powerful as a randomized controlled trial if that experience is based on thousands of patients.

Although the trans-oral circular stapler technique described by Wittgrove and Clark (perhaps one of the first NOTES applications) was revolutionary, we chose to perform the gastrojejunostomy manually – why? Simply stated, the leak rate described (3–4%) was significantly higher than our experience with the hand-sewn anastomosis in the open procedure (0%) [13]. However, this anastomosis was not the most challenging aspect of this procedure. There were multiple obstacles to performing a "classic" gastric bypass without compromise, especially in the formation of the gastric pouch.

Preoperative evaluation and optimization of the patient is extensive and should be discussed elsewhere in this book. Preparation of the surgeon and surgical team is no less important and begins with a clear understanding of the procedure and alternatives depending on the individual's anatomic challenges. What if there are multiple adhesions? What if the liver is exceptionally large? What if there is malrotation of the intestine? What if a stapler misfires?

The steps of the operation and solutions to the challenges one might encounter should be orchestrated well in advance in one's "mental rehearsal" of the operation prior to stepping into the operating room.

Fig. 3.45 Setting, Positioning and Trocar Placement

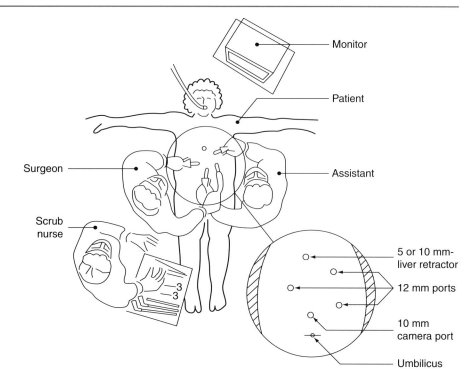

Preparation

Setting, Positioning, and the Surgical Team
- The patient is placed supine with two monitors at the right and left head of the bed.
- The surgeon stands to the right of the patient, while the assistant (also the camera operator) stands to the left of the patient. In this way, potential complications related to lithotomy position are avoided, while optimizing ergonomics for the surgeon. Less time is spent positioning the patient; potential pressure points are limited.
- A single 34 Fr orogastric tube is placed by the anesthesiologist after induction of anesthesia. This tube serves to decompress the stomach, size, and orient the gastric pouch and calibrate the gastrojejunostomy.

> By using a single tube, we avoid the potential complication of stapling across a smaller NG tube and eliminate an extra step for the anesthesiologist.

- Initial entry and insufflation is accomplished through a 12 mm left subcostal "optical" trocar. The left subcostal location allows for safe entry without prior insufflation due to the support provided by the thorax and allows for more accurate positioning of the supraumbilical camera port.

> One of the most important aspects of this, or any laparoscopic technique is proper location and orientation of the port sites. Even more critical in the morbidly obese patient; the ports must be placed according to "intra-abdominal" landmarks, rather than "external" landmarks commonly referred to in surgical texts. As the abdominal wall thickness can often exceed 10 cm, the point of entry on the skin will have little relation to the point of entry at the peritoneum.

- A total of (4) 12 mm ports are placed according to (Fig. 3.45). This allows the surgeon to triangulate the objective providing a more natural visual orientation. The liver retractor is not placed at this time as it is not needed and can get in the way during small bowel dissection.

Surgical Technique

Initial survey includes visualization of the esophageal hiatus and survey of omental adhesions. If the liver is too large to see the esophageal hiatus, a laparoscopic gastric bypass (or a sleeve gastrectomy for that matter)

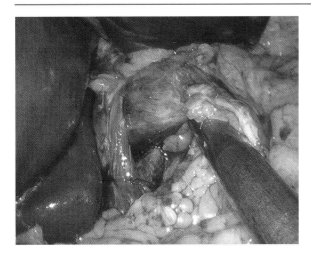

Fig. 3.46 Closure of a hiatal hernia with posterior hiatoplasty

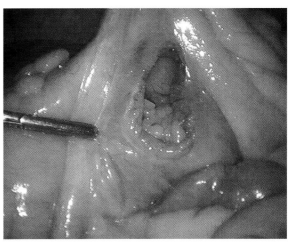

Fig. 3.47 Window in mesocolon (above of the ligament of Treitz) for the retro-colic Roux limb

cannot be done and the surgeon must make a decision to abort the procedure, stage the operation, or convert to open. If a hiatal hernia is found, one must plan to repair it in order to make a more precise gastric pouch and to clearly identify the esophagogastric junction (Fig. 3.46).

The gastrocolic omentum is entered to make sure there is a clear retro-gastric path for stapling the stomach and avoiding damage to the pancreas or splenic vessels. Dissection here can save time in formation of the gastric pouch. If there are omental adhesions preventing cephalad displacement of the omentum, a supra-mesocolic approach to the ligament of Treitz avoids unnecessary adhesion-lysis. This is also helpful when a very large, heavy omentum is encountered; avoiding potential bleeding caused by excessive mobilization.

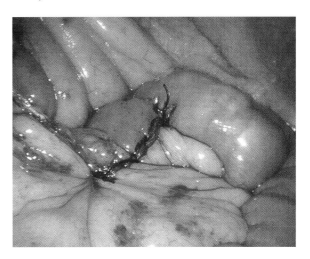

Fig. 3.48 Closure of mesenterial defects

There has been much discussion regarding the incidence of internal hernias following laparoscopic gastric bypass. Most feel that an ante-colic Roux limb is safer in this regard. Our own publications have shown an unusually high incidence of bowel obstruction and unreliability of radiographic imaging studies (20% false negative) in the diagnosis of internal hernias [14].

The rationale for the retro-colic route (Fig. 3.47) is as follows:

1. The incidence is currently less than 0.1% now that we use a continuous, permanent suture to close Petersen's space, the mesocolon and jejunojejunostomy defects.

2. Bleeding and inefficiency is associated with division of the omentum as well as increased tension on the gastrojejunostomy with the ante-colic method.
3. One still must close the large Petersen's hernia defect in the ante-colic method.

The advantages of the antegastric approach: First, it is easier to visualize and suture. Second, it is easier to revise, in the case of persistent marginal or perforated marginal ulcers and third, it is easier to visualize and suture.

In the end it does not matter which method you employ as long as the incidence of internal hernia/bowel obstruction is low and your center can properly take care of such complications (Fig. 3.48).

- After the Roux limb has been created, the jejunojejunostomy has been accomplished and the potential internal hernia defects have been closed, the liver retractor is now placed. A single 5 mm instrument introduced in the sub-xiphoid region will provide excellent exposure in most cases.

> If the liver is exceptionally large, displacement to the right of the patient, rather than lifting it anteriorly will often suffice.

- The angle of His is now exposed, removing the fat pad that obscures the hiatus and proximal stomach. This allows for a more precise formation of the gastric pouch.
- Approximately 5 cm distal to the GE junction along the lesser curve, a perigastric dissection is performed until the lesser sac is reached. This allows for the first linear cutter stapler to be introduced from the right trocar, horizontal to the axis of the stomach.
- The 34 Fr orogastric tube, which had been "parked" at the GE junction, is now advanced and provides a template for subsequent vertical firings of the linear cutter stapler introduced from the left subcostal trocar.

> Care must be taken not to staple the lower esophagus as one nears the angle of His or a leak will occur here.

- One must also strive to be precise in eliminating as much fundus from the gastric pouch as possible in order to limit subsequent dilation, weight recidivism, and marginal ulceration.

> Correct orientation and size of the pouch cannot be over emphasized. The use of an esophageal retractor or "gold-finger" can aid this dissection by exposing the posterior GE junction and moving the fundus laterally, so as not to leave too wide a pouch. Complete division of the stomach pouch is essential and can best be achieved through sharp rather than blunt dissection.

- The Roux limb usually lies in close approximation to the inferior portion of the pouch. One must be careful not to leave a "candy cane" afferent limb in

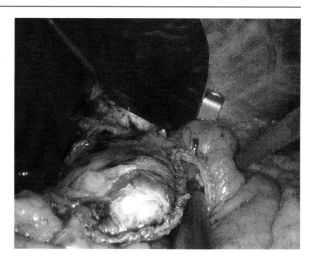

Fig. 3.49 Creation of the gastric pouch. Retraction the angle of His with an esophageal retractor to complete division of the stomach pouch

order to avoid mesenteric tension. This can lead to "unexplained" post-operative nausea and pain. If necessary, some of the Roux limb can be sacrificed by taking more of the small bowel mesentery, close to the bowel wall, and excising the ischemic tip.
- A two-layer, continuous, absorbable suture line incorporating the gastric staple line is performed using the 34 Fr orogastric tube (1.2 cm diameter) as a guide.
- Visual inspection, rather than a provocative leak test, is employed. A negative leak test is not always reliable and should never prevent a surgeon from re-exploration if clinically indicated.
- Precise, safe dissection/creation of the gastric pouch is probably more important (and difficult) to master as opposed to the manual suturing (which every bariatric surgeon should have proficiency in) (Fig. 3.49).
- By utilizing the optical trocars, the 12 mm ports do not require fascial closure.
- Routine drainage and post-operative UGI studies, advisable early in the learning curve, have little benefit once competency has been achieved. The best test for a post-operative leak is re-exploration.

Complications

The only way to avoid complications in surgery is not to operate. The combination of a morbidly obese patient, a complex and often, lengthy operation, and inexperienced surgeons and centers is a formula for disaster. However, even with the most intense proctoring and knowledge of the existing literature is not enough to avoid the inevitable. It is through one's disasters, some avoidable, others not, by which we gain the experience to deal with them and, hopefully, avoid them in the future.

Operative complications are often preventable, but only in retrospect. Every bariatric surgeon will staple across an NG tube (some more than once), or will cause an inadvertent enterotomy, or bleeding, not usually through carelessness, but by virtue of the complex system of variables by which we must function. One can prepare for the inevitable, but only partially. It is these times by which a surgeon is judged, not when the routine is achieved, but when the unexpected happens – what will you do now? It is during these times that humility should prevail along with the recognition that you alone must take responsibility for the occurrence and, more importantly, fix the problem.

Post-operative complications are usually a result of denial. Denial that something is wrong leads to a delay in returning to the operating room, increasing the effect of the complication several fold. Unexplained tachycardia, pain, or a deterioration of a patient's clinical status in the immediate post-operative period require an exploration – period. A CT scan, an UGI, repeat examinations will lead to unnecessary delays in intervention and suboptimal outcomes.

Bowel Obstruction
Bowel obstruction, either due to an internal hernia or unrelated adhesions is a surgical emergency because of potential distension of the gastric remnant. Attempts at percutaneous placement of a gastrostomy tube should only be considered when an operating room is not readily available. Decompression and relief of the obstruction is curative.

Hemorrhage
Bleeding can either be intra-luminal or extra-luminal and can present a diagnostic dilemma. Endoscopic control of bleeding from the gastric pouch or gastrojejunostomy can be useful, but other sources require operative intervention. Simply over sewing all staple and suture lines is preferable to searching for the bleeding site, which invariably will have stopped by the time of exploration.

Marginal Ulceration
The late complication of marginal ulcer can present with chronic pain, bleeding, or perforation. Conservative treatment with proton pump inhibitors and endoscopic coagulation is often successful. However, one must be vigilant for the occasional gastrogastric fistula as a potential cause. Surgical intervention for intractable or perforated ulcers is preferably accomplished laparoscopic. In the case of a perforated ulcer, an omental patch with adequate drainage and placement of a gastrostomy tube for enteral feedings is all that is required. Intractable ulcers present a challenge; requiring complete revision of the gastrojejunal anastomosis and possibly a reduction of the size of the gastric pouch.

Appropriate recognition and control of surgical disasters is what defines us as surgeons and demonstrates our dedication to our profession and patient care. Minimally invasive approaches to surgical disasters are not initially comfortable for the novice surgeon. However, it is our opinion that the advantages of these techniques in elective surgery also apply in this setting: better visualization, less inflammatory response, and avoidance of wound issues.

Revision Procedures

Although the pathophysiology of the disease of obesity is still under debate, there is consensus as to its chronic and recurring nature. Weight recidivism along with comorbid conditions is relatively common and adds to the complexity of postoperative management. A strategy and honest risk assessment must be made on an individual basis with consideration of the primary operation, potential benefits for the patient, and experience of the surgical team.

The first question in this process requires an in-depth analysis of the patient, his/her environment, and the original procedure. Did the patient fail the operation, or did the operation fail the patient? Nutritional and psychological counseling, ongoing in most bariatric practices should be reinforced or reintroduced as required. Concurrently, evaluation of the surgical anatomy with contrast and endoscopic examinations are complimentary as well as updated nutritional analysis to determine the need for correction of malabsorptive issues.

Patients that present with complications of the gastric bypass such as recurring gastrojejunal stenosis or marginal ulceration need to be evaluated for the potential of a gastrogastric fistula or enlarged gastric pouch. Patients with longstanding symptoms will often respond temporarily to usual acid blockade with proton-pump inhibitors, but at the time of surgery will have chronically perforating marginal ulcers requiring major revision. Occasionally, it will be bile-reflux as a result of a shortened Roux limb causing chronic pain and/or reflux symptomatology.

Revision of the gastrojejunostomy without attention to causation will result in recurrence; therefore, these patients will often require revision of the gastric pouch and anastomosis. This is the only way to certify there is no connection between the pouch and remnant reliably. Bile reflux is much easier to treat, simply by extending the Roux limb.

Occasionally, there will be patients whose nutritional deficiencies defy supplementation. Usually in the case of distal or long-limb gastric bypass, the etiology of the malabsorptive syndromes is not clear. Fat, protein, carbohydrate, and micronutrient deficiencies appear independent of each other as well as irrespective of total enteric and bypassed limb lengths. The individual response to redirecting biliopancreatic secretions along with alterations in intestinal motility is probably responsible for this unpredictable response in the host. Fortunately, most of these patients do well with conversion to standard proximal gastric bypass anatomy.

Perhaps the most challenging of issues is the patient with appropriate anatomy and inadequate initial weight loss or recidivism of weight. Almost inconceivable, the adaptive ability of the human organism both psychosocially and physiologically cannot be underestimated. Despite our best efforts, the disease of obesity sometimes prevails and presents frustration for both the patient and surgeon.

Seldom will thorough evaluation of the anatomy after gastric bypass result in a perfect situation. There is room for improvement after mostly every operation. However, subtle changes in anatomy will not result in long-term success. Therefore, endoscopic treatments such as the use of sclerosing agents or suturing devices have not shown significant long-term success.

Operative solutions such as banding, adjustable or static, gastroplasty or adding malabsorption has resulted in both significant weight loss as well as comorbidity resolution. However, the price is that of higher complications, especially related to staple failure.

The advantages of minimally invasive techniques in primary bariatric surgery also apply to revision surgery. Emphasis on technique, limiting blood loss, preserving blood supply, and anatomic awareness are even more important in revision procedures. There can be

no compromise as the margin for error is narrow in this population.

3.3   Surgical Technique by Antonio Iannelli (France)

Antonio Iannelli

Introduction

LRYGBP is currently considered the gold standard for the surgical treatment of morbid obesity. The recent epidemic of obesity as well as the application of the laparoscopic technique to bariatric surgery has dramatically increased the interest for LRYGBP and the whole field of bariatric surgery. After the first description of the laparoscopic technique for RYGBP by Witgrove more than 10 years ago [1], the technique of RYGBP under laparoscopy has been refined and is now widely used in the current surgical practice in the majority of bariatric centers. This is mainly because of the several advantages inherent to the laparoscopic approach as compared to the standard open technique [2]. However, the laparoscopic procedure is technically challenging as it includes the laparoscopic dissection, creation of digestive anastomoses, suturing, and knotting. In addition, the thick abdominal wall, the reduced intraoperative space because of the intraperitoneal fat and an enlarged liver in the case of central obesity further complicate the procedure. Finally the morbidly obese patient often has some associated conditions such as diabetes, sleep apnoea, and hypertension that render him or her a critical patient under all points of view.

> Although the laparoscopic approach offers several advantages, it remains an approach and the surgical technique must remain the same as in the standard open approach, adhering strictly to the principles that are widely accepted for this procedure.

Whenever the surgeon feels that going on under laparoscopy may impair the correct fashioning of the gastric pouch or any other step of the procedure he or she should not hesitate to convert to open surgery to correctly perform the procedure in order to lower the rate of postoperative complications and obtain good long-term functional results.

This chapter deals with the current technique that the author uses for LRYGBP based on a personal experience of more than 250 cases including the pitfalls and some tricks that may help the young laparoscopic surgeon approaching the field of advanced laparoscopic bariatric surgery.

Preparation

Setting, Positioning, and the Surgical Team

- The patient is put under general anesthesia and oro-tracheal intubation on his back on the operating table and he or she is secured to the operating table with legs closed.
- Pneumatic compressions for the inferior limbs can be used to reduce the incidence of phlebothrombosis, but it is not yet part of our set up.
- The patient is draped in a standard fashion with the surgeon standing on the right side of the patient with the camera man by his or her right side, the first assistant and the scrub nurse in front of the operating surgeon.
- For all the cases a laparoscopic aspiration system, a harmonic shears device, bipolar coagulation forceps, and monopolar hook are used.

Installation of the Pneumoperitoneum and Trocar Placement

- The pneumoperitoneum is established in the left hypochondrium first at 14 mmHg. The cannulas are introduced as shown in (Fig. 3.50).
- For this advanced laparoscopic technique in the morbidly obese a standard umbilical minilaparotomic approach should be preferred.

Surgical Technique [3–8]

Roux-en-Y Loop

- The procedure starts with the identification of the duodeno-jejunal angle. To the scope the greater omentum is lifted up in the supramesocolic space allowing the identification of the meso of the transverse colon that is easily identified as its yellow color is different from the one of the greater omentum.

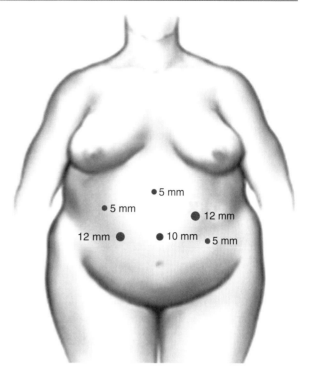

Fig. 3.50 Trocar placement

- The assistant pulls the meso of the transverse colon upward and the surgeon easily identifies the duodeno-jejunal angle.

> In difficult cases the patient is put in the Trendelenburg position to allow the small bowel to fall into the lower abdomen.

- Fifty cm are measured from the duodeno-jejunal angle by a two hands technique with a 50-cm long tape. Measures should always be done with a tape until the surgeon has hands on experience to avoid too short bowel segments.

  A trick to speed measuring of the small bowel is to leave the distal end of the tape outside the abdomen while the proximal extremity is introduced through the operating port of the right hand of the surgeon. In this way the tape is kept continuously under tension. The bowel must not be stretched during the measure.
- At this step of the procedure the small bowel is divided by means of an endostapler with a white cartridge.
- The assistant holds the biliopancreatic limb (proximal) that is always on the left of the operating field.

- The operating surgeon measures the alimentary limb up to 150 cm as previously indicated.
- The assistant holds the distal part of the alimentary limb while the operating surgeon sutures the alimentary limb to the cut end of the biliopancreatic limb (15 cm long monocryl 2/0 suture Ethicon) avoiding the creation of a cul de sac (blind loop) at the level of the biliopancreatic limb that may enlarge with time.

> Failing to identify the proximal and distal part of the alimentary limb correctly may lead to a rotation of 180°C.

- Two short enterotomies are done close to the stay suture to allow the introduction of the endostapler with a white cartridge. The enterotomies must be done on the outer side of the V.
- The stapler with a white cartridge is introduced, fired, and retrieved. The resulted enterotomy is closed with a running suture (25 cm long of monocryl 2/0 Ethicon) that is secured to the stay suture placed at the beginning of the construction of the Roux-en-Y loop.
- At this stage the pitfall is the incomplete closure of the enterotomy that may happen if the two enterotomies are done in the medial aspect of the V or if the Roux-en-Y loop is constructed without the stay suture. In this last case a suture should always be placed where the enterotomy ends and the running suture should be started at the opposite corner. In any case it is strongly recommended to inspect the posterior aspect of the suture before starting the second step of the procedure.

Creation of the Gastric Pouch

This step of the procedure starts with the retraction of the liver. The patient is put in the Trendelenburg position and the liver is retracted with a Nathanson liver retractor. The use of this device may be extremely difficult especially in very obese patients with a very thick abdominal wall. To the scope it is useful to have different sizes of the device at hand. If the introduction of the Nathanson device fails, a fan retractor or the endoscopic forceps can be used. In any case the abdominal wall should be lifted to avoid any pressure on the epigastrium by the retraction system that inev-itably impairs the field of vision at this stage of the procedure. The patient with a liver that covers the stomach entirely and occupies the complete left hypochondrium represents a truly difficult situation. In this case, the surgeon may decide not to perform the LRYGBP at the time of exploration and to eventually reoperate on him or her after an appropriate loss of weight. Another option is to do a different procedure such as a RYGBP with a horizontal pouch that avoids the need to go up to the gastric cardia. The gastric pouch is sleeved some months later when the patient has achieved a consistent weight loss [9]. A sleeve gastrectomy can be an option but it is in no way easier [10]. These difficult cases should be identified preoperatively and avoided if wide experience has not been yet acquired. Male gender, android obesity (apple shaped), metabolic syndrome, and recent increase of weight are good parameters to consider before undertaking surgery. In any doubtful situation an abdominal CT scan should be done to evaluate the size of the liver and its consistency. A short course of preoperative diet may help in reducing the size and the consistency of the liver, and help the surgeon perform the LRYGBP.

- Before starting dissection of the stomach, the nasogastric tube should be removed as it may be inadvertently stapled.
- The angle of His is dissected first. The fat pad at the gastric cardia is dissected allowing the identification of the angle of His. There is no need to remove the fat pad that may be used later as an anatomical landmark during the creation of the gastric pouch. On the contrary it is mandatory to partially dissect it in order to identify the angle of His which is the only way to fashion the gastric pouch as it is recommended.
- The second and third vessels on the lesser curvature are identified and the third vessel is divided with the harmonic shears.

> The second vessel may also be divided in order to obtain a micro pouch that guarantees a true restriction and does not dilate over time.

- Dissection is carried out close to the stomach and all vessels are carefully divided with the harmonic shears.

> It is important to stress that this is not a blunt dissection. Any bleeding can be easily controlled by means of the bipolar coagulation. The Latarjet nerve along the lesser curvature can be spared but this is only for fun and elegant surgical technique purposes as there is no evidence that its division may give rise to any postoperative complication.

- A wide window should be obtained. Dissection has to be carried out behind the stomach at the level of the bursa omentalis.
- The stomach is divided horizontally with an endostapler with a blue cartridge introduced through the port of the left hand of the operating surgeon. The division of the stomach is done 2 cm from the esophagogastric junction.

> If the division is done lower, the resultant gastric pouch is generally too large. This happens because the posterior gastric folds are generally missed and the desired vertical tube, in reality, is a large gastric pouch. This is evident on postoperative upper GI series. Large pouches dilate very much according to the Laplace's law especially if the gastric fundus is included in the pouch, as it is thin and prone to dilation. Another reason to avoid pouches including the fundus is the secretion of a hormone from the gastric fundus, ghrelin, that controls the feeling of hunger [10].

- Once the stomach is divided horizontally, the dissection is carried out through the bursa omentalis to identify the left pillar crus of the diaphragm and to join the angle of His posteriorly. There is no need to divide any short gastric vessels as the stomach is stapled at the angle of His. However, sometimes the operative field is extremely limited and the division of the first short gastric vessel allows a better vision rendering the identification of the left pillar and the angle of His easier.

> Care must be taken in patients with hiatal hernia as a consistent considerable part of the posterior gastric wall can be missed.

- Then the stapler with a blue cartridge is introduced into the port in the upper left quadrant and positioned perpendicularly to the previous staple line. The fat pad can be used as an anatomical landmark: as long as it remains medial to the stapler there is no danger of stapling the esophagus.
- Depending on the size of the stapler two or three vertical applications of the stapler are needed. The 60-mm long cartridge simplifies and fastens the procedure as the consecutive staple lines can be more easily put along the same line avoiding the zigzag effect that may occur when shorter cartridges are used.

> With the 60-mm long stapler, two applications are enough and the second application is only partial. If several vertical applications of the stapler are used the pouch is generally too large or the posterior dissection has not been carried out effectively.

- The stapler suture can be reinforced with buttress material such as Seamguard (Gore, Flagstaff) that seems to reduce the occurrence of bleeding from the staple line.

Gastrojejunal Anastomosis

This is a crucial step of the procedure as most of the immediate postoperative complications occur at the level of this anastomosis. There are different options to fashion this anastomosis: circular stapled, linear stapled with hand-sewn closure of the anterior aspect of the suture, and completely hand sewn. The preference of the author is to perform a completely hand-sewn gastrojejunal anastomosis for several reasons. First, the hand-sewn anastomosis has a low incidence of stenosis when fashioned in one layer of absorbable suture (monocryl 2/0 Ethicon) and virtually no bleeding. The circular stapled anastomosis requires the cooperation of the anesthesiologist and seems to be quite time-consuming. Furthermore, the circular stapled anastomosis requires a distinct stapler and an additional cartridge for the linear stapler that increases the costs of the procedure substantially.

The staple line may bleed and the rate of stenosis is not negligible. The linear stapled anastomosis is simple but it completely eliminates the restriction component that is obtained with the calibration of the anastomosis.

- The small bowel is fastened to the gastric pouch with a 25-cm long suture (2/0 monocryl Ethicon) with the staple line of the small bowel orientated toward the spleen. The alimentary loop is taken up to the stomach in an antecolic antegastric fashion.
- The greater omentum is divided if too thick in order to avoid additional tension on the gastrojejunal suture.

> The trans mesocolic route is associated with an increased risk of internal hernia and the retrogastric route is technically demanding with no real advantage over the antegastric route. Furthermore, in case of leak the gastrojejunal anastomosis is inaccessible.

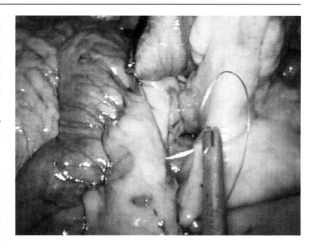

Fig. 3.51 Closure of the mesenteric defects

- A 1-cm long gastrotomy on the posterior aspect of the gastric pouch close to the 25 cm suture, and an enterotomy of the same length are done and the posterior layer of the anastomosis is completed.
- Gastrotomy is better done on the posterior aspect of the stomach, as fashioning the gastrojejunal anastomosis at the level of the anterior aspect of a small pouch may be more challenging and even not possible.
- Any fat pad at the level of the suture line must be removed as this may impair the correct fashioning of the suture. Care is taken to take large bites of tissue and complete the right corner (liver side) of the anastomosis while the assistant pulls on the suture toward the spleen.
- The anterior layer is started either on the right or left side of the anastomosis with a 25-cm long monofilament suture (2/0 monocryl Ethicon) that is tied to the previous suture.
- The anastomosis is tested with a methylene blue and air tested through a nasogastric tube. Interestingly the air leak test is more sensitive than the methylene blue test.

Closure of the Mesenteric Defects

Mesenteric defects exist whatever surgical technique is used. In fact, whenever a small bowel loop is taken to the upper mesocolic space a defect at the level of the mesentery and another between the mesocolon and the mesentery is created. The transmesocolic defect can be avoided passing the alimentary loop antecolic.

- Closure of the defects is done with non-absorbable running sutures. The mesenteric defect appears as a V with the apex pointing to the root of the mesentery. A running suture is started at the level of the apex and continued up to the anastomosis. Care must be taken to avoid asymmetric sutures and the kinking of the anastomosis. The intermesenterico-colic defect or Petersen's space is easily identified by lifting the transverse mesocolon that exposes the space between the mesocolon and the mesentery of the alimentary loop. The suture is started at the apex of the V that points downward and is continued up to the tenia of the transverse colon (Fig. 3.51).

> Failure to close the defects exposes the patient to the occurrence of an internal hernia. This complication may occur at any time during the patient's life and can be life-threatening. On the other hand, the closure of the defects implies a rigorous surgical technique to obtain a tight approximation of the two edges of each defect, as partial closures can be even more dangerous. This suture may give rise to a bleeding in the mesentery and/or mesocolon that can be managed with a transfixing suture.

End of the Procedure

- At the end of the procedure a drain may be placed at the level of the gastrojejunostomy. The author's preference is to leave an abdominal drain only in revision surgery as in this case the risk of leak is increased compared to a procedure on a patient with an intact stomach.
- The cannulas are removed under visual control as bleeding at port site is more common than one would think. On the other hand, no fascial closure is used for the port sites as port site complications are rare in the obese patient and never occurred in the author's experience.
- The skin incisions are approximated with absorbable subcutaneous sutures.

Postoperative Management

- All patients have subcutaneous low molecular heparin (0,6 Lovenox) started on the day before surgery and continued for 4 weeks.
- Upper gastrointestinal series with water-soluble contrast swallow are done on day 2 and patients are started on an oral diet if the contrast passed through the bowel and there was no evidence of leak.
- Patients are generally discharged on day 5 after having received a thorough diet counseling by a dedicated nutritionist.
- Proton pomp inhibitors are systematically given for 4 weeks postoperatively and vitamin tablets lifelong.
- Patients are seen on an outpatient basis at 1, 3, 6, 12, and 18 months postoperatively and yearly thereafter by the surgeon and the nutritionist.
- A regular psychiatric follow-up is advised for all patients.

3.4 Surgical Technique by Sayeed Ikramuddin (USA)

Gintaras Antanavicius and Sayeed Ikramuddin

Introduction

Laparoscopic Roux-en-Y gastric bypass (RYGBP) has been performed since 1994 and a variety of techniques are being put forth. All of them demonstrate success. We prefer the antecolic, antegastric, and linear stapler anastomosis technique fashioned over a 30 Fr endoscope. Over the years, we have learned that the best tool to optimize the outcome is perioperative weight loss.

Preparation

Setting, Positioning, and the Surgical Team

- We recommend using a table capable of supporting at least 800 lb and capable of a steep reverse Trendelenburg position. A steep reverse Trendelenburg position is essential to provide exposure of the upper abdomen.
- The patient is positioned supine with both arms outward. Sometimes, the right arm may be tucked in to facilitate access when suturing the small bowel anastomosis and mesenteric defects.
- The foot board must be secured firmly to prevent the patient from sliding during the operation.
- Pneumatic compression devices must be functioning before induction of the anesthesia.
- All of our patients receive prophylactic antibiotics and Lovenox for Deep Vein Thrombosis prophylaxis in the preoperative area.

The patient shifts on the table during operation: Stop operation, take off the drapes, and secure the patient appropriately to the bed. It is always a good idea to test the operating room table with the steep reverse Trendelenburg position before prepping the patient.

Foot skin ischemia or necrosis: Use soft padding before taping the patient's feet to the foot board. Elevate calves slightly on a pillow.

Port Placement

- The ports should be placed accurately. We use a six-port technique.
- A Veress needle (Ethicon Endo-Surgery, Inc, Cincinnati, OH, USA) is used to establish pneumoperitoneum in the left upper quadrant mid-clavicular line [1].
- The first port – 5 mm trocar – is placed, a 45 degree laparoscope is inserted and an abdominal exploration is performed.

- The second port – 12 mm trocar – is usually placed under visual control about 15–20 cm below the xiphoid at the midline, to the right. This ensures visualization of the hiatus. A 10 mm, 45° laparoscope is inserted into this port.
- The patient then is placed into a steep reverse Trendelenburg position.
- Next, two working ports are positioned into the right upper quadrant at least 5 cm apart – the 5 mm trocar is placed into the midclavicular line and the 12 mm trocar slightly medial and caudad.
- An additional 5-mm port is inserted into the right flank for the liver retractor. The best place for the liver retractor port is the area around the liver edge.
- The sixth port – 5 mm trocar – is then placed into the left flank for additional retraction used by an assistant.

Significant adhesions due to previous surgery: In this case, it is probably safer to start the operation using the open Hasson technique. We typically use the right lateral abdomen, so we can use this port as one of the working ports. If the patient has severe adhesions, consideration for open surgery should be taken.

Working ports are too close together: Ports too close together may have an effect on ergonomics. Place an additional port.

Liver is too large: Add an additional subxiphoid liver retractor port or convert to open operation.

Surgical Technique

Creation of the Gastric Pouch

- Using laparoscopic scissors, the angle of His is cleared from adhesions. This facilitates stapling and visualizing of the last stapling load of the gastric pouch. At this stage of the operation, look for a hiatal hernia.

Bleeding during dissection: Dissection must be done carefully and very gently. The diaphragmatic artery and vein may start bleeding significantly if injured. The bleeding can be stopped by using a Harmonic dissector, but this would significantly prolong the case and may decrease visualization when creating the pouch.

- The gastric pouch must be 15–20 cm² in size [2–11]. We start with the opening of an avascular portion of the gastrohepatic ligament using the Harmonic dissector.
- Visualization of the posterior stomach and vessels in the lesser curvature must be ensured. We use a surgical stapler with 60-mm blue cartridges with 3.5 mm staples, along with Gore Seamguard staple line reinforcement material [12–14].
- The stapler must be directed at a 90 degree angle toward the lesser curvature of the stomach, about 2 cm distal to the gastroesophageal junction and the Seamguard must cover vascular and fatty tissue in the lesser curvature area.
- Remove the OG tube!
- Subsequent applications of staplers without Seamguard are oriented toward the angle of His and parallel to the lesser curvature.
- Typically, a total of three loads are adequate to create the pouch.

Stapled nasogastric tube: Always remember to ask the anesthesia team to remove the nasogastric tube before starting any stapling through the tissues.

Bleeding during stapling: A Seamguard seems to reduce the possibility of bleeding from the first staple line at the lesser curvature level. If it still bleeds, you may need to reinforce your staple line with clips or place a stitch. In general, light oozing from the gastric pouch side may be stopped using piece of topical hemostatic agent, such as Surgicel (Johnson & Johnson, Brunswick, NJ, USA). Bleeding from the gastric remnant side is generally controlled using a nonabsorbable running stitch over the staple line.

Incomplete division of the stomach with a possible gastrogastric fistula formation in the future: Ensure good visualization of the angle of His during stapling.

Size of the pouch: If the sizing is not accurate, the pouch becomes too small or too big. In case of a slightly bigger pouch, one may want to consider taking more tissue at the time of suturing the G-J anastomosis. Sometimes trimming the pouch with an additional staple load may be required. If the pouch is too small, then suturing the G-J anastomosis becomes very difficult.

Consideration of circular stapler use or a hand-sewn anastomosis should be taken.

Hiatal hernia encountered: Hiatal hernia must be repaired before the gastric pouch is created. If done in reverse order, the pouch size will be difficult to assess and the pouch may disappear into the mediastinum after the last staple load. During mobilization and dissection of the hiatal hernia, special attention must be taken to the gastric pouch blood supply. A vascular pedicle to the proximal lesser curvature must be preserved.

- The new gastric pouch is cleansed of surrounding fatty tissue using a harmonic dissector. This ensures a good quality of G-J anastomosis when suturing, thus decreasing the possibility of a leak.

Creation of Gastrojejunal Anastomosis
- To expose the ligament of Treitz, the table is leveled and the omentum is reflected over the transverse colon into the upper compartment of the abdomen. Elevating the transverse colon mesentery with a grasper usually gives adequate exposure of the ligament of Treitz.

The omentum is not mobile: Inspect the pelvis for adhesions and take them down. Divide the omentum or make a window.

- We measure a 100 cm BP limb using graspers [15–19]. The bowel is positioned from the medial side to the patient's left while measuring the limb. The proximal part of the bowel is held by an assistant
- The distal part is held by the operating surgeon. A Penrose drain is then inserted into the abdomen. Using a Maryland dissector, it is passed through the mesentery just below the small bowel. The loop is then firmly held in place by the assistant (Fig. 3.52).

Misinterpretation of proximal and distal part of the small bowel: This is a major problem since it can lead to the creation of "Roux and O anastomosis." If there is any doubt, remeasure the BP limb from the ligament of Treitz and never lose your view on the small bowel while manipulating it.

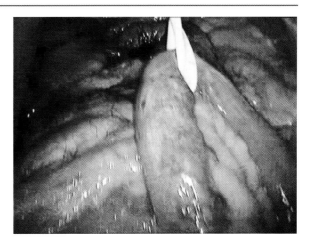

Fig. 3.52 The chosen intestinal loop is secured with a Penrose drain

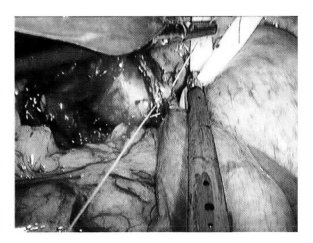

Fig. 3.53 Beginning of the back row of the G-J anastomosis with an Endo Stitch suturing device

- To create the gastrojejunal (G-J) anastomosis gently pulls the small bowel loop with a Penrose drain up to the gastric pouch. The omentum is rolled back into a normal anatomical position to ensure that there is no tension on the small bowel loop. This maneuver is best performed with the patient positioned out of the reverse Trendelenburg position.
- We begin the G-J anastomosis with a back row of a layer of a running seromuscular nonabsorbable suture. Using an Endo Stitch 10 mm suturing device, we start the back row at the antimesenteric border of the small bowel loop, where the Penrose is attached and the very proximal part of the pouch at the angle of His (Fig. 3.53).

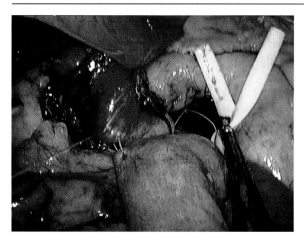

Fig. 3.54 Back row of the G-J anastomosis completed

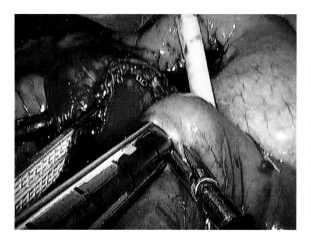

Fig. 3.55 Inserting the linear stapler for the G-J anastomosis

- The seromuscular layer is then continued along the posterior aspect of the pouch and along the Roux limb parallel to the mesentery (Fig. 3.54).

> Care must be taken to leave enough tissue for suturing subsequent layers of the anastomosis later.

- Using a Harmonic dissector, a gastrotomy in the gastric pouch and an enterotomy in the Roux limb are made.
- A blue load stapler is then used to make an anastomosis between the gastric pouch and the Roux limb. Typically, the anastomosis is made no more than 1.5 cm in length (Fig. 3.55).

- A white load (vascular) staple load is then used to separate the small bowel Roux limb from the BP limb. A Penrose drain should be pulled out before firing the stapler to avoid drain incorporation into the staple line.
- The gastrojejunostomy is finished by oversewing the remaining defect with two layers – the seromucosal inner row using the Connell type running stitch with an absorbable suture [20–22] and the seromuscular outer row using a simple running stitch with a nonabsorbable suture.
- At the time when the inner layer is almost finished, we typically proceed with an upper endoscopy. A 30 Fr endoscope is advanced through the anastomosis under direct visualization and is used as a stent to finish the anastomosis.

> *Loop won't reach*: Take the patient out of the reverse Trendelenburg position and pull the omentum to the right. If that does not work, go more distal on the small bowel. If it still does not work, go retrocolic after dividing the small bowel.
> *Bleeding during suturing*: Avoid vessels while suturing. Tightening stitches and holding the suture under tension usually helps.
> *Roux limb perforation while advancing stapler into bowel loop for G-J anastomosis*: To avoid this problem, make sure that you staple your G-J anastomosis before separating the Roux limb from the biliopancreatic limb.

- For the leak test [23] a bowel clamp is placed distally from the tip of the endoscope to ensure complete occlusion of the Roux limb. Air is insufflated via the endoscope into the bowel lumen, while at the same time irrigation is used to put the G-J anastomosis under saline. The anastomosis must be water tight and no bubbling must be observed.

> *Bubbling observed during the leak test*: One must find the area of the leak and additional stitches should be placed until the leak test is negative. If multiple stitches do not resolve the problem, place sutures at the heel of the anastomosis. If that still does not work, take down the anastomosis and redo it. Never rely on fibrin sealant products such as Tisseel alone.

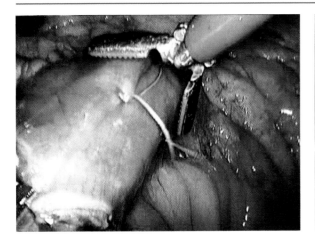

Fig. 3.56 Inserting the linear stapler for the enteroenteral anastomosis

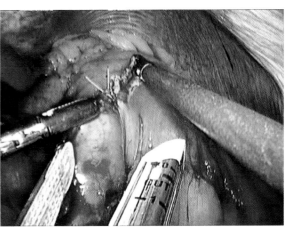

Fig. 3.57 Closing the jejunojejunostomy with a linear stapler (white cartridge)

Creation of the Jejunojejunal (J-J) Anastomosis

- The correct positioning of the Roux limb and BP limb must be confirmed to avoid Roux and O configuration. The Roux limb is measured to be 150 cm [24–29] and the small bowel loop is approximated to the BP limb. The Roux limb should lay in a "C"-shaped position.
- At the site of the planned enteroenterostomy, we sew an antimesenteric border of the Roux limb to the antimesenteric border of the BP limb.
- A Harmonic dissector is used to make enterotomies in both limbs. The location of the enterotomies is important and requires special attention. We excise the corner of the end of the BP limb and make a small opening into the corresponding Roux/common channel limb. It is important to make the Roux enterotomy about 1 cm proximal to the corresponding enterotomy in the BP limb. A 60-mm white cartridge load in the Endo GIA surgical stapler is used to create a jejunojejunal anastomosis (Fig. 3.56) [30].
- The stapler is fully inserted into the small bowel and fired. To decrease the tension at the heel of the jejunojejunal anastomosis we typically place an additional stitch.
- We re-approximate the opening of the new common channel with one stitch and rotate the jejunojejunostomy by 90° so that the BP part comes closer to the midline (Fig. 3.57).
- We then close the opening with a white load Endo GIA surgical stapling device. Care must be taken to minimize the amount of bowel in the staple line to

ensure an adequate diameter of the remaining small bowel lumen in the area of closure.

> *Incorrect positioning of the distal and the proximal part of the Roux limb*: This would create significant kinking of the small bowel. The anastomosis must be redone.
>
> *Diameter of the small bowel in the area of closure is less than 1.5 cm*: The patient may experience obstruction symptoms. The anastomosis needs to be redone or enteroenterostomy should be considered.
>
> *Mucosa is visible at the staple line*: Always carefully inspect all staple lines. If there is any doubt of a staple misfire or inadequate closure, always reinforce the staple line with Lembert-type additional stitches. You may use 250 cc of Metylene blue to check for a leak.

- A nonabsorbable suture is used to close the J-J mesenteric defect [31–34]. We begin the closure with an anti-obstruction stitch and run it down to the mesentery until the defect is completely closed (Fig. 3.58).
- *Petersen's defect*: The opening between the transverse mesocolon and Roux limb mesentery is typically closed with a running nonabsorbable suture. Special attention is taken to close the root of the mesenteric defect.
- Fibrin sealant – Tisseel™ is used to cover all anastomotic sites [35].

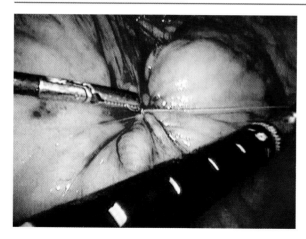

Fig. 3.58 Closing the mesenterial openings for the jejunojejunostomy

- We typically do not place drains into the abdomen.

  Typically we do not close the port site fascia located above the umbilicus, since we use noncutting, dilating trocars.

- Skin is closed using staples.

Postoperative Care

- After the operation, patients are usually transferred to the regular floor. The next day patients undergo routine upper gastrointestinal study with contrast. A bariatric clear liquid diet is started after the contrast study, assuming that patient is making appropriate progress clinically. Typically, patients are discharged on day 2 after the procedure.

Revision Procedures

Laparoscopic Roux-en-Y gastric bypass (RYGBP) has been successful in achieving a majority of our patients' weight loss goals [36, 37]. In some reports up to 29% of RYGBP patients will suffer weight regain or other complications requiring redo operations [38, 39]. The most common indication for redo operations is pouch enlargement, followed by staple line dehiscence with gasto-gastric (GG) fistula or non-healing marginal ulcers. Other, less common, indications would include gastrojejunal

(GJ) stricture, jejunojejunal (JJ) stricture, and dilated GJ anastomosis. Redo operations have higher risks to develop postoperative complications [40]. Although by some reports it is a feasible operation [3], it requires significant expertise to achieve acceptable results.

Open or laparoscopic approaches could be used depending on the clinical scenario and previous surgical history. Upper gastrointestinal contrast study and endoscopy are of paramount importance to identify the anatomy [41].

Operating room set up, table set up, and port placement is identical as in primary operations.

It is always a good idea to start with exploration and identify the anatomy before even starting dissection in the pouch area. At any time during laparoscopic surgery, if there is no progress or progress is minimal, the operation should be converted to open.

Recreation of the Gastric Pouch

- First the old pouch is dissected and the anatomical situation is identified. Using laparoscopic scissors and/or a Harmonic scalper, the liver is cleared from adhesions to identify the pouch.
- Tedious dissection is continued until all anatomical landmarks and structures are identified, especially the pouch, gastric remnant, and Roux limb (Fig. 3.59). During dissection, we concentrate our attention to the posterior wall of the pouch to assure that dissection is not in a false lumen.

  Bleeding during dissection: Dissection must be done carefully and very gently. Most of the times bleeding can be stopped with piece of topical hemostatic agent, such as Surgicel® (Johnson & Johnson, Brunswick, NJ, USA).
  Injuring other organs (pancreas, liver, spleen) during dissection: The severity of the injury should be addressed immediately. In case of mild injury, under controlled circumstances, the laparoscopic approach could be continued. If a more severe injury jeopardizes the patient's safety, convert to open.

- The new gastric pouch must be small – 15 to 20 cm² in size. The stapling of the stomach is identical as in primary operations. The staple line should go through healthy tissues. Most of the time we use 60 mm green cartridge load staples due to tissue thickness.

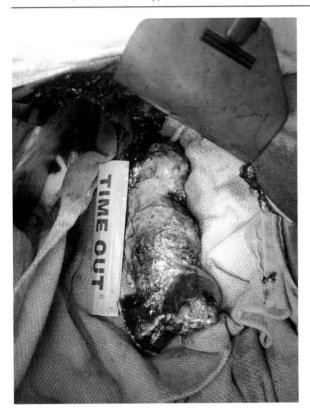

Fig. 3.59 View of the open redo operation with long (9 cm) and dilated gastric pouch

GG fistula: Make sure gastric remnant site is stapled off. Often partial gastrectomy/fundectomy has to be performed.

Size of the pouch: If the pouch becomes too small, consider circular stapler or hand-sewn GJ anastomosis.

Pouch ischemia: During mobilization and dissection special attention must be taken to the gastric pouch blood supply. Vascular pedicle to the proximal lesser curvature must be preserved. If pouch becomes ischemic, esophagojejunostomy must be considered.

Creation of Gastrojejunal Anastomosis

- The anastomosis is created identically as in primary operations. Before creating the anastomosis, the proximal part of the Roux limb is resected at the level of healthy tissues.

Roux limb won't reach: Take the patient out of the reverse Trendelenburg position and pull the omentum to the right. Consider dividing the omentum. If that does not work, go retrocolic.

- Endoscopic leak test [42] is no different than in the primary operation.
- If the redo operation was performed due to the GJ problem, the operation is finished.

Creation of a Jejunojejunal (J-J) Anastomosis

- If the operation was performed due to JJ obstruction, we prefer to bring the loop of the common channel up and to connect it to the Roux limb. Typically, two 60 mm white cartridge loads are used to create jejunojejunal anastomosis. Care must be taken to minimize the amount of bowel in the staple line to ensure an adequate blood supply and diameter of remaining small bowel lumen in the area of closure.

Diameter of the small bowel in the area of closure is too small: Consider hand-sewn anastomosis or resect the affected segment of the small bowel completely and create a new side-to-side enteroenteral anastomosis.

Significant bowel distention due to obstruction: Consider G tube placement to keep bowel decompressed in the postoperative period.

- At the end of the redo operation we always leave one or two drains, depending on the difficulty of dissection during operation.

Postoperative Care

After operation, patients are usually transferred to the regular floor. The next day, patients undergo routine upper gastrointestinal study with contrast just like in primary operations. A bariatric clear liquid diet is started typically after the contrast study, assuming that patient is clinically making appropriate progress. We are more cautious with advancing diet especially if the dissection was very difficult. Typically, patients stay in the hospital for a day or two longer than in primary operations. Drains are removed before discharge unless output is still significant.

3.5   Surgical Technique by Rudolf Weiner (Germany)

Rudolf Weiner

Introduction

In surgical therapy of obesity, the proximal gastric bypass is an established procedure worldwide with extensive long-term experience. Adding metabolic diseases to the list of indications for surgical procedures of the stomach has only begun. Laparoscopic techniques (MIS, minimally invasive surgery) have succeeded in lowering postoperative morbidity and mortality significantly as compared to the "open" era of laparotomy. The introduction of MIS techniques has helped spread bariatric surgery, which is well accepted by the affected patients.

Performing primary gastric bypass surgery for weight loss laparoscopic is standard today. Introduction and feasibility studies for NOTES (Natural Orifice Transluminal Endoscopic Surgery) are imminent, but the pathophysiological principles of bariatric surgery will not change fundamentally. The large variety indicates that there is no ideal technique. The antecolic and antegastric approach is much easier than the retrocolic and retrogastral pathway. The Roux-en-Y shape has proven to avoid bile reflux well. The proximal gastric bypass results in less cases of malnutrition, especially concerning protein metabolism, than the distal variation. For these reasons, the proximal antecolic approach is the most frequently performed technique of all gastric bypass procedures worldwide.

Preparation

Setting, Positioning, and the Surgical Team
- You stand between the patient's spread legs, which is ergonomically best ("French position").
- Unless you have a voice-controlled camera, you will need an assistant to guide it (Fig. 3.60).
- A pneumatic liver retractor on the patient's left side holds the left hepatic lobe constantly.
- The scrub nurse stands left to the surgeon.

Creating the Pneumoperitoneum
The camera trocar is positioned in the left upper abdomen for all stomach procedures. Place it at least 15 cm, but not further than 20 cm from the lymphoid (Fig. 3.61). The umbilicus is not helpful for trocar placement, as it can be situated very far downwards, especially in males. Creation of the pneumoperitoneum enlargens the distance between lymphoid and the umbilicus even more. Creation of the pneumoperitoneum is usually also done from there.

> *Mistake*: Using the umbilicus as a guideline results in trocars too far away from the hiatus.
> *Solution*: Additional trocars in the epigastrium.

In case of an extremely thick abdominal wall (gynoid type of fat distribution), try the following techniques:
- Double-click technique with an extra long Veress needle
- Use of a screw or an optic trocar under visual control of the camera

We prefer the double-click method for primary procedures and have not seen any complications in 4,000 patients that lead to a conversion or termination of the procedure. In secondary procedures (after surgery in the upper abdomen, peritonitis or with preoperatively diagnosed extreme hepatomegaly) we perform open laparoscopy infraumbilically (Hasson technique).
- After reaching an intraabdominal pressure of 15 mmHg, insert dilatation trocars or single-use trocars. To maintain pressure, always use high volume insufflators in bariatric surgery with a pumping volume of 40 L/min or more.
- Further trocar placement is performed under visual control and after bringing the patient into an anti-Trendelenburg position, because gravity will cause the internal organs to move in caudal direction. This also improves ventilation in extreme obesity. Number, size, and localization of the trocars vary depending on the procedure, five are usually sufficient. Linear staplers require 12 mm trocars.
- Match the length of the trocars to the thickness of the abdominal wall. Trocars are never inserted before the patient is in an anti-Trendelenburg position and always under visual control.
- Lateral trocars need to cover longer distances to the hiatus.

Surgical Technique
- Begin every laparoscopic procedure with an inspection of the abdominal cavity.
  Mistake: Failure to see, e.g., an ovarian cancer.

Fig. 3.60 Setting of the surgical team for laparoscopic stomach surgery

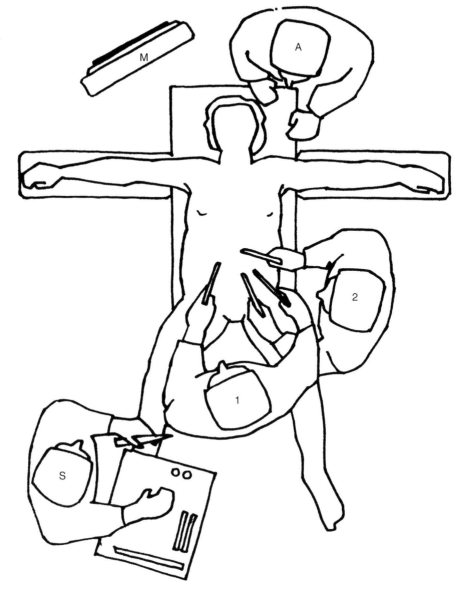

• Next display the left crus of diaphragm and mark it. It will help determine the shape of the pouch.

Mistake: Unreduced large hiatus hernia with parts of the stomach in the mediastinum; large pouch.
   Solution: Consequent identification of the left (spleen-) side of the GE junction.

Solution: A 360° inspection of the abdominal cave. Also check for adhesions.
   Mistake: Stomach resection and massive adhesions of the small intestine.
   Prevention: Inspection and test of the availability of the oral (later the alimentary) loop.
   Solution: Sleeve gastrectomy in case of a "frozen" intestine.

• First indentify the angle of His. Hiatus hernias are always reduced to avoid creating a too large pouch.

• Begin creating the gastric pouch at the lesser curvature 2 cm below the GE junction. The left gastric artery supplies the pouch with blood and must be spared to avoid hemorrhage and impaired blood supply of the pouch.

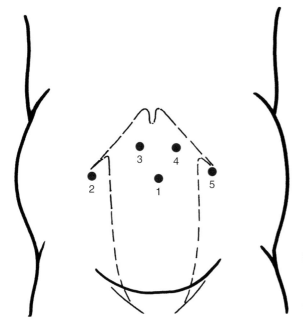

Fig. 3.61 Trocar positions in the upper abdomen for gastric bypass. Liver retractor on the right side, babcock forceps on the left side, camera trocar in the middle (next to the middle line), two working trocars

Mistake: Contact of the active part of the ultrasound scanner with the left gastric artery.

Prevention: Dissection strictly close to the stomach wall.

Solution: Creation of a micropouch.

- Transsect the stomach horizontally with the linear stapler (3.5 mm staples). Dissection is performed in a triangular shape (Fig. 3.62) toward the left crus of diaphragm. Cut the fundus off completely to shut off the production site of the enterohormone ghrelin from the passage of food and to prevent later dilatation.

Mistake: Take great care to avoid an incomplete transsection of the stomach (Fig. 3.63), as this can lead to gastrogastral fistulation.

Prevention: Probing a potential gastric bridge with a flexible instrument to rule out a connection.

Solution: Second resection.

Mistake: Massive hemorrhage from stapler sutures (this is the most frequent complication).

Prevention: This can be reduced by using stapler seam reinforcement. Hemorrhage with the need of blood transfusion occurs in 8% of all procedures. If you use stapler seam reinforcements or sew over the stapler seams you can avoid later leaks and hemorrhage.

Solution: If it bleeds nevertheless, you must place a running suture over the stapler seam.

- When the stomach is cut completely, identify Treitz's arch. If the greater omentum is very fatty, it must be cut.
- Measure 40–50 cm from there and move the Roux loop into the upper abdomen.

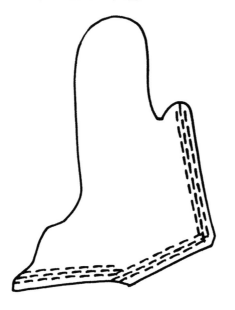

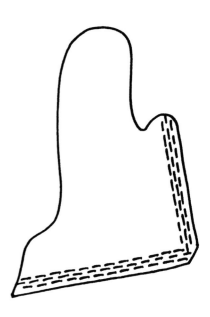

Fig. 3.62 Triangular gastric pouch

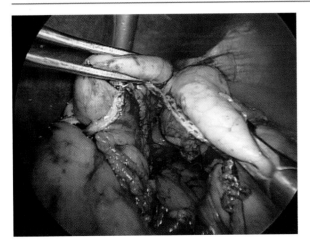

Fig. 3.63 Gastrogastral fistula – incompletely cut stomach

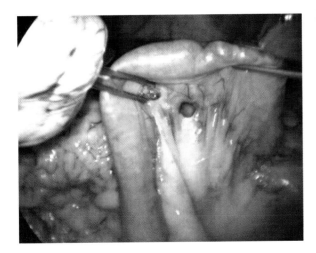

Fig. 3.64 Small mesenterial opening for transsection of the intestine (prevents kinking)

Mistake: Confusion of the loops.
   Prevention: Consequent definite identification of Treitz's arch.
   Solution: Immediate correction, as cardiac arrest might result from the overly distended stomach.
   Important: Short biliodigestive loops are hardly accessible in revision procedures.

• After cutting an opening into the mesentery (Fig. 3.64), you can already proceed to cutting the intestine (white cartridge).

Mistake: Potential herniation, rotation, twisting, or kinking of the enteroanastomosis due to skeletonization.
   Prevention: Small opening close to the intestine.
   Solution: Fastening the enteroanastomosis with non absorbable suture (Brolin stich)

• For the antecolic approach and if the omentum is very fatty, cut the pars libera to release tension at the anastomosis.

Mistake: Impaired blood supply and necrosis of the omentum.
   Prevention: Sagittal transsection without severing blood vessels.
   Solution: A second resection of the omentum (rare: 1 in more than 1,000 cases).

• The performance of a gastric bypass with one anastomosis in Billroth-II manner is only done exceptionally because of the high risk of bile reflux. The alimentary loop is brought up to the stomach in the following ways, whereby rotations must be avoided:
   – Antecolic–antegastric: technically the most simple, the longest distance is favored
   – Retrocolic–retrogastric: technically demanding, shortest distance
   – Retrocolic–antegastric: technically more difficult than antecolic–antegastric, but with no major gain of length.

Mistake: The loop is too short.
   Prevention: Initial test of the availability of the loop for connection to the pouch.
   Solution: Sleeve-shaped pouch and/or skeletonization of the alimentary loop or retrocolic-retrogastric approach.

• After creating the pouch, place a stay suture between the lateral pouch (toward the spleen) (Fig. 3.65) and the alimentary loop.

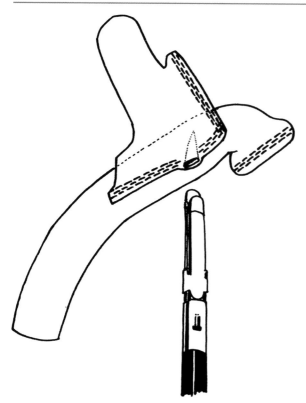

Fig. 3.65 Fastening the alimentary loop sideways to avoid severe dumping syndrome postoperatively

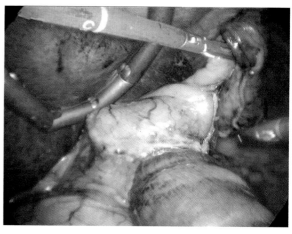

Fig. 3.66 Resecting the tip of the alimentary segment to reduce pouch size

• Open the gastric pouch and the alimentary loop with a cautery hook, scissors, an ultrasound cutter or the ligasure system.

Mistake No 1: Posterior perforation.
   Prevention: Careful incision of a tensed caudal stay suture.
   Solution: Suturing the defect after detection with the methylene blue test.
   Mistake No 2: The distance to the end of the alimentary loop is too long.
   Prevention: Measuring the distance.
   Solution: Resection of the blind loop (Fig. 3.66).

• Insert a calibration probe before you close the openings in stomach and intestine.

Mistake: Stenosis of an anastomosis immediately after surgery is a technical mistake.
   Prevention: Place an 8-mm tube over the anastomosis to prevent suturing through the posterior wall while suturing the anterior side.
   Solution: If the posterior wall is sutured, the suture must be undone.

• Test the anastomosis for tightness with methylene blue or gas.

Mistake: Anastomosis too far cranially, a distal pouch reservoir develops with spill-phenomenon; anastomosis too far caudally, high risk of a dumping syndrome.
   Prevention: Placing the loop onto the second stapler seam.
   Solution: Adaptation to shape and size of the pouch.

• Fasten the alimentary loop parallel to the pouch.

Mistake: Twisted loop ("blue loop").
   Prevention: Moving the loop under visual control, the mesentery shows to the left, the biliodigestive loop is on the left side.
   Solution: Removal and correction.

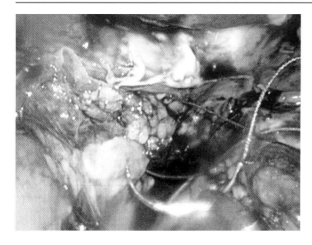

Fig. 3.67 Suturing a leak at the backside of the pouch, identified by methylene blue leakage

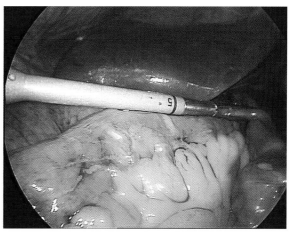

Fig. 3.68 Measuring the intestine with marked instruments in a halfway stretched position (Storz, Germany)

> *Mistake*: The test is not performed, inspection not thorough.
>   *Prevention*: Careful testing; rinse with water to detect even small amounts of blue from the posterior wall.
>   *Solution*: Suture (Fig. 3.67) and test again.

- In primary procedures gastrojejunostomy is performed as a combined technique with a linear anastomosis of the posterior wall and hand sutures in the anterior wall. In revision and switch procedures the entire anastomosis is created by hand.
- After finishing the anastomosis measure the efferent loop with instruments measuring tape (Fig. 3.68). Measurement is performed with the intestine unstretched and on the mesenterial side. In patients with a BMI between 40 and 50 the alimentary segment should be 120–150 cm long. In patients with a BMI over 50 you might consider a long-limb bypass with 200 cm.

> *Mistake*: Unnoticed perforation of the small intestine with the graspers.
>   *Prevention*: Use atraumatic instruments and always work under visual control.
>   *Solution*: Suture all openings rigorously.

- Create a side-to-side enteroenteral anastomosis with linear staplers.

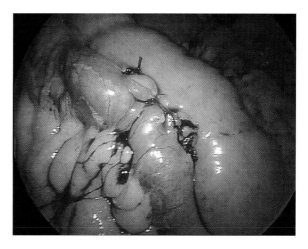

Fig. 3.69 Closing the openings of the enteroenteral anastomosis with a running vicryl suture

- Close the openings for the staplers with an absorbable running suture (Fig. 3.69).

> *Mistake No 1*: Breakdown of the suture.
>   *Prevention*: Rigorous closure of the seams and final inspection from all sides.
>   *Solution*: Suturing, timely revision.
>   *Mistake No 2*: Stenosis.
>   *Prevention*: No constriction of the intestine when closing the openings.
>   *Solution*: Undo the sutures, insert a linear stapler in the opposite direction.

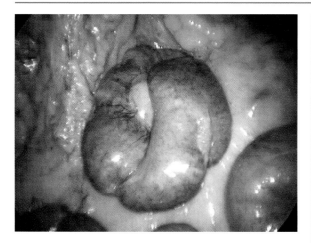

Fig. 3.70 Petersen's hernia after antecolic gastric bypass

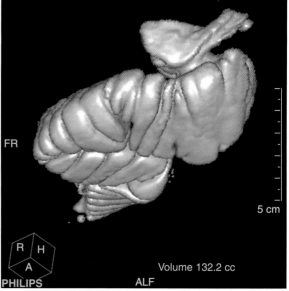

Fig. 3.72 Dilatation of the alimentary loop as seen in a virtual MRI scan; total volume of pouch and dilatated segment: 185 cm³

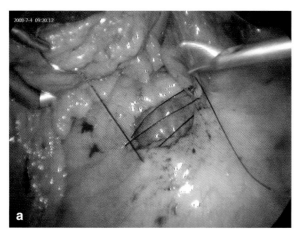

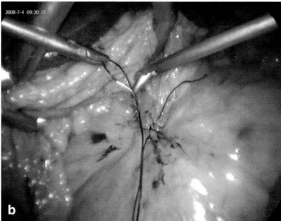

Fig. 3.71 (**a**) Closure of the mesenterial openings and of Petersen's space with non absorbable material; prepared sutures. (**b**) Complete closure of Petersen's space

- Close the openings in the mesentery with non absorbable sutures (Fig. 3.70a and b) to prevent Petersen's hernia (Fig. 3.71).

Mistake: Openings in the mesentery are not all closed with non absorbable single sutures. Herniations of intestinal loops through openings in the mesentery are potential late complications. The highest risk comes with the retrocolic gastric bypass. Diagnosis is best made with revision procedure or a CT scan.

Prevention: Consequent closure with non absorbable material.

Solution: Relaparoscopy in case of pain in the left upper abdomen. CT scan, X-ray, and other diagnostic measures are only helpful if an ileus is present. Reinforcement of the pouch with a ring to prevent dilatation of the alimentary loop (Figs. 3.72 and 3.73) is an option for revision procedures with growing popularity.

Mistake: Stenosis through the ring.

Prevention: Calibration with a probe; 6.5 cm circumference.

Solution: Revision resection of the too large pouch and blind loop.

Remember: Any tachycardia (over 120 bpm) is a reason to consider a revision procedure.

Remember: Closing the mesentery is standard for retro- and antecolic gastric bypass.

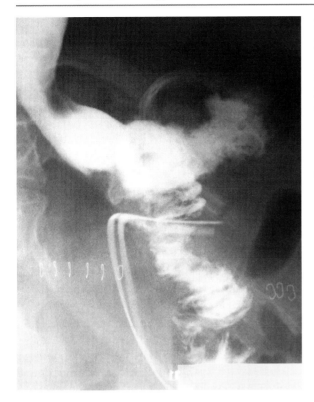

Fig. 3.73 Rare X-ray of a broken gastroenterostomy with drain in place

Conclusion

To perform gastric bypass surgery safely, all potential complications must be ruled out. The procedure must follow standards. Every movement is defined; everyone in the theater knows them exactly. This is the only way to minimize these risks and to reduce general risks through speedy proceedings.

Revision rates are low (under 2%) following this technique. A breakdown of the anastomosis is seen in less than 1% of the primary bypasses (no previous stomach surgery) and can end lethally if diagnosed too late. In large series breakdown rates are below 0.1%. This complication is especially dangerous and potentially life-threatening for patients with morbid obesity. Many times, tachycardia is the only symptom. Immediate relaparoscopy has a good prospect of success.

In extreme obesity (BMI over 60) a stepwise treatment should be considered. Sleeve gastrectomy is a procedure that can reduce the patient's risk for the following procedure. There are no sufficient data as to how stable sleeve gastrectomy is as a stand-alone procedure. Surgical intervention in extreme obesity is

high risk surgery that requires good training and preparation. Technical equipment, facilities, and aftercare must be optimized and guaranteed according to the standards. Bariatric surgery must be a focus point in a clinic to ensure a sufficient number of procedures. Qualification of centers for bariatric surgery is an important tool to improve quality of bariatric surgery in Germany.

3.6   Surgical Technique by Manuel Garcia-Caballero (Spain)

Manuel Garcia-Caballero

Introduction

Setting, Positioning, and the Surgical Team
- We perform the procedure standing between the legs of the patient.

  This is the easier and more ergonomic way for performing the different steps of the procedure. However, measuring the intestine is more comfortably done standing on the right side of the patient [1].

- We create the pneumoperitoneum through the left subcostal space. The Veress needle is inserted at the middle point of the subcostal space, sliding over the periosteum of the rib.

  Experience gained from operating incisional hernias with multiple intra-abdominal adhesions shows that this region is usually almost free of adhesions; injury of organs is virtually impossible. We also find this to be a safe and easy place in superobese patients.

- The first trocar (10 mm) is introduced through the line between the xiphoid and umbilicus at a point according to the size of the patient. Taking the xiphoid as a reference, it is either placed in the middle or, in shorter patients, closer to the umbilicus. The camera is introduced here.
- The second trocar (12 mm) is positioned 5 cm to the right side of the first (from the view of the surgeon) and at the same level.

- Then the third trocar (12 mm) is inserted 5 cm to the left side of the first one, and again at the same level.
- The fourth (10 mm) is inserted into the right flank at the lower edge of the liver (internal view control) and serves to allow the introduction of the liver retractor.
- The fifth trocar (5 mm) is positioned in a left subcostal position, and is approximately 10 cm away from the second trocar.
- Finally, the sixth trocar (5 mm) is positioned on the right side at umbilicus level and approximately 15 cm down from the third trocar.

Trocar placement plays a central role in avoiding bleeding complications as well as facilitating the procedure. Although we have fixed places for each of the six trocars we use, the exact position is determined only after the pneumoperitoneum is created. The final position can also change depending on the angle formed by the ribs. In patients whose angle is closed, we put all the trocars lower, trying to enlarge the distance between them to allow for more comfortable maneuvers during the operation.

Surgical Technique

- For the first step we operate from the right side of the patient and the camera is moved from the center to the right (third trocar in the description above)
- We proceed to identifying the Treitz ligament
- Then we measure between 1.5 and 3 m jejunum distally from the Treitz ligament (depending on the BMI and the age of the patient).
- Once this point distally from Treitz has been localized, a soft penrose drainage is passed around the small intestine to localize the intestinal loop for the anastomosis.

Standing on the right side of the patient, changing the camera to the 12 mm trocar localized in the middle of the right subcostal space, and placing the two intestine graspers in triangle position, we identify the jejunal loop that will be anastomosed to the gastric pouch. The length of the loop is determined according to BMI and age of the patient [2–6]. So, we tailor the bypass limb according to the necessities of each patient directly, given that in this procedure an alimentary limb does not exist (besides the biliopancreatic limb and the common channel), as in other bariatric procedures. This is a central advantage, because, there is no anti-physiologic effect of the alimentary bolus being in contact with intestinal mucosa without biliopancreatic secretion. So, when we say that we excluded some cm of the intestinal transit that is a real exclusion since the nutrients have no possibility of being absorbed as it happens in the alimentary limb. That could be the reason why a randomized control trial has demonstrated the superiority of the gastric bypass with a single anastomosis over the two anastomoses as in the Roux-en-Y gastric bypass [7]. Another factor we have observed that influences the results of the one-anastomosis bypass is age. Diarrhea and weight loss of older patients last longer than those of young patients. Our interpretation of this clinical fact is that the efferent intestinal loop adapts quicker in the young, but slower in older patients. For the same BMI we measure 20 cm less in old patients and 20 cm more in young, in an attempt to compensate the digestive and nutritional effects of the intestinal adaptation process [8]. Clinical data after correcting the length of the excluded intestine are not available yet, but support our pathophysiological deductions. This is the most important decision in this procedure (length of the excluded intestine) since the gastric pouch always has the same size.

- Then we return to the position between the patient's legs and insert the camera into the central trocar.

Dissection in the angle of His facilitates firing the last endostapler correctly and thus finishing transsection of the stomach.

- Then we move to the esophago-gastric junction to prepare a window in the angle of His there. This

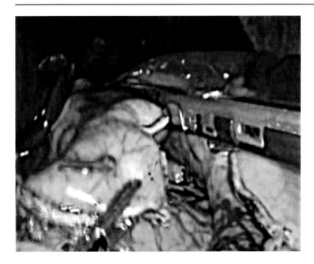

Fig. 3.74 Creating the gastric pouch

allows access to the posterior wall of the stomach which will facilitate the introduction of the last stapler in the creation of the gastric pouch.

- Afterward, we move to the lesser curvature and identify a point at the "crow's foot" level
- As close as possible to the gastric serosa, we start by making a hole in order to gain access to the posterior wall of the stomach. Once we come to the posterior stomach wall we introduce a 45 mm linear stapler, 3.5 mm blue cartridge (Covidien) and transect the stomach horizontally.

To access the posterior part of the stomach, we choose the lower point in order to obtain a long pouch that facilitates an easy gastrojejunal anastomosis and to perform the anti-reflux mechanism for minimizing the contact of the biliopancreatic secretion with the stomach mucosa, the main criticism concerning this type of anastomosis.

- Then we commence the vertical stomach transection (Fig. 3.74) which progresses until the esophageal–gastric junction has been reached, using a 1 cm nasogastric tube placed in the lesser curvature of the stomach as a guide. We use two or three 60 mm EndoGhia, 3.5 mm blue cartridges (Covidien®) to complete transsection of the stomach. An additional 30 or 45 mm EndoGhia, 3.5 mm blue cartridge (Covidien), is sometimes needed.

We create a narrow gastric pouch with the stapler, using a 1 cm diameter nasogastric tube as a guide. The pouch is a prolongation of the esophagus. That means that we transect the stomach just at the esophago–gastric junction, but within the gastric wall in order to avoid esophageal fistulas.

- After creating the gastric pouch, we approximate the jejunal loop prepared as first step of the procedure to the gastric pouch with the help of a grasper.
- When both are in position side by side, we fix the jejunum to the staple line of the gastric pouch with six to ten sutures using an Endostitch (Covidien), *thus creating an anti-reflux mechanism which keeps biliopancreatic secretion away from the anastomosis.*

To construct the anti-reflux mechanism, we suture the gastric pouch to the intestinal loop latero-laterally for around 10 cm first. The latero-lateral gastrojejunal anastomosis is performed with the lineal stapler to avoid stenosis, using a 30-mm endostapler. The holes used for introducing the endostapler are always closed with single sutures, also to prevent stenosis.

- When both are fixed, we anastomose the gastric pouch to the jejunal loop using a 30 mm linear stapler, 3.5 mm blue cartridge (Covidien) (the final diameter of the anastomosis is around 20 mm). The gastric and jejunal holes are closed using four to six single sutures.

The anastomosis is reinforced by placing two additional stitches up and down the suture line.

- We place a suture between the afferent intestinal loop and the excluded gastric body and a second suture between the efferent loop and the antrum so as to "unload" the anastomosis. It must be oriented appropriately in direction of the gastrointestinal transit to avoid the pass of biliopancreatic secretion to the gastric pouch, as part of the anti-reflux mechanism (Fig. 3.75).

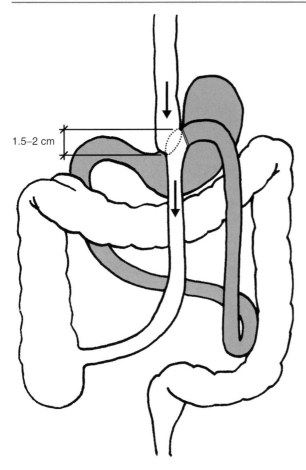

1.5–2 cm

Fig. 3.75 Diagram of a one-anastomosis gastric bypass

> The anastomosis is always sealed with fibrin glue; we have a leakage/fistula rate of zero since we adopted this practice in April 2003.

• To check whether the anastomosis is securely closed, we put it under saline and inject 60–100 mL of air through the nasogastric tube. There should be no air bubbles seen escaping from the anastomosis. Finally we seal the single anastomosis by using 2 mL of fibrin glue (Tissucol).

Difficult Situations and Intraoperative Complications

So far we have never experienced intra-operative disaster in more than 7 years of performing this procedure. One important reason is that the procedure is uncomplicated, very physiological, and requires only minimal anatomical changes. It is performed without interrupting the intestinal continuity and, hence, without opening the mesenterium and the possibility of internal hernia. In summary, in Roux-en-Y gastric bypass the global complication rates are between 20% and 25% [9, 10] in comparison to one-anastomosis gastric bypass around 5% in the first 209 cases [3], and reduced to 3% after the learning curve [5].

Inaccessible Angle of His

We have aborted two interventions. In one case of truncal obesity (34-years old, 1.95 m, 178 kg, BMI = 47) it was due to the impossibility of accessing the angle of His, and in general of moving the stomach wall due to fat invasion. We decided to use other methods to reduce the weight of the patient in order to reduce the risk of complications. The second case was a superobese with previous surgery secondary to peritonitis after appendicitis that fixed part of the small bowel to the pubic bone and the right colon. After trying for more than 1 h without significant advance we decided to do the same as in the previous case to avoid fatal complications.

No Retrogastric Cavity

• The main intra-operative difficulty in some patients is the non existence of a retrogastric cavity which impedes the creation of the gastric pouch. Sometimes it is impossible to introduce a nasogastric tube due to the size of the stomach. Orientation is so difficult that the endostapler could be directed inadequately toward the lesser curvature, resulting in a blind gastric pouch. A solution in these cases is to use an endostapler of 30 or 45 mm and to proceed slowly until the anatomy is clear enough.

Positioning the Jaws of the Stapler Within Stomach and Jejunum

Another difficult intraoperative situation is the anastomosis. The adequate direction of both branches of the endostapler in stomach and jejunum is necessary to avoid perforation of the wall. Another possibility is the failure to close the holes with suture. In both cases the bubbles arising in a test for tightness permit identification and correction of the defect.

Revision Procedures

Personally none of our cases have needed reoperation during these 7 years. However other surgeons that learn with us have reported cases of patients with excessive weight loss in Mexico and Italy. Finally they informed us about the conversion to Roux-en-Y gastric bypass or reduction of the length of the excluded intestine.

References

3.2   Surgical Technique

1. Mason EE, Ito C (1967) Gastric bypass in obesity. Surg Clin North Am 47:1845–1852
2. Santry HP, Gillen DL, Lauderdale DS (2005) Trends in bariatric surgical procedures. JAMA 294(15):1909–1917
3. Demaria EJ, Jamal MK (2005) Surgical options for obesity. Gastroenterol Clin North Am 34(1):127–142
4. Andrew CG, Hanna W, Look D et al (2006) Early results after laparoscopic roux-en-Y gastric bypass: Effect of the learning curve. Can J Surg 49(6):417–421
5. Nguyen NT, Goldman C, Rosenquist CJ et al (2001) Laparoscopic versus open gastric bypass: a randomized study of outcomes, quality of life, and costs. Ann Surg 234(3):279–289
6. Wittgrove AC, Clark GW, Tremblay LJ (1994) Laparoscopic gastric bypass, Roux-en-Y: preliminary report of five cases. Obes Surg 4:353–357
7. dela Torre RA, Scott JS (1999) Laparoscopic Roux-en-Y gastric bypass: a totally intra-abdominal approach: technique and preliminary report. Obes Surg 9:492–498
8. Schauer PR, Ikramuddin S, Gourash W et al (2000) Outcomes after laparoscopic Roux-en-Y gastric bypass for morbid obesity. Ann Surg 232:515–529
9. Higa KD, Boone KB, Ho T et al (2000) Laparoscopic Roux-en-Y gastric bypass for morbid obesity: technique and preliminary results of our first 400 patients. Arch Surg 9: 1029–1033
10. Choban PS, Flancbaum L (2002) The effect of Roux limb lengths on outcome after Roux-en-Y gastric bypass: a prospective, randomized clinical trial. Obes Surg 12(4):540–545
11. Champion JK, Williams M (2003) Small bowel obstruction and internal hernias after laparoscopic Roux-en-Y gastric bypass. Obes Surg 13(4):596–600
12. Higa KD, Ho T, Boone KB (2003) Internal hernias after laparoscopic Roux-en-Y gastric bypass: incidence, treatment and prevention. Obes Surg 13(3):350–354
13. Wittgrove AC, Clark GW, Schubert KR (1996) Laparoscopic gastric bypass, Roux-en-Y: technique and results in 75 patients with 3–30 month follow-up. Obes Surg 6: 500–504
14. Higa K, Ho T, Boone K (2003) Internal hernias after laparoscopic Roux-en-Y gastric bypass: incidence, treatment and prevention. Obes Surg 13:350–354

3.3   Surgical Technique

1. Wittgrove AC, Clark GW, Tremblay LJ (1994) Laparoscopic gastric bypass, Roux-en-Y: preliminary report of five cases. Obes Surg 4:353–357
2. Nguyen NT, Goldman C, Rosenquist CJ, Arango A, Cole CJ, Lee SJ, Wolfe BM (2001) Laparoscopic versus open gastric bypass: a randomized study of outcomes, quality of life, and costs. Ann Surg 234(3):279–289; discussion 289–291
3. Iannelli A, Sejor E, Mouremble O, Nataf S, Gugenheim J (2006) Leak of the bypassed stomach after laparoscopic gastric bypass, presenting as abdominal wall cellulites. Obes Surg 16:924–927
4. Iannelli A, Facchiano E, Gugenheim J (2006) Internal hernia after laparoscopic Roux-en-Y gastric bypass for morbid obesity. Obes Surg 16:1265–1271
5. Iannelli A, Piche T, Novellas S, Gugenheim J (2006) Small bowel diverticulitis of Roux-en-Y loop: a rare complication of laparoscopic Roux-en-Y gastric bypass. Obes Surg; 16 (9):1249–1251
6. Iannelli A, Addeo P, Dahman M, Senni Buratti M, Ben Amor I, Piche T, Gugenheim J (2007) Laparoscopic conversion of vertical banded gastroplasty with an antireflux wrap into Roux en Y gastric bypass. Obes Surg 17:901–904
7. Iannelli A, Senni Buratti M, Novellas S, Dahman M, Ben Amor I, Facchiano E, Addeo P, Gugenheim J (2007) Internal hernia as a complication of laparoscopic Roux-en-Y gastric bypass for morbid obesity. Obes Surg 17:1283–1286
8. Iannelli A, Amato D, Addeo P, Senni Buratti M, Damhan M, Ben Amor I, Sejor E, Facchiano E, Gugenheim J (2008) Laparoscopic conversion of vertical banded gastroplasty (Mason MacLean) into Roux en Y gastric bypass. Obes Surg 18:43–46
9. Nguyen NT, Longoria M, Gelfand DV, Sabio A, Wilson SE (2005) Staged laparoscopic Roux-en-Y: a novel two-stage bariatric operation as an alternative in the super-obese with massively enlarged liver. Obes Surg 15(7):1077–1081
10. Iannelli A, Dainese R, Piche T, Facchiano E, Gugenheim J (2008) Laparoscopic Sleeve gastrectomy for morbid obesity. World J Gastroenterol 14:821–827

3.4   Surgical Technique

1. Schwartz ML, Drew RL, Andersen JN (2003) Induction of pneumoperitoneum in morbidly obese patients. Obes Surg 13(4):601–604
2. Madan AK, Harper JL, Tichansky DS (2007) Techniques of laparoscopic gastric bypass: on-line survey of American Society for Bariatric Surgery practicing surgeons. Surg Obes Relat Dis 4(2):166–172
3. Nishie A, Brown B, Barloon T, Kuehn D, Samuel I (2007) Comparison of size of proximal gastric pouch and short-term weight loss following routine upper gastrointestinal contrast study after laparoscopic Roux-en-Y gastric bypass. Obes Surg 17(9):1183–1188
4. Roberts K, Duffy A, Kaufman J, Burrell M, Dziura J, Bell R (2007) Size matters: gastric pouch size correlates with weight loss after laparoscopic Roux-en-Y gastric bypass. Surg Endosc 21(8):1397–1402. Epub 2007 Mar 1
5. Madan AK, Tichansky DS, Phillips JC (2007) Does pouch size matter? Obes Surg 17(3):317–320
6. Williams MD, Champion JK (2004) Linear technique of laparoscopic Roux-en-Y gastric bypass. Surg Technol Int 13:101–105. Review.

7. Sugerman HJ (2001) Bariatric surgery for severe obesity. J Assoc Acad Minor Phys 12(3):129–136. Review.

8. Flanagan L (1996) Measurement of functional pouch volume following the gastric bypass procedure. Obes Surg 6(1): 38–43

9. Flickinger EG, Sinar DR, Swanson M (1987) Gastric bypass. Gastroenterol Clin North Am. 16(2):283–292

10. Andersen T, Pedersen BH (1984) Pouch volume, stoma diameter, and clinical outcome after gastroplasty for morbid obesity. A prospective study. Scand J Gastroenterol 19(5): 643–649

11. Horowitz M, Cook DJ, Collins PJ, Harding PE, Hooper MJ, Walsh JF, Shearman DJ (1982) Measurement of gastric emptying after gastric bypass surgery using radionuclides. Br J Surg 69(11):655–657

12. Miller KA, Pump A (2007) Use of bioabsorbable staple reinforcement material in gastric bypass: a prospective randomized clinical trial. Surg Obes Relat Dis 3(4):417–421; discussion 422. Epub 2007 Jun 12

13. Nguyen NT, Longoria M, Chalifoux S, Wilson SE (2005) Bioabsorbable staple line reinforcement for laparoscopic gastrointestinal surgery. Surg Technol Int 14:107–111

14. Consten EC, Gagner M, Pomp A, Inabnet WB (2004) Decreased bleeding after laparoscopic sleeve gastrectomy with or without duodenal switch for morbid obesity using a stapled buttressed absorbable polymer membrane. Obes Surg 14(10):1360–1366

15. Inabnet WB, Quinn T, Gagner M, Urban M, Pomp A (2005). Laparoscopic Roux-en-Y gastric bypass in patients with BMI <50: a prospective randomized trial comparing short and long limb lengths. Obes Surg 15(1):51–57.

16. Leifsson BG, Gislason HG (2005) Laparoscopic Roux-en-Y gastric bypass with 2-metre long biliopancreatic limb for morbid obesity: technique and experience with the first 150 patients. Obes Surg. 15(1):35–42

17. Skroubis G, Sakellaropoulos G, Pouggouras K, Mead N, Nikiforidis G, Kalfarentzos F (2002) Comparison of nutritional deficiencies after Roux-en-Y gastric bypass and after biliopancreatic diversion with Roux-en-Y gastric bypass. Obes Surg 12(4):551–558

18. Murr MM, Balsiger BM, Kennedy FP, Mai JL, Sarr MG (1999) Malabsorptive procedures for severe obesity: comparison of pancreaticobiliary bypass and very very long limb Roux-en-Y gastric bypass. J Gastrointest Surg 3(6):607–612

19. Brolin RE, Kenler HA, Gorman JH, Cody RP (1992) Long-limb gastric bypass in the superobese. A prospective randomized study. Ann Surg 215(4):387–395

20. Patel C, Van Dam J, Curet M, Morton JM, Banerjee S (2008) Use of flexible endoscopic scissors to cut obstructing suture material in gastric bypass patients. Obes Surg 18(3):336–339

21. Frezza EE, Herbert H, Ford R (2007) Wachtel MS. Endoscopic suture removal at gastrojejunal anastomosis after Roux-en-Y gastric bypass to prevent marginal ulceration. Surg Obes Relat Dis 3(6):619–622

22. Sacks BC, Mattar SG, Qureshi FG, Eid GM, Collins JL, Barinas-Mitchell EJ, Schauer PR, Ramanathan RC (2006) Incidence of marginal ulcers and the use of absorbable anastomotic sutures in laparoscopic Roux-en-Y gastric bypass. Surg Obes Relat Dis. 2(1):11–16

23. Sekhar N, Torquati A, Lutfi R, Richards WO (2006) Endoscopic evaluation of the gastrojejunostomy in laparoscopic gastric bypass. A series of 340 patients without postoperative leak. Surg Endosc 20(2):199–201. Epub 2005 Dec 5

24. Lee WJ, Wang W, Lee YC, Huang MT, Ser KH, Chen JC (2008) Laparoscopic mini-gastric bypass: experience with tailored bypass limb according to body weight. Obes Surg 18(3):294–299

25. Ciovica R, Takata M, Vittinghoff E, Lin F, Posselt AM, Rabl C, Stein HJ, Campos GM (2008) The impact of roux limb length on weight loss after gastric bypass. Obes Surg 18(1):5–10. Epub 2007 Dec 7

26. Christou NV, Look D, Maclean LD (2006) Weight gain after short- and long-limb gastric bypass in patients followed for longer than 10 years. Ann Surg 44(5):734–740

27. Nelson WK, Fatima J, Houghton SG, Thompson GB, Kendrick ML, Mai JL, Kennel KA, Sarr MG (2006) The malabsorptive very, very long limb Roux-en-Y gastric bypass for super obesity: results in 257 patients. Surgery. 140(4):517–522, discussion 522–533. Epub 2006 Sep 1

28. Lee S, Sahagian KG, Schriver JP (2006) Relationship between varying Roux limb lengths and weight loss in gastric bypass. Curr Surg 63(4):259–263

29. Brolin RE, Kenler HA, Gorman JH, Cody RP (1992) Long-limb gastric bypass in the superobese. A prospective randomized study. Ann Surg 215(4):387–395

30. Frantzides CT, Zeni TM, Madan AK, Zografakis JG, Moore RE, Laguna L (2006) Laparoscopic Roux-en-Y Gastric bypass utilizing the triple stapling technique. JSLS 10(2):176–179

31. Steele KE, Prokopowicz GP, Magnuson T, Lidor A, Schweitzer M (2008) Laparoscopic antecolic Roux-En-Y gastric bypass with closure of internal defects leads to fewer internal hernias than the retrocolic approach. Surg Endosc 22(9):2056–2061

32. Higa K, Boone K, Arteaga González I, López-Tomassetti Fernández E (2007) Mesenteric closure in laparoscopic gastric bypass: surgical technique and literature review. Cir Esp 82(2):77–88. Review. Spanish

33. Iannelli A, Facchiano E, Gugenheim J (2006) Internal hernia after laparoscopic Roux-en-Y gastric bypass for morbid obesity. Obes Surg 16(10):1265–12671

34. Cho M, Pinto D, Carrodeguas L, Lascano C, Soto F, Whipple O, Simpfendorfer C, Gonzalvo JP, Zundel N, Szomstein S, Rosenthal RJ (2006) Frequency and management of internal hernias after laparoscopic antecolic antegastric Roux-en-Y gastric bypass without division of the small bowel mesentery or closure of mesenteric defects: review of 1400 consecutive cases. Surg Obes Relat Dis 2(2):87–91

35. Silecchia G, Boru CE, Mouiel J, Rossi M, Anselmino M, Tacchino RM, Foco M, Gaspari AL, Gentileschi P, Morino M, Toppino M, Basso N (2006) Clinical evaluation of fibrin glue in the prevention of anastomotic leak and internal hernia after laparoscopic gastric bypass: preliminary results of a prospective, randomized multicenter trial. Obes Surg 16(2):125–131

36. Buchwald H, Avidor Y, Braunwald E et al (2004) Bariatric surgery: a systematic review and meta-analysis. JAMA 292(14):1724–1737

37. Buchwald H, Estok R, Fahrbach K et al (2007) Trends in mortality in bariatric surgery: a systematic review and meta-analysis. Surgery 142(4):621–632; discussion 632–635

38. Khaitan L, Van Sickle K, Gonzalez R et al (2005) Laparoscopic revision of bariatric procedures: is it feasible? Am Surg 71(1):6–10; discussion 10–12

39. Christou NV, Look D, Maclean LD (2006) Weight gain after short- and long-limb gastric bypass in patients followed for longer than 10 years. Ann Surg 244(5):734–740

40. Schwartz RW, Strodel WE, Simpson WS, Griffen WO, Jr (1988). Gastric bypass revision: lessons learned from 920 cases. Surgery 104(4):806–812

41. Brethauer SA, Nfonsam V, Sherman V et al (2006) Endoscopy and upper gastrointestinal contrast studies are complementary in evaluation of weight regain after bariatric surgery. Surg Obes Relat Dis 2(6):643–648; discussion 649–650

42. Sekhar N, Torquati A, Lutfi R, Richards WO (2006) Endoscopic evaluation of the gastrojejunostomy in laparoscopic gastric bypass. A series of 340 patients without postoperative leak. Surg Endosc 20(2):199–201

3.6 Surgical Technique

1. García-Caballero M, Carbajo M (2004) One anastomosis gastric bypass: a simple, safe and efficient surgical procedure for treating morbid obesity. Nutr Hosp 19:372–375

2. García-Caballero M (2005) Surgery to modify nutritional behaviour. Nutr Hosp 20:2–4

3. Carbajo M, García-Caballero M, Toledano M, Osorio D, García-Lanza C, Carmona JA (2005) One-anastomosis gastric bypass by laparoscopy: results of the first 209 patients. Obes Surg 15:398–404

4. Garcia-Caballero M, Carbajo M, Martinez-Moreno JM, Sarria M, Osorio D, Carmona JA (2005) Drain erosion and gastro-jejunal fistula after one-anastomosis gastric bypass: endoscopic occlusion by fibrin sealant. Obes Surg 15:719–722

5. García-Caballero M, Ortiz J (2007) One-anastomosis gastric bypass by laparoscopy (BAGUA) with robotic assistance: experience in 600 patients. Obes Surg 17:1046

6. Lee WJ, Wang W, Lee YC, Huang MT, Ser KH, Chen JC (2008) Laparoscopic mini-gastric bypass: experience with tailored bypass limb according to body weight. Obes Surg 18:294–299

7. Lee WJ, Yu PJ, Wang W, Chen TC, Wei PL, Huang MT (2005) Laparoscopic Roux-en-Y versus mini-gastric bypass for the treatment of morbid obesity: a prospective randomized controlled clinical trial. Ann Surg 242:20–28

8. García-Caballero M, Fernández JL, Ruiz J, Muñoz M, Núñez de Castro I (1996) Middle term intestinal adaptation after massive distal small bowel resection in oral feeding dogs. Nutr Hosp 11:265–273

9. Suter M, Giusti V, Heraief E, Zysset F, Calmes JM (2003) Laparoscopic Roux-en-Y gastric bypass: initial 2-year experience. Surg Endosc 17:603–609

10. Papasavas PK, Caushaj PF, McCormick JT, Quinlin RF, Hayetian FD, Maurer J, Kelly JJ, Gagne DJ (2003) Laparoscopic management of complications following laparoscopic Roux-en-Y gastric bypass for morbid obesity. Surg Endosc 17:610–614

Further Reading

3   Proximal (Classic) Gastric Bypass

Ballesta C, Berindoague R, Cabrera M, Palau M, Gonzales M (2008) Management of anastomotic leaks after laparoscopic Roux-en-Y gastric bypass. Obes Surg 18:623–630

Chin PL, Ali M, Francis K, LePort PC (2009) Adjustable gastric band placed around gastric pouch as revision operation for failed gastric bypass. Surg Obes Relat Dis 5(1):38–42

Decker GA, DiBaise JK, Leighton JA, Swain JM, Crowell MD (2007) Nausea, bloating and abdominal pain in the Rouy-en-Y gastric bypass patient: more questions than answers. Obes Surg 17:1529–1533

Fleser PS, Villalba M (2003) Afferent limb volvulus and perforation of the bypassed stomach as a complication of Roux-en-Y gastric bypass. Obes Surg 13(3):453–446

Goitein D, Papasavas PK, Gagne DJ, Caushaj PF (2005) Late perforation of the jejuno-jejunal anastomosis after laparoscopic Roux-en-Y gastric bypass. Obes Surg 15(6):880–882

Pitt T, Brethauer S, Sherman V, Udomsawaengsup S, Metz M, Chikunguwo S, Chand B. Schauer P (2008) Diagnostic laparoscopy for chronic abdominal pain after gastric bypass. Surg Obes Relat Dis 4(3):394–398

Kellogg TA, Bantle JP, Leslie DB, Redmond JB, Slusarek B, Swan T, Buchwald H, Ikramuddin S (2008) Postgastric bypass hyperinsulinemic hypoglycaemia syndrome: characterization and response to a modified diet. Postgastric bypass hyperinsulinemic hypoglycaemia syndrome: characterization and response to a modified diet. Surg Obes Relat Dis 4(4):492–499

Koppman, JS, Gandsas A (2008) Small bowel obstruction after laparoscopic Roux-en-Ygastric bypass: a review of 9,527 patients. J Am Coll Surg 206(3):571–584

Korenkov M, Goh P, Yucel N, Troidl H (2003) Laparoscopic gastric bypass for morbid obesity with linear gastroenterostomy. Obes Surg 13(3):360–363

Madan AK, Kuykendall SJ 4th, Ternovits CA, Tichansky DS (2005) Mallory-Weiss tear after laparoscopic Roux-en-Y gastric bypass. Surg Obes Relat Dis 1(5):500–502

Marshall SJ, Srivastava A, Gupta SK, Rossi TR, DeBord JR (2003) Roux-en-Y gastric bypass leak complications. Arch Surg 138:520–524

Nguen T. Ninh, De Maria Eric J, Ikramuddin S, Hutter M (2008) Anastomotic leaks after laparoscopic gatsric bypass. In: The sages manual. A practical guide to bariatric surgery, Springer, New York, pp 193–197

Rundall BK, Denlinger CE, Parrino GP, Foley EF, Jones DR (2005) Laparoscopic gastric bypass complicated by gastric pouch necrosis: considerations in gastroesophageal reconstruction. J Gastrointest Surg 9(7):938–940

Service GJ, Thompson GB, Service FJ, Andrews JC, Collazo-Clavell ML, Lloyd RV (2005) Hyperinsulinemic hypoglycemia with nesidioblastosis after gastric bypass surgery. N Engl J Med 353:249–254

Tucker ON, Szomstein S, Rosenthal RJ (2007) Surgical management of gastro-gastric fistula after divided laparoscopic Roux-en-Y gastric bypass for morbid obesity. J Gastrointest Surg 11(12):1673–1679

Yu J, Turner MA, Cho S-R, Fulcher AS, DeMaria EJ, Kellum JM, Sugerman HJ (2004) Normal anatomy and complications after gastric bypass surgery: helical CT findings. Radiology 231:753–760

Zerey M, Sigmon LB, Kuwada TS, Heniford BT, Sing RF (2008) Bleeding duodenal ulcer after Roux-en-Y gastric bypass surgery. JAOA 108:25–27

Sleeve Gastrectomy

Michael Korenkov, Phillipe Mognol, David Nocca,
Andrés Sánchez-Pernaute, Elia Pérez-Aguirre,
Miguel Angel Rubio, and Antonio Torres García

Introduction

The aim of the procedure is to restrict the size of the stomach by cutting the stomach vertically alongside the lesser curvature and to shut off the production of ghrelin through a complete removal of the gastric fundus (Fig. 4.1). This procedure can stand alone or be the first step of a duodenal switch procedure in high risk patients.

M. Korenkov
Abteilung für Allgemein- und Visceralchirurgie,
Klinikum Werra-Meissner, Akademisches Lehrkrankenhaus der
Universität Göttingen, Elsa-Brendström-Straße 1,
37269 Eschwege, Germany
e-mail: michael.korenkov@klinikum-wm.de

P. Mognol (✉)
Service de Chirurgie, Générale A, Hôpital Bichat, 46 rue Henri
Huchard, 75877 Paris, Cedex 18, France
e-mail: philippe.mognol@bch.ap-hop-paris.fr

D. Nocca
Department of Digestive Surgery Pr Fabre, Hopital Saint Eloi,
University Hospital of Montpellier, Avenue Bertin SANS,
34000 Montpellier, France
e-mail: d.nocca@wanadoo.fr

A. Sánchez-Pernaute
Servicio de Cirugía 2, 3a planta, ala Sur, Hospital Clínico San
Carlos, c/Martín Lago s/n, 28040 Madrid, Spain
e-mail: asanchezp.hcsc@salud.madrid.org,
penaute@yahoo.com

E. Pérez-Aguirre • M.A. Rubio • A.T.García
Servicio de Cirugía 2, 3a planta, ala Sur, Hospital Clínico San
Carlos, c/Martín Lago s/n, 28040 Madrid, Spain

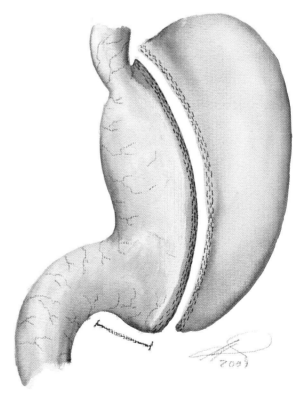

Fig. 4.1 Sleeve gastrectomy

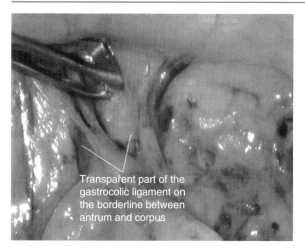

Fig. 4.2 Beginning dissection close to the stomach wall

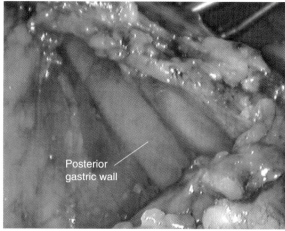

Fig. 4.3 Transsecting the omental bursa near the greater curvature

Preparation

Setting, Positioning, and the Surgical Team

The following aspects are similar to those for classic gastric bypass surgery (see p. 54):

- Positioning the patient
- Setting of the surgical team
- Creation of the pneumoperitoneum
- Positioning the trocars

Surgical Technique

This procedure is technically simple, but nevertheless bears the risk for serious intraoperative complications.

Step 1 – Dissection of the Stomach Close to the Greater Curvature

- Begin dissection between the antrum and the corpus near the greater curvature (Fig. 4.2).
- Grasp the stomach's distal end with a grasper (preferably a babcock forceps; right working trocar) and pull it to the right and cranial.
- Pull the greater omentum with a second grasper (not mandatory, but recommendable) (left additional trocar) to the opposite side.
- Cut a small opening into the transparent part of the gastrocolic ligament close to the stomach wall with the endoscopic scissor. Then detach the greater omentum from the stomach with ultrasound scissors, working in cranial direction (Fig. 4.3). Move the two graspers upward following the level of dissection.

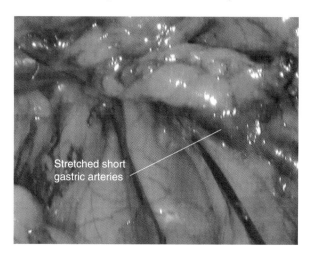

Fig. 4.4 Showing the short gastric arteries

Dissection is done easily and without major technical difficulties up to the level of the lower end of the spleen. From now on the situation can be a little more confusing due to more massive fat tissue. We recommend tilting the table to the left; gravity will help to keep the spleen out of the way. If adhesions between the spleen and the stomach exist, a rough handling of the stomach can lead to diffuse hemorrhage from the spleen.

Step 2 – Cutting the Short Gastric Arteries and Mobilization of the Fundus

- Continue dissecting in the same direction. The short gastric arteries are also cut with the ultrasound scissors (Fig. 4.4).

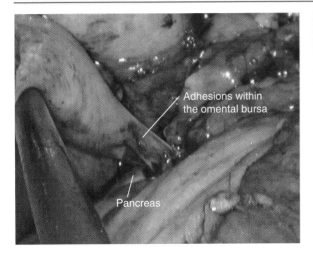

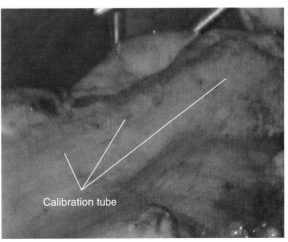

Fig. 4.5 Adhesions within the omental bursa

Fig. 4.6 Placing the calibration probe into the stomach

- Now the fundus is dissected. It is very important to mobilize it all the way up to the angle of His. Dissect the left crus of diaphragm first.
- Then pull the fundus with a babcock forceps (right working trocar) toward the liver.
- Next tense the tissue between the left crus and the angle of His; the latter is now clearly visible.

In very obese patients with massive intraabdominal fat tissue it can be somewhat difficult to identify structures clearly. It is helpful to pull the already skeletonized and mobile fundus toward the liver hilum (babcock forceps, right working trocar) and the greater omentum downward with the other grasper (left additional trocar). We believe it to be very important to detach the left crus of diaphragm completely from the backside of the stomach.

Step 3 – Mobilizing the Backside of the Stomach

- After mobilizing the greater curvature completely, pull the stomach toward the liver with the babcock forceps (left additional trocar), flipping it to remove all adhesions with the greater omentum (Fig. 4.5). This step is very important for a trouble-free transsection of the stomach along the greater curvature later. Remaining adhesions might lead to an incomplete resection of the stomach fundus.

- Cut the adhesions with the ultrasound cutter or, if they are thin and transparent, with scissors without electricity. Take care to not injure the left stomach arteries or even the celiac trunk! Only very thin and transparent adhesion may be cut quickly; thick adhesions containing fat tissue must be cut very carefully and in small portions at a time.

Step 4 – Transsection of the Stomach

This step is technically simple, but where exactly to begin cutting is still a matter of discussion. Some authors recommend beginning between the antrum and the corpus. This way the antrum remains intact and gastric emptying is undisturbed. The antrum itself also has thick muscle layers. Stapling here requires staplers with 4.8 mm cartridge, which do not always close blood vessels sufficiently. This may lead to heavy diffuse hemorrhage with the need of laborious suturing.

Some authors begin transsection close to the pylorus, thereby also performing a partial resection of the antrum. Result of this technique is permanently impaired gastric emptying. Supporters of this technique welcome this, as it leads to a marked restriction of food intake and successful weight loss.

We perform a small partial resection of the antrum (cutting 4 cm away from pylorus) to produce mildly impaired gastric emptying; long-term results, however, are not available yet.

- Insert a calibration probe (we use an 18-mm probe, 57 Fr) into the stomach before transsecting (Fig. 4.6).
- This step is mandatory. Resection without a calibration probe can lead to postoperative stenosis of the

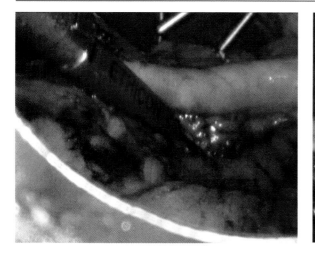

Fig. 4.7 Beginning the transsection of the stomach with the linear stapler (green cartridge)

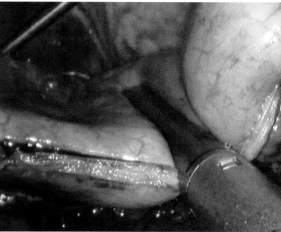

Fig. 4.8 Continuing transsection of the stomach (green cartridge)

gastric sleeve with irreversible obstruction or an intraoperative injury of the esophagus.

- After determining the starting point for dissection, insert the first Endo-GIA stapler and cut. When using an angled Endo-GIA, insert the stapler always through the left working trocar.
- Tense the stomach between two babcock forceps (left additional trocar and right working trocar) to facilitate the placement of the stapler. A straight linear stapler for the first cut is inserted through the right working trocar (Fig. 4.7), the following staplers are inserted through the left working trocar.

Many authors recommend stapling the corpus with 4.8 mm staples (green) and the fundus with 3.5 mm staples (blue). To prevent hemorrhage from the stapler suture use staple line reinforcement. We use a 60-mm linear stapler with a green cartridge without staple line reinforcement for the entire stomach. We suture diffuse hemorrhage or use a coagulation suction tube with ultrashort monopolar electricity (Figs. 4.8 and 4.9)

- Cutting the stomach usually can be done quickly and without any major difficulties. When positioning the last cartridge take special care to not injure the esophagus.

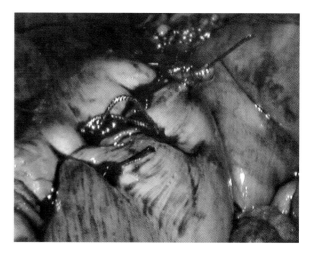

Fig. 4.9 Suturing a bleeding stapler suture line by hand

Position the last stapler cartridge parallel to the left crus of diaphragm.

Step 5 – Retrieving the Specimen

The specimen is placed into a retrieval bag (extra large) and removed (Fig. 4.10).

- The size of the specimen requires the enlargement of the trocar channel, an incision of about 1.5–2 cm is sufficient.

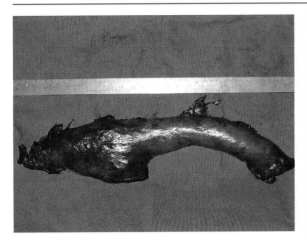

Fig. 4.10 Gastric sleeve specimen

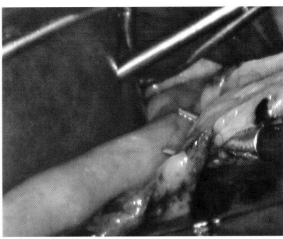

Fig. 4.11 Arching fat tissue with the endodissector before transsection

- After retrieving the specimen, remove the calibration tube and check the stapler suture again for hemorrhage. If no bleeding occurs, the procedure is finished.

Difficult situations and Intraoperative Complications

Endoscopic sleeve gastrectomy is a comparatively simple procedure. But it too has a potential for difficult intraoperative situations, some of which can already arise during the first steps.

Massive Hemorrhage During Skeletonization of the Greater Curvature from the Greater Omentum or the Short Gastric Arteries

Predisposing factors: Cutting through fat tissue without having dissected the tip of the scissors first or rough handling of the stomach during dissection.

Prevention: Hemorrhage usually stems from gastroepiploic vessels or the short gastric vessels during dissection of the greater curvature.

A bleeding from the gastroepiploic vessels can be avoided by beginning dissection close to the greater curvature in the vessel-free, transparent region of the gastrocolic ligament. This way, the gastroepiploic vessels are out of the line of dissection until up to the splenic artery.

Dissection of the stomach is usually done with ultrasound scissors. The preparation of the opening in the gastrocolic ligament is uncomplicated.

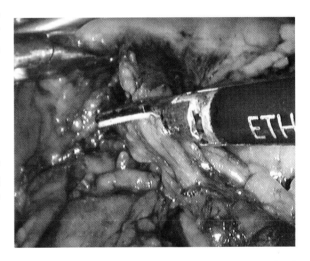

Fig. 4.12 Skeletonization of the greater curvature. The tip of the ultrasound cutter is visible

When the opening is finished and the path for dissection is clearly visible, the surgeons tend to cut more and more farther up in order to save time. If a blood vessel is injured this way, the bleeding can be stopped easily, but more time is lost than gained.

We recommend dissecting short "bridges" of tissue before cutting (Fig. 4.11). Create a small opening with the endodissector or the ultrasound scissors (without electricity) (blunt dissection). Then position the scissors showing the tips (Fig. 4.12). Only then electricity is applied to cut.

Hemorrhage from the short gastric arteries can be the result of rough handling of the stomach during dissection.

Management: Stopping *hemorrhage from the greater omentum* is simple. The bleeding spot is grasped with an endodissector, and then the bleeding can be stopped with the ultrasound scissors, the bipolar grasper, or an endoclip.

Hemorrhage from the short gastric arteries, however, can lead to serious intraoperative problems in some cases. If it is massive, efforts to grasp the bleeding spot can result in an injury of the spleen, which worsens the situation. Efficient management of this situation requires good and coordinated teamwork of surgeon, assistant, and scrub nurse.

- The assistant must keep the operating area dry using an aspirator (left additional trocar), as you as the surgeon take hold of the bleeding vessel with an atraumatic grasper or the endodissector. Use two graspers (left and right working trocar).
- Perform hemostasis following your preferred method.

> It is advisable to have two graspers for hemostasis and an aspirator at hand before starting dissection around the short gastric arteries. Never coagulate untargeted or grasp "blindly."

Diffuse Hemorrhage While Skeletonizing the Greater Curvature Due To a Spleen Injury

Predisposing factors: Perisplenitis with substantial adhesions between the splenic capsule and the greater omentum or a confusing operation area due to hemorrhage from the short gastric arteries and the greater omentum.

Prevention: This complication is very rare during laparoscopic surgery, but in cases of severe perisplenitis it can happen. Make sure there are no such adhesions before beginning dissection the stomach. If there are massive adhesions, remove them first.

When dissecting the greater omentum around the spleen, grasp the omentum and pull it toward the spleen first, then pull the stomach into the other direction.

When stopping hemorrhage from the greater omentum, avoid pulling it too hard toward the stomach.

Management: The most frequent spleen injury during a surgical procedure is an accidental removal of serous

membrane, with resulting diffuse hemorrhage. Hemostasis can be achieved with an argon-plasma-beamer or the intraoperative application of fibrin glue. We prefer the argon-plasma-beamer. The coagulated area can be reinforced with a hemostyptic-containing thrombin and fibrinogen.

Revision Procedures

Revision procedures after sleeve gastrectomy are performed because of postoperative complications such as breakdown of stapler sutures, dilatation of the sleeve stomach, refractory gastroesophageal reflux, or because of insufficient weight loss.

Revision Procedures Due To Postoperative Complications

Complications requiring a revision procedure are a broken stapler seam with diffuse or local peritonitis and an intraabdominal abscess, the result of an infected hematoma.

Broken Stapler Suture

Diagnostic procedures in a patient with reduced overall condition and abdominal pain reveal a broken stapler suture.

Predisposing factors: We differentiate between high and lower leaks, depending on the location. Reasons can be impaired blood supply in the proximal segment of the stomach or a faulty stapler. High leaks are usually caused by impaired blood supply, because the fundus is less well perfused than other parts of the stomach. Lower leaks are usually the result of a faulty stapler.

Prevention: Proficient bariatric surgeons perform this procedure quickly, but still must always take time to carefully inspect the stapler sutures. Problems concerning the sutures and blood supply are very often the cause of postoperative complications.

> At the slightest suspicion of impaired blood supply or a weak stapler suture, sew the suspicious area over immediately. The weak part can also be reinforced with a pedicled segment of the greater omentum.

Management: In some patients in a good condition and with limited inflammation, broad band antibiosis and food restriction will help. Much more often however, a broken stapler suture requires surgical revision. The extent of the procedure depends on the individual findings, ranging from a simple suture up to more complex procedures to close the leak. If the leak is located in the lower or middle part of the stomach, sewing the leak over and reinforcing the seam with a pedicled segment of the greater omentum is usually sufficient. Therapy of a leak in the proximal part of the stomach is very much more difficult and can get the surgeon into serious trouble at times. Difficulties arise if inspection reveals that no safe suture can be created. The extent of the perifocal inflammation and the distance to the GE-junction are of great importance for therapeutical decisions.

> The farther proximal the leak is located, the more difficult is therapy.

The extent of the procedure can be estimated before operating by localizing the leakage. If the leak is far proximal, the insertion of a stent is the best option. If this is not possible or fails to resolve the problem, a surgical procedure is performed. It is rarely possible to sew a large proximal leak over successfully.

The leak can be sealed with a Roux segment, which is pulled up. If this fails, the last possibility is the removal of the gastric sleeve, closure of the esophagus, creation of a jejunostoma, and possibly a cervical esophageal fistula. The closed esophagus can be drained with a soft nasoesophageal tube. This procedure is associated with high lethality.

Marked Subphrenic Abscess

Diagnostic procedures in a patient with reduced overall condition after surgery reveal no leakage, but a large subphrenic abscess is seen on the left side.

Predisposing factors: Subphrenic hematoma.

Prevention: This complication is extremely rare, but a larger amount of blood located underneath the diaphragm can lead to inflammation and abscess formation.

Management: In case of a subdiaphragmatic abscess without any sign of leakage, abscess drainage is the method of choice. If this fails, a laparoscopic procedure is performed to remove it.

Persistent Agonizing Heartburn and Regurgitation After Sleeve Gastrectomy; Proton Pump Inhibitors Are Ineffective

Predisposing factors: Some patients experience persistent refractory gastroesophageal reflux after sleeve gastrectomy. The exact reason for this undesirable situation is not known. Possible explanations include the slowed passage of food and a functional pyloric obstruction.

Prevention: As the underlying causes are not completely understood, it is difficult to give advice on prevention. Begin dissection at least 4 to 6 cm away from the pylorus.

Management: If a patient suffers intolerably, gastric bypass surgery can be considered in some cases.

Persistent Dysphagia, Heartburn, and Regurgitation, a Water-Soluble Contrast Swallow Reveals a Long Distance Stenosis Between Antrum and Fundus

Predisposing factors: Reasons for a long distance stricture are a restriction of the lumen of the gastric sleeve (if the stapler was positioned incorrectly because the position of the calibration probe was not checked before cutting) and an ischemic stomach wall due to impaired blood supply. Clinically inapparent breakdown of a stapler seam can also be responsible. If the stenosis is located at the gastric notch, faulty positioning of the stapler is the reason. A more proximal stenosis is usually of ischemic or inflammatory origin.

Prevention: Before firing the first stapler cartridge make sure the calibration probe is inserted far enough down into the stomach. Sometimes the tip is moved upward accidentally, which can lead to stenosis, if the stapler is not positioned correctly before firing. Make sure the calibration probe is positioned correctly first.

Management: A clinically relevant stenosis can be treated in several different ways. If possible, try dilatation or bouginage of the stenosis, which is sufficient in some cases. If these measures fail to improve the situation, a surgical procedure is performed, most frequently a transformation into a gastric bypass. Some authors report successful therapy of long distance stenosis with seromyotomy.

Revision Procedures Due To Inadequate Weight Loss

Revision procedures due to inadequate weight loss are performed rarely, because sleeve gastrectomy is often performed as a first step before biliopancreatic switch or duodenal switch surgery. If a sleeve gastrectomy is performed as an independent procedure, expect a dilatation of the gastric sleeve.

Revision procedures after sleeve gastrectomy include a conversion into a duodenal switch or a gastric bypass.

Some authors reduce the size of the dilated stomach by repeating the original procedure to create a new, smaller sleeve.

In some cases, patients experience refractory gastro-esophageal reflux after sleeve gastrectomy, which requires the conversion into a duodenal switch or a gastric bypass.

4.1 Surgical Technique by Phillipe Mognol (France)

Phillipe Mognol

Introduction

Laparoscopic sleeve gastrectomy (LSG) is currently gaining ground as an alternative bariatric operation.

LSG involves a longitudinal resection of the stomach on the greater curvature from the antrum to the angle of His.

Despite its reputation to be an easier and safer procedure than much more complex procedures like gastric bypass or duodenal switch, LSG is associated with significant morbidity and mortality. Most of them are probably due to technical difficulty.

There are two different techniques for the LSG. They differ in that in one stapling is performed after full devascularization and mobilization of the gastric greater curve, whereas in the other stapling is performed as soon as the lesser sac is entered; the greater curve is devascularized after full completion of the sleeve.

Preparation

Setting, Positioning, and the Surgical Team

- Gastrectomy is performed laparoscopic using in the French position (legs abducted with the surgeon standing between the patient's legs).

  We think that LSG should always be considered a first procedure until we have long-term results about it as a sole procedure. Therefore the laparoscopic approach should always be preferred.

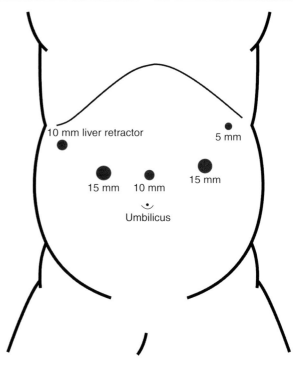

Fig. 4.13 Trocar placement for sleeve gastrectomy

- The operation is performed under general anesthesia. Pneumoperitoneum (17 mmHg) is obtained through a Veress needle.
- The procedure requires five trocars (Fig. 4.13):
  - One trocar 10 mm for the liver retractor in the right flank
  - One trocar 10 mm (camera) is placed 10–15 cm subxiphoidally 1 cm to the left of the median line
  - Two 15-mm trocars are placed in the left and right anterior axillary line 3–4 cm under the costal margin
  - One 5-mm trocar is placed 2 cm below the left costal margin in the left flank.

Surgical Technique

- Dissection begins on the greater curvature 3 cm to 6 cm proximal to the pylorus.
- The gastroepiploic vessels along the greater curvature of the stomach are divided using the Harmonic Scalpel (Ethicon Endo-surgery, Cincinnati, OH, USA) or Ligasure (ValleyLab, Boulder, CO,USA) (Fig. 4.14).
- After the lesser sac is entered, dissection is continued in cephalad direction, the lower pole of the spleen is reached quickly (Figs. 4.15 and 4.16).

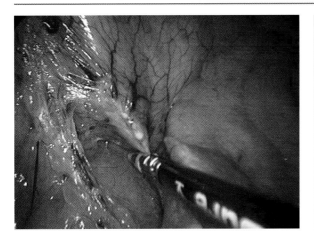

Fig. 4.14 Beginning dissection by cutting the gastroepiploic vessels at the greater curvature with the ligasure

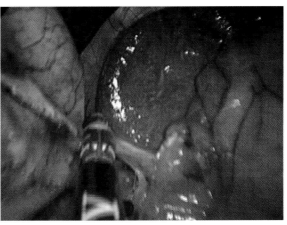

Fig. 4.17 At the level of the spleen, the short gastric vessels must be coagulated separately, i.e., with the ligasure

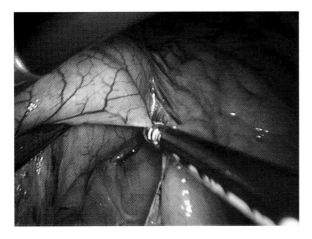

Fig. 4.15 Opening the omental bursa and dissecting alongside the greater curvature toward the lower pole of the spleen

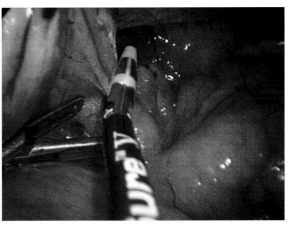

Fig. 4.18 To avoid hemorrhage from the spleen or the short gastric arteries, dissect very cautiously, especially in extremely obese patients. It might be helpful to remove any retrogastric adhesions to obtain a better view

- At the level of the spleen, the short gastric vessels must be coagulated separately, by using the Ligasure (ValleyLab, Boulder, CO, USA (Figs. 4.17 and 4.18).
- Dissection reaches the root of the left crus of diaphragm (Figs. 4.19, 4.20a and b).

> At this point it could be useful to remove fat tissue around to the stomach to allow good exposure of the left crus (Fig. 4.21a and b).

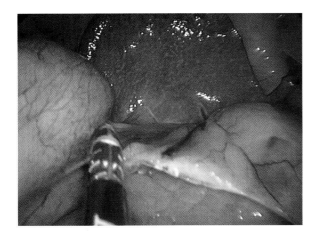

Fig. 4.16 The lower pole of the spleen is reached quickly

- Any adhesions on the posterior gastric wall should be divided respecting the left gastric vessels to allow complete mobilization of the stomach before stapling (Fig. 4.22a–d).

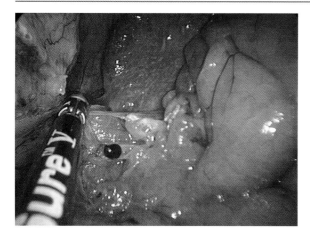

Fig. 4.19 The gastrosplenic ligament is cut with the Ligasure

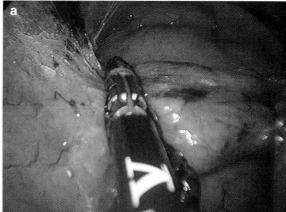

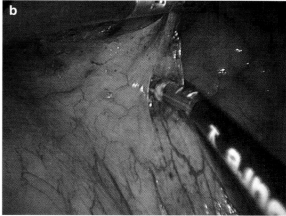

Fig. 4.21 (a, b) Removal of fat pads around the GE junction facilitates dissection of the left crus of diaphragm

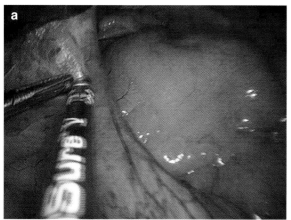

Left crus

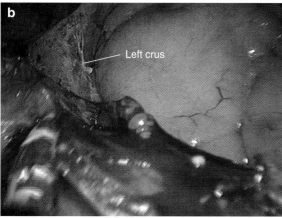

Fig. 4.20 (a, b) The left crus of diaphragm must be displayed completely when cutting the gastrosplenic ligament

- The short gastric vessels and the greater curvature ligaments (gastrosplenic and gastrocolic) are divided using ultrasonic dissection to complete the resection. A good exposure should be attempted before transsecting the stomach.

- Insert the linear stapler (green cartridge) through the left 15-mm trocar (Figs. 4.23 and 4.24).
- Before you continue stapling, the anesthetist inserts a 32-French gastric tube into the stomach (Fig. 4.25).
- The stapler is then positioned to push the nasogastric tube loosely against the lesser curvature and oriented so that the tip of the devascularized stomach lies between the jaws; the tip of the instrument is oriented toward and just to the left of the visible endings of the lesser curvature vessels (Figs. 4.26 and 4.27).
- The instrument is fired, reloaded, and the maneuver repeated.
- Finally, after five or six firings of the stapler, the greater curvature is detached completely from the stomach (Fig. 4.28).
- A 15-mm retrieval bag is used to remove the sleeve gastrectomy specimen (Fig. 4.29).
- The gastric suture line is then electrocoagulated to prevent bleeding from the stapler suture (Fig. 4.30).

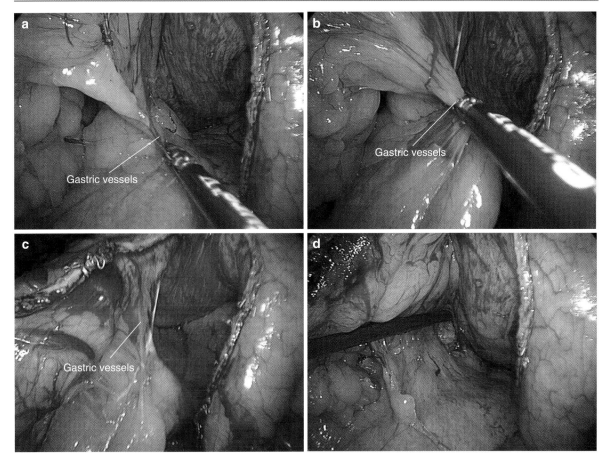

Fig. 4.22 (**a–d**) Any adhesions on the posterior gastric wall should be divided respecting the left gastric vessels (**a–c**) to allow complete mobilization of the stomach before stapling (**d**)

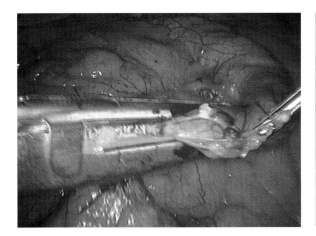

Fig. 4.23 The first linear stapler (green cartridge) is positioned between antrum and corpus

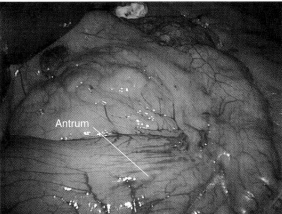

Fig. 4.24 View after firing the first stapler

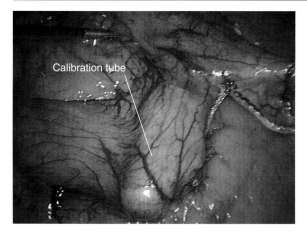

Fig. 4.25 Before you continue stapling, the anesthetist inserts a 32-French gastric tube into the stomach

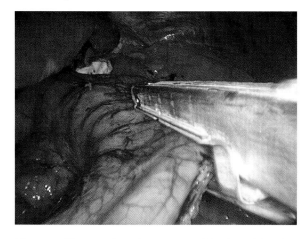

Fig. 4.26 The second stapler (green cartridge) is positioned to push the naso-gastric tube loosely against the lesser curvature; the jaws must be placed a little medial to the visible ends of the vessels of the lesser curvature

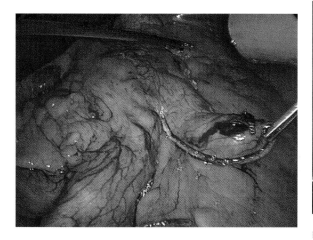

Fig. 4.27 View after firing the second stapler

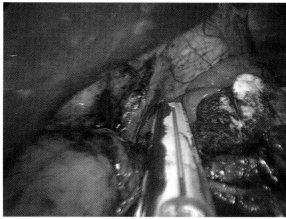

Fig. 4.28 Firing the last stapler

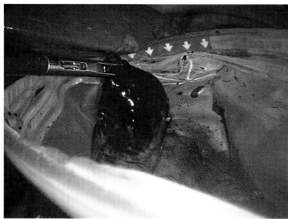

Fig. 4.29 The specimen is placed into an extra large retrieval bag

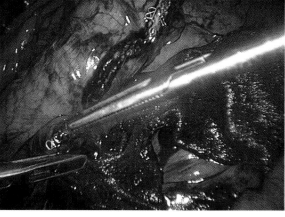

Fig. 4.30 Electrocoagulating diffuse hemorrhage from the stapler suture

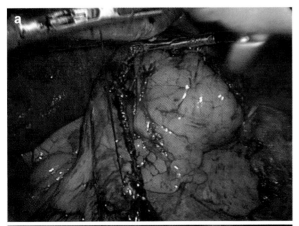

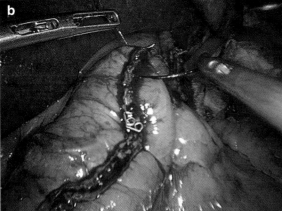

Fig. 4.31 (**a, b**) The whole stapler line is overstitched by absorbable running sutures. This is done to prevent insufficiency of the stapler line and bleeding

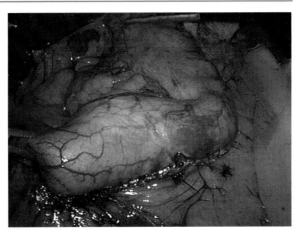

Fig. 4.32 An instillation of saline with methylene blue by the anesthetist through a nasogastric tube placed after withdrawal of the bougie is used to exclude leaks of the suture-line and to measure gastric capacity. For this purpose, we block the flow into the duodenum transiently with a long intestinal forceps at the pyloric channel

- The whole stapler line is overstitched by absorbable running sutures. This is done to prevent insufficiency of the stapler line and bleeding (Fig. 4.31a and b).
- An instillation of saline with methylene blue by the anesthetist through a nasogastric tube placed after withdrawal of the bougie is used to exclude leaks of the suture-line and to measure gastric capacity. For this purpose, we block the flow into the duodenum transiently with a long intestinal forceps at the pyloric channel (Fig. 4.32).
- A Jackson-Pratt drain is placed alongside the stapler line and a nasogastric tube is left in place (Fig. 4.33 a and b).
- The patient is taken to the recovery room and from there back to his/her room.

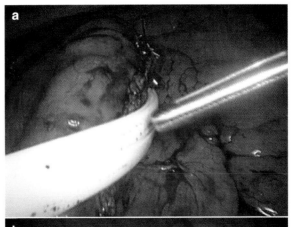

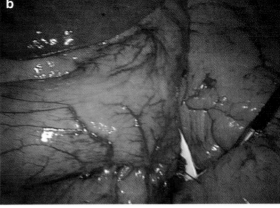

Fig. 4.33 (**a, b**) A Jackson-Pratt drain is placed alongside the stapler line, the nasogastric tube is left in place

- A water-soluble contrast swallow is performed on the second postoperative day. The GI study excludes leaks or strictures. Oral fluid intake is allowed if no leakage is demonstrated.
- Patients are discharged after removal of the drain.

Difficult Situations and Intraoperative Complications

Fistulas

A high risk location for fistulas is located at the level of the antrum where the gastric wall is very thick.

> We think that at this level a green cartridge (4.8-mm staples) should be used to allow safe stapling of the thick stomach. We use 60 mm green cartridge for the two first stomach stapler sutures.

After that gastric tubulization is continued by dividing the gastric corpus toward the angle of His, applying – three to four cartridges of a 3.8-mm 60 mm linear stapler (blue cartridge).

The second one is located at the level of the angle of His.

To avoid fistula at this level we think that the angle of His and the greater curvature must be completely freed up to the left crus of diaphragm to allow safe stapling at this level.

To avoid staple line dehiscence, the stapler line is reinforced by a running suture using absorbable material.

When sleeve gastrectomy is performed as a redo procedure after laparoscopic gastric banding or VBG, fragility and thickness of the gastric wall due to fibrosis created after contact with a silicone band and previous dissection could be important. We think that in this case a green cartridge (4.8-mm staples) should be used to allow safe stapling of the thick stomach.

Stricture or Stenosis

The other risk of complication after sleeve-gastrectomy is stricture or stenosis. To avoid this type of complication a calibration tube should be used during stomach transsection. This tube diameter should be between 32 and 40 French. Before the second or third firing the surgeon should rule out stenosis at the angle between the oblique antrum stapler line and the vertical stapler line

parallel to the lesser curve. Correct positioning of the gastric tube prevents stricture at this level.

Bleeding

The principal causes of intraoperative bleeding are: splenic trauma, dissection of short gastric vessels, and bleeding from the stapler line.

To avoid bleeding from the spleen or the short gastric vessels, dissection should be performed carefully at this point especially in super-obese patients. To allow good exposition at this point, it could be useful to perform dissection of the retrogastric adhesion at the upper part of the stomach or perhaps in some cases to staple the stomach first to allow correct mobilization of the stomach.

Methods that could be used to reinforce the stapler line (to avoid leak/bleeding):
- Fibrin glue (Tisseel VH, Baxter, Deer.eld, IL, USA)
- A running suture using absorbable material
- Seamguard, Bioseamguard® (Gore, Newark, DE, USA).

To avoid bleeding from the stapler line, the surgeon could use:
- Electrocoagulation of the stapler line
- A running suture using absorbable material or separate stitches
- Seamguard, Bioseamguard (Gore, Newark, DE, USA)

Leakage

Leaks are major complications after LSG.

Leaks could be treated with total parenteral nutrition and strict oral restriction mainly if the drain has not been removed. If reoperation is required, a suture with or without plication with omentum and drainage could be attempted.

Coated self-expandable stents have been proposed as an alternative therapeutic option for the management of GE junction leaks after LSG with good results in terms of morbidity and survival.

In the worst case patients could develop gastric dehiscence with generalized peritonitis, sepsis, and shock, requiring operation such as total gastrectomy of the remnant stomach with Roux in Y esophago-jejunostomy reconstruction as a last chance in a life-saving procedure. If the leak is at the bottom part of the gastric sleeve, a Roux-en-Y gastric bypass could be attempted with resection of the part of the gastric sleeve with the leak sites and gastrojejunostomy.

Another possibility to avoid performing an anasto-mosis in patients with generalized peritonitis and shock is to perform a total remnant gastrectomy with closure of the duodenum and the esophagus with an oro-gastric tube to drain salivary secretion and an alimentary jejunos-tomy. In these cases the patient is reoperated 4 months later to perform a Roux in Y esophago-jejunostomy.

Stricture

Stricture could be treated by endoscopic dilatation with a through-the-scope endoscopic balloon.

Another possibility to treat stricture of the gastric tube is to convert the sleeve gastrectomy to a Roux-en-Y gastric bypass.

Revision Procedures

Sleeve gastrectomy could be performed as a redo proce-dure. It has been published as a rescue procedure after failed gastric banding and after dilatation of the gastric pouch after duodenal switch and Roux-en-Y gastric bypass. We have also performed sleeve gastrectomy in obese patients with previous Nissen procedure.

In all these cases, we think that the surgeon should use the green cartridge to staple thick tissue. And we also think that dissection of the left crus should be attempted even if it could be very difficult because of adhesions after the previous procedure.

We experienced good results in terms of weight loss in patients undergoing re-sleeve of the dilated gastric pouch after failed RYGB. In these cases the main cause of RYGB failure should be a dilated gastric pouch.

Sleeve gastrectomy has been initially described as a first-step procedure before more complex procedures such as duodenal switch and gastric bypass in super-obese patients.

Since these first reports, sleeve gastrectomy has changed to an isolated bariatric procedure. In literature the percentage of patients requiring a second-step pro-cedure after initial sleeve gastrectomy for insufficient weight loss varies from 10% to 70%.

The average BMI loss after LSG is 20 kg/m^2; we think that the percentage of patients who will require a second-step procedure will mostly depend on the ini-tial BMI. Super (BMI > 50 kg/m^2) and super-super-obese (BMI > 60 kg/m^2) patients will probably require a second-step procedure. This could either be a duode-nal switch or a Roux-en-Y gastric bypass. It seems that

this second stage procedure should be performed within 1 year after the first step when maximum weight loss is achieved.

LSG reduces the operative risk (ASA score) and major obesity-related co-morbidities in super-obese patients undergoing two-stage procedure.

For converting LSG to RYGB, we stapled the gas-tric sleeve horizontally, tube and then we create the gastrojejunal anastomosis with a circular stapler using the trans-oral technique for anvil placement. If the gas-tric tube is dilated, it could be necessary to re-sleeve the stomach. The results in terms of weight loss are very good and allow in our experience a BMI reduc-tion of 10 to 20 kg/m^2 depending on the initial BMI at the time of the second-step procedure.

4.2 Surgical Technique by David Nocca (France)

David Nocca

Introduction

Laparoscopic sleeve gastrectomy (LSG) is performed in our institution since 2005 in a prospective French trial. This procedure is indicated to treat morbid obesity or superobesity. Nowadays there is no consensual oper-ative technique described today, even if there are more and more LSG performed throughout the world. The key points of this operation however, are well known:

- The fundus has to be removed completely
- Any posterior attachments or adhesions of the stom-ach have to be removed
- The size of the gastric bougie may be the same than for VBG procedure (32 to 36 French)
- The distance between the pylorus and the first staple line depends on the concept of conserving the antrum in order to facilitate gastric emptying. In that case, 8 to 10 cm are enough to place the first stapler suture, parallel to the lesser curvature.

Description of the LSG with Conservation of the Antrum

- All the patients receive perioperative deep vein thrombosis prophylaxis using low molecular weight heparin.

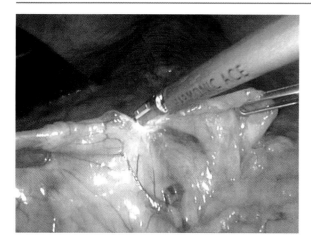

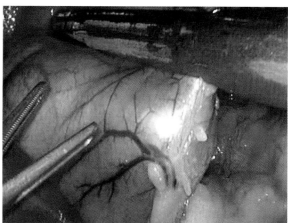

Fig. 4.34 Beginning dissection by cutting the gastrocolic ligament

Fig. 4.35 The tip of the calibration tube helps find the starting point for the transsection of the stomach

- The patient is placed in a Lloyd-Davis position with the upper abdomen upright (Lazy chair position).
- The pneumoperitoneum is obtained by an open Hassan technique or with a Veress needle.
- Five to six trocars are inserted in a classic gastric laparoscopy configuration. The retraction of the left liver is obtained by a 5–10 mm trocar in the subxiphoid position.
- The first step is the dissection of the gastrocolic ligament in vicinity of the stomach and thereby entering the omental bursa (Fig. 4.34). This step is performed by using the ultrasonic scalpel (Ace????). Dissection along the lower part of the greater curvature stops 10 cm from the pylorus. Dissection along the upper part of the greater curvature progresses toward the angle of His.
- All the posterior adhesions or attachments of the stomach have to be removed. A calibration tube of 36 French is placed trans-orally along the lesser curvature to perform a controlled vertical gastrectomy.
- *Sleeve gastrectomy is started where the calibration tube makes contact with the greater curvature*! The Resection is performed parallel to the lesser curvature in contact to the calibration tube (Fig. 4.35). It requires staplers (green or gold) capable of stapling the thick tissue of the stomach to prevent dehiscence of the stapler line.
- The transsection line runs parallel to the lesser curvature close to where the blood vessels of the small curvature enter the stomach wall (Fig. 4.36).
- The stapler line may be reinforced with a running suture or with adding absorbable material such as Bioseamguard (Gore). The stapler line is checked

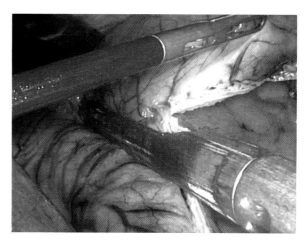

Fig. 4.36 The transsection line runs parallel to the lesser curvature close to where the blood vessels of the small curvature enter the stomach wall

for leakage by injecting methylene blue through a gastric tube.
- A suction drain (Redon type) of 16 mm is left in contact to the stomach.

Postoperative Care

- Two days after the procedure, a water-soluble contrast swallow is performed to exclude fistulas on the stapler line or stenosis. If the sleeve gastrectomy is confirmed watertight, the orogastric tube is removed and the patient is started on a liquid diet.
- The patient is mobilized to the chair on the first postoperative day.

Fig. 4.37 Sleeve gastrectomy as a first step before gastric bypass or duodenal switch surgery

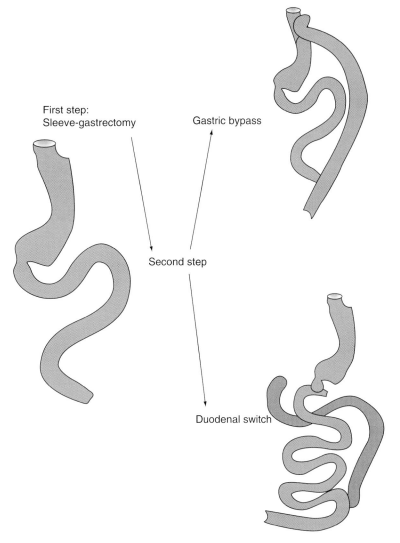

First step:
Sleeve-gastrectomy

Gastric bypass

Second step

Duodenal switch

4.3   Surgical Technique by Andrés Sánchez-Pernaute (Spain)

Andrés Sánchez-Pernaute, Elia Pérez-Aguirre, Miguel Angel Rubio, and Antonio Torres García

Introduction

Sleeve gastrectomy is basically the removal of the greater curvature, after which a small sleeve remains with a capacity of 80–150 mL.

This technique was developed in the late twentieth century as an innovative treatment of extreme obesity. It was introduced as a first-step procedure for high-risk patients. After a certain weight loss, they were all meant to undergo a second, malabsorptive procedure, such as gastric bypass or duodenal switch (Fig. 4.37) [1–3].

Surgeons soon noted, however, that many patients experienced substantial weight loss after sleeve gastrectomy [4] that they managed to keep their weight down [5] and also succeeded in improving their obesity-related comorbidities [6–8]. The possibility of offering sleeve gastrectomy as a stand-alone procedure for the treatment of extreme obesity was considered [9]. Most groups must admit that it is not a purely restrictive procedure, because it differs in various aspects from classic gastroplasty techniques, such as the vertical or the adjustable gastric band [10, 11]. The differences seem to be related to hormone production, especially that of ghrelin, whose secretion is shut off with resection of the gastric fundus. But other aspects might be involved, too [12, 13]. We accept the following indications for sleeve gastrectomy:

- BMI over 60, as a first-step procedure before a duodenal switch
- Age over 65
- Patients with comorbidities that might worsen with a biliopancreatic diversion, such as liver cirrhosis
- Very young patients who wish a "second chance" to avoid a malabsorptive procedure

It is very important to consider the indication for every case very carefully, as there are slight modifications in surgical technique.

Surgical Technique

Setting, Positioning, and the Surgical Team

- Sleeve gastrectomy is performed laparoscopic.
- The patient is in an anti-Trendelenburg position with spread legs.
- You as the surgeon stand between the patient's legs.
- For the first access to the abdomen we use the Endopath-Xcel-Bladeless-Trokar (Ethicon, USA). It is inserted under visual control two fingers above the umbilicus and 3–4 cm toward the left side of the patient through the rectus abdominis muscle.
- Create a pneumoperitoneum with a pressure between 14 and 18 mmHg.
- Now insert three more trocars:
  - A 5 mm trocar subxiphoidally for the left hand grasper
  - A 10 mm trocar just below the left costal arch on the anterior axillary line for the ultrasound cutter or the linear stapler
  - A 12–15-mm trocar for the live retractor, the linear stapler and the specimen bag.

  A fifth trocar can be placed in the left upper quadrant, if necessary; it can assist in pulling the omentum out of the way during dissection of the short gastric arteries and the stomach (Fig. 4.38).

- We use a 30° laparoscope for the entire procedure.

Surgical Technique

- After accessing the abdomen, identify the pylorus.
- Pull the stomach wall upward with the left hand grasper to spread out the branches of the gastroepi-

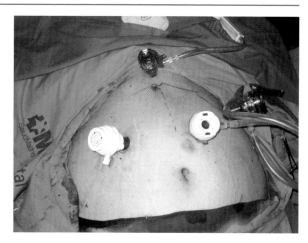

Fig. 4.38 Trocar placement for sleeve gastrectomy as performed by Sánchez-Pernaute

ploic artery. At this probably uncomplicated point cut the gastric vessels close to the stomach wall to create access to the retrogastric space (Fig. 4.39).
- Continue dissecting upward, holding the stomach up to cut the gastric vessels with ultrasound scissors.
- Cut the short gastric arteries, too, as well as some of the posterior vessels, until the fundus is completely mobilized and the left crus of diaphragm is dissected.

  Sometimes the stomach is stuck to the spleen in the upper part of the gastric fundus. Dissecting the short gastric arteries can cause injury of the spleen capsule. Do not try to stop an eventually bothersome hemorrhage immediately, but proceed to dissecting the gastric arteries. This reduces tension to the capsule and should lead to a spontaneous stop of the hemorrhage.

- Cut all adhesions at the posterior wall of the stomach in order to mobilize the stomach completely (Fig. 4.40).
- Now turn to the lower part of the greater curvature. Continue dissection of the gastroepiploic arteries downward stopping 6–8 cm proximal to the pylorus. The idea is to create the gastric sleeve that includes the antrum.
- Insert a 54 Fr gastric tube orally to splint the stomach. This way you make sure the sleeve is not too tight, as this could impair food intake. It should not be too wide, either, so as to guarantee food restriction.

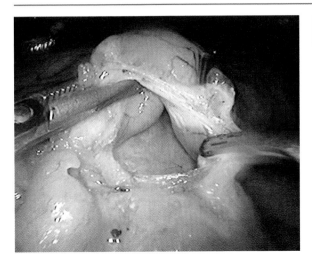

Fig. 4.39 The retrogastric space is accessible after cutting the branches of the gastroepiploic artery

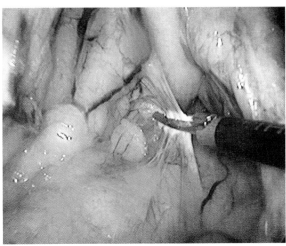

Fig. 4.40 Removing adhesions at the posterior stomach wall to completely mobilize the organ

Surgical indication should determine the correct size of the sleeve: Patients receiving sleeve gastrectomy as a stand-alone procedure and who have contraindications for a second procedure, should have a thinner calibration tube. Patients, for whom sleeve gastrectomy is just the first step before a malabsorptive procedure, should never be restricted too much. If a gastric bypass is planned as a second step, the sleeve must not be tighter than it needs to be for a duodenal switch. If the calibration tube cannot be inserted far enough into the stomach, a gastroscopy should be performed to rule out serious problems. The endoscope is a substitute for the calibration tube. If gastroscopy fails and a "blind" transsection of the stomach has to be performed, use the fat pad around the left gastric arteries as a landmark and make sure to keep the stapler away from it.

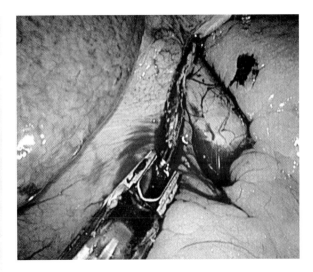

Fig. 4.41 Hemostasis at the stapler suture with clips

- Before you insert the stapler, the anesthetist gives the patient a bolus of butylscopolamine to relax the smooth musculature of the stomach and to stretch the organ as much as possible. This makes it easier to handle and the final size of the finished pouch can be estimated more precisely.
- Insert a 45-mm linear stapler (Endo-GIA Roticulator, USA) through the 15-mm trocar. A green cartridge is used best, because the stomach wall is thicker around the antrum.

As the staples are longer (4.8 mm), they can grasp more tissue, but allow for less control of hemorrhage; bleeding is stopped with a cautery hook, clips, or single sutures (Fig. 4.41).

- Insert the first stapler through the left hand trocar as well as the second one, which could also be inserted through the right hand trocar, depending on the individual anatomical situation. Rotation and articulation of the tip of the instrument make it very flexible.

- Do not position the stapler too close to the calibration tube, as this can result in tension on the stapler line and impair the tightness of the seam. It would also lead to a sleeve that is too thin, which can promote food congestion.
- You can use Seamguard (W.L. Gore, USA) to reinforce the stapler line [14].
- Usually five to eight cartridges for the 60-mm instrument (blue cartridge, 3.5 mm staples) are sufficient to complete sleeve gastrectomy.

It is very important to maintain constant traction of the posterior wall of the stomach, so that the anterior and the posterior wall form a symmetrical sleeve without twists. Sometimes the staples do not take hold of the entire stomach wall and the seam reopens after the stapler is removed. In this case a running suture should be placed by hand. We use 000 prolene or PDS, as monofil sutures are easier to handle laparoscopic. For single sutures we use 00 Ethibond.

- After completing sleeve gastrectomy, remove the resected stomach from the abdomen with a specimen bag (Endo catch II, United States Surgical, Tyco healthcare Group, USA) through the 15 mm trocar.
- Remove the calibration tube and inject methylene blue to test for tightness of the sutures through an orally inserted gastric tube.
- Inspect the stapler sutures and the gastric vessels carefully for hemorrhage.

We usually apply fibrin glue (Tisseel, Baxter, USA). Sometimes we place a TachoSil-patch onto the seam (Nycomed, Schweiz), which consists of a collagen sponge coated with human coagulation factor (Fig. 4.42).

- Three to four TachoSil patches cover the stapler suture to secure hemostasis and reduce the risk of leakage.
- Place a vacuum drain on the left side.
- Check all openings for hemorrhage while removing the trocars. The opening for the 15 mm trocar is covered with a patch to avoid later herniation (Bard Ventralex Hernia Patch, C.R. Bard, USA) (Fig. 4.43).
- The patient can drink the next day and leave hospital after 2–3 days.

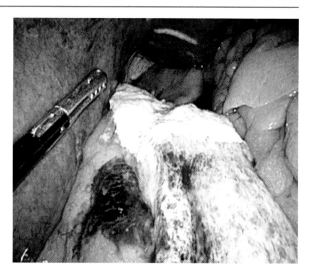

Fig. 4.42 TachoSil-patches on the stapler suture

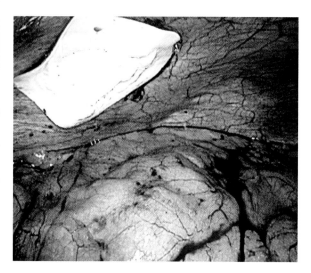

Fig 4.43 Preventing herniation at the trocar channel: mesh plug over the 15-mm opening

Complications

Complications in sleeve gastrectomy are
- Intraluminal or intrabdominal hemorrhage
- Breakdown of the stapler suture
- Stricture of the gastric sleeve

Late complications are stricture or dilatation of the gastric sleeve [15].

Postoperative hemorrhage can have the following sources:
- Stapler suture
- Cut blood vessels

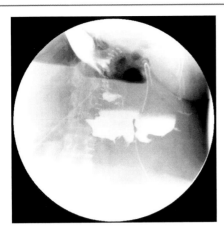

Fig. 4.44 Massive leakage of the upper part of the stapler suture after sleeve gastrectomy

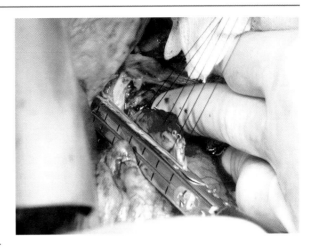

Fig. 4.45 Perforation of the upper part of the stapler suture is closed with another linear stapler

- Gastric branches of the gastroepiploic vessel in the greater omentum
- Short gastric arteries above the spleen hilus

Postoperative hemorrhage from the spleen is very rare. We place a drain routinely to detect postoperative hemorrhage early. Relevant hemorrhage requires a revision procedure, preferably laparoscopic.

An *intraluminal hemorrhage* leads to hematemsis or melena; in these cases a gastroscopy is performed and hemostasis achieved with electrocautery or injection of adrenalin.

Breakdown of the stapler suture is seen in 0–5% of all cases. The antrum has a thicker wall and sometimes the staples do not take hold of all the layers completely. The upper part of the sleeve is also less well supplied with blood, which increases the risk for an ischemic breakdown. We have never experienced the breakdown of a stapler suture after sleeve gastrectomy, but we have seen four cases of dehiscence of the gastric sleeve after duodenal switch surgery. In two cases the leakage was in the antrum, the other two in the upper part of the sleeve. The two cases of distal perforation were treated conservatively; the abdominal drain worked well. The cases of perforation in the upper part were revised. In one case, a preexisting vertical gastroplasty had been changed into a duodenal switch. A water-soluble contrast swallow revealed massive extravasation requiring surgical revision (Fig. 4.44).

In the second case the patient experienced sudden abdominal pain; a CT scan was performed. Pneumoperitoneum and clinical signs of peritonitis lead to a surgical revision. A breakdown in the upper part of the stapler suture was found and closed with a linear stapler (Fig. 4.45).

We do not routinely suture the stapler sutures, but in these cases we used a 000 prolene suture. The new suture must be placed very carefully so as not to impair gastric passage. A calibration tube is recommended.

Proximal leaks can be a serious problem. If the reason is ischemia of the gastric sleeve and peritonitis develops, the new suture is doomed to break down again. If the gastric sleeve is too tight below the perforation, gastric juices and saliva will rather flow into the abdominal cave than through the operated stomach. This difficult situation may end in total gastrectomy [16]. The defect can otherwise be patched with a self-expanding stent [17] or surgically be drained into a jejunal Roux loop [18].

If a patient vomits after having begun fluid intake, a water-soluble contrast swallow must be performed to rule out *stricture of the gastric sleeve*. If a stenosis is revealed, the patient can undergo an endoscopic dilatation or the implantation of a removable stent. Stenosis as a late complication is treated the same way.

Revision Procedures

In bariatric surgery, all procedures that become necessary because of inadequate weight loss or medium or late complications are referred to as revision procedures.

As sleeve gastrectomy is a restrictive procedure, there is no way to restore the original anatomical situation, although dilatation of the stomach results in near-normal circumstances in the long run. This long-term dilatation is also mainly responsible for inadequate weight loss after sleeve gastrectomy [19].

Some authors favor a repeated sleeve gastrectomy [20], as the blame for failure is laid on a too wide sleeve. Usually a large antrum is the cause; it can easily be narrowed laparoscopic.

Other authors prefer the placement of an adjustable gastric band [21, 22], which can be a good solution in the rare cases in which a part of the gastric fundus, usually posterior, was accidentally left behind.

We believe that after failure of a restrictive procedure a malabsorptive technique, such as a Roux-en-Y gastric bypass or a duodenal switch should be considered to achieve the desired weight loss. In patients after sleeve gastrectomy as a first-step procedure (high BMI), a duodenal switch with a short common channel (50 cm) is performed. Young patients, who received sleeve gastrectomy as a "second chance," are offered a duodenal switch or a gastric bypass. The duodenal switch poses less intraoperative difficulties, because it is performed within a previously untouched area where less adhesions are to be expected. The antrum is mobilized up to the pylorus. Dissection is continued to the duodenum up to the gastroduodenal artery, where the duodenum is cut. Blood supply for the lesser curvature remains untouched.

There are, however, absolute contraindications for a bypass, such as liver cirrhosis, as well as relative contraindications, such as advanced age. In these cases one of the other before mentioned procedures, such as repeated sleeve gastrectomy or implantation of an adjustable gastric band, should be performed.

Late complications of sleeve gastrectomy are caused by *gastric sleeve stricture*, usually located at the gastric notch. The stapler changes direction here during resection and the cut can accidentally have been directed toward the lesser curvature instead of running parallel (Fig. 4.46).

The stomach looks like an hourglass or a diabolo (Fig. 4.47).

Patients with a stricture of the gastric sleeve present food intolerance and vomiting. If left untreated, hypovitaminosis and deficiency symptoms ensue. Just as in early stenosis, endoscopic dilatation should be tried first. If this fails, however, a revision procedure must be contemplated. Gastric bypass is the first choice for these patients.

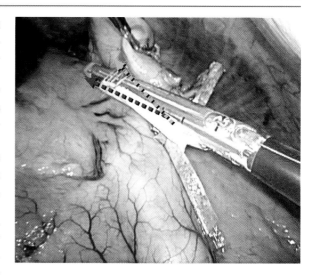

Fig. 4.46 Cutting the antrum, if the stapler was accidentally directed toward the lesser curvature (*red arrow*). The gastric sleeve is then close to the gastric notch, the resulting stenosis is very troublesome for the patient

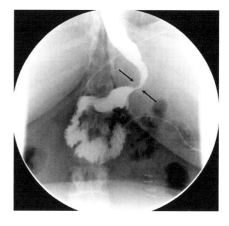

Fig. 4.47 X-ray of an hourglass stomach

Other complications and unsolved problems, such as severe gastroesophageal reflux, are regarded individually, but usually treated in the same way.

There are many different treatment options for extreme obesity today. Sleeve gastrectomy is not purely restrictive, but the exact mechanism of this procedure is not yet fully understood. Impaired hormone secretion, distension of the stomach wall, receptors within the stomach wall, etc., all contribute in various degrees to satisfying weight loss and successful treatment of comorbidities. The good results have changed the procedure from being merely the first step of a more complex operation to a complete and stand-alone treatment for extreme obesity.

References

4.3 Surgical Technique

1. Regan JP, Inabnet WB, Gagner M, Pomp A (2003) Early experience with two-stage laparoscopic Roux-en-Y gastric bypass as an alternative in the super-super obese patient. Obes Surg 13(6):861–864
2. Mognol P, Chosidow D, Marmuse JP (2005) Laparoscopic sleeve gastrectomy as an initial bariatric operation for high-risk patients: initial results in 10 patients. Obes Surg 15(7):1030–1033
3. Nguyen NT, Longoria M, Gelfand DV et al (2005) Staged laparoscopic Roux-en-Y: a novel two-stage bariatric operation as an alternative in the super-obese with massively enlarged liver. Obes Surg 15(7):1077–1081
4. Moon Han S, Kim WW, Oh JH (2005) Results of laparoscopic sleeve gastrectomy (LSG) at 1 year in morbidly obese Korean patients. Obes Surg 15(10):1469–1475
5. Mognol P, Chosidow D, Marmuse JP (2006) Laparoscopic sleeve gastrectomy (LSG): review of a new bariatric procedure and initial results. Surg Technol Int 15:47–52
6. Gan SS, Talbot ML, Jorgensen JO (2007) Efficacy of surgery in the management of obesity-related type 2 diabetes mellitus. ANZ J Surg 77(11):958–962
7. McCloskey CA, Ramani GV, Mathier MA et al (2007) Bariatric surgery improves cardiac function in morbidly obese patients with severe cardiomyopathy. Surg Obes Relat Dis 3(5):503–507
8. Vidal J, Ibarzabal A, Nicolau J et al (2007) Short-term effects of sleeve gastrectomy on type 2 diabetes mellitus in severely obese subjects. Obes Surg 17(8):1069–1074
9. Tucker ON, Szomstein S, Rosenthal RJ (2008) Indications for sleeve gastrectomy as a primary procedure for weight loss in the morbidly obese. J Gastrointest Surg 12(4):662–667
10. Melissas J, Koukouraki S, Askoxylakis J et al (2007) Sleeve gastrectomy: a restrictive procedure? Obes Surg 17(1):57–62
11. Himpens J, Dapri G, Cadiere GB (2006) A prospective randomized study between laparoscopic gastric banding and laparoscopic isolated sleeve gastrectomy: results after 1 and 3 years. Obes Surg 16(11):1450–1456
12. Sabench Pereferrer F, Hernandez Gonzalez M, Feliu Rovira A et al (2008) Influence of sleeve gastrectomy on several experimental models of obesity: metabolic and hormonal implications. Obes Surg 18(1):97–108
13. Langer FB, Reza Hoda MA, Bohdjalian A et al (2005) Sleeve gastrectomy and gastric banding: effects on plasma ghrelin levels. Obes Surg 15(7):1024–1029
14. Consten EC, Gagner M, Pomp A, Inabnet WB (2004) Decreased bleeding after laparoscopic sleeve gastrectomy with or without duodenal switch for morbid obesity using a stapled buttressed absorbable polymer membrane. Obes Surg 14(10):1360–1366
15. Lalor PF, Tucker ON, Szomstein S, Rosenthal RJ (2008). Complications after laparoscopic sleeve gastrectomy. Surg Obes Relat Dis 4(1):33–38
16. Serra C, Baltasar A, Perez N et al (2006) Total gastrectomy for complications of the duodenal switch, with reversal. Obes Surg 16(8):1082–1086
17. Serra C, Baltasar A, Andreo L et al (2007) Treatment of gastric leaks with coated self-expanding stents after sleeve gastrectomy. Obes Surg 17(7):866–872
18. Baltasar A, Bou R, Bengochea M et al (2007) Use of a Roux limb to correct esophagogastric junction fistulas after sleeve gastrectomy. Obes Surg 17(10):1408–1410
19. Langer FB, Bohdjalian A, Felberbauer FX et al (2006) Does gastric dilatation limit the success of sleeve gastrectomy as a sole operation for morbid obesity? Obes Surg 16(2):166–171
20. Baltasar A, Serra C, Perez N et al (2006) Re-sleeve gastrectomy. Obes Surg 16(11):1535–1538
21. Ueda K, Gagner M, Milone L et al (2007) Sleeve gastrectomy with wrapping using polytetrafluoroethylene to prevent gastric enlargement in a porcine model. Surg Obes Relat Dis.
22. Gumbs AA, Pomp A, Gagner M (2007) Revisional bariatric surgery for inadequate weight loss. Obes Surg 17(9):1137–1145

Further Reading

4.1 Surgical Technique

Akkary E, Duffy A, Bell R (2008) Deciphering the sleeve: technique, indications, efficacy, and safety of sleeve gastrectomy. Obes Surg 18(10):1323–1329

Arias E, Martinez PR, Li VKM, Szomstein S, Rosenthal RJ (2009) Mid-term follow-up after sleeve gastrectomy as a final approach for morbid obesity. Obes Surg 2009; 19(5):544–548

Baltasar A, Serra C, Bengochea M, Bou R, Andreo L (2008) Use of Roux limb as remedial surgery for sleeve gastrectomy fistulas. Surg Obes Relat Dis 4(6):759–763.

Dapri G, Cadiere GB, Himpens J (2009) Laparoscopic seromyotomy for long stenosis after sleeve gastrectomy with or without duodenal switch. Obes Surg 19(4):495–499

Deitel M, Crosby RD, Gagner M (2008) The First International Consensus Summit for Sleeve Gastrectomy, New York City, October 25–27, 2007. Obes Surg 18:487–496

Frezza EE, Reddy S, Gee LL, Wachtel MS (2008) Complications after sleeve gastrectomy for morbid obesity. Obes Surg 19(6):684–687

Gumbs AA, Gagner M, Dakin G, Pomp A (2007) Sleeve gastrectomy for morbid obesity. Obes Surg 17(7):962–969

Lalor PF, Tucker ON, Szomstein S, Rosenthal RJ (2008) Complications after laparoscopic sleeve gastrectomy. Surg Obes Relat Dis 4(1):33–38

Santoro S (2007) Technical aspects in sleeve gastrectomy. Obes Surg 17(11):1534–1535

Biliopancreatic Diversion with Duodenal Switch

5

Michael Korenkov, Laurent Biertho,
Rudolf Steffen, Michael Gagner, Nelson Trelles,
Philippe Topart, Guillaume Becouarn,
Ernesto Di Betta, and Francesco Mittempergher

M. Korenkov
Abteilung für Allgemein- und Visceralchirurgie,
Klinikum Werra-Meissner, Akademisches Lehrkrankenhaus der
Universität Göttingen, Elsa-Brendström-Straße 1,
37269 Eschwege, Germany
e-mail: michael.korenkov@klinikum-wm.de

L. Biertho
Department of Surgery, Laparoscopic and Bariatric Surgery,
Laval University, Hospital Laval, Quebec City, Quebec, Canada
e-mail: laurentbiertho@hotmail.com

R. Steffen
Facharzt FMH für Chirurgie, Brunngasse 14,
3011 Bern, Switzerland
e-mail: steffen.rudolf@bluewin.ch

M. Gagner
Department of Surgery, Mount Sinai Medical Center,
4300 Alton Road, Miami Beach, FL 33140, USA
e-mail: mgagner@msmc.com,
gagner.michel@gmail.com,

N. Trelles (✉)
Department of Surgery, Mount Sinai Medical Center,
4300 Alton Road, Miami Beach, FL 33140, USA

P. Topart • G. Becouarn
Société de Chirurgie Viscérale,
140 Avenue De Lattre de Tassigny, 49000 Angers, France
e-mail: philippetopart@orange.fr

E.D. Betta
Department of Surgery – 1 Chirurgia Generale, Spedali Civili,
P. le Spedali Civili 2, 25123 Brescia, Italy
e-mail: fmitt@libero.it

F. Mittempergher
Department of General Surgery,
Spedali Civili, P. le Spedali Civili 2, 25133 Brescia, Italy
e-mail: edibetta@libero.it

Introduction

The aims of the procedure are to restrict the size of the stomach through a vertical gastric resection, to shut off the production of ghrelin by removing the fundus completely (gastric sleeve) and to produce malabsorption by separating the small intestine into an alimentary and a biliopancreatic segment. Both segments run parallel, this way digestive juices (bile, pancreatic juice) and food meet only where the segments are connected to form the so-called common channel. The anastomosis is between 50 and 100 cm from the ileocecal valve.

This procedure is considered to be the most difficult of all bariatric procedures, because of the extent of surgical intervention and because it is mostly performed in super-obese patients. Therefore it also has the greatest potential for serious intraoperative and postoperative complications (Fig. 5.1).

Preparation

Setting, Positioning, and the Surgical Team
- Positioning of the patient and the surgical team as well as the creation of the pneumoperitoneum are similar to gastric bypass surgery (see page 54). It is advisable to add shoulder rests.
- Position the trocars as you would for gastric bypass surgery, only 2–3 cm lower.

M. Korenkov (ed.), *Bariatric Surgery*,
DOI 10.1007/978-3-642-16245-9_5, © Springer-Verlag Berlin Heidelberg 2012

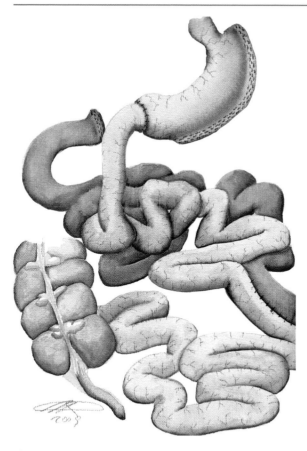

Fig 5.1 Duodenal switch with sleeve gastrectomy

Surgical Technique

Step 1 – Creating a Gastric Sleeve

- After performing sleeve gastrectomy (see Chap. 4), stop to decide whether to proceed or to finish the procedure as a first step to BPD-DS.
- If you decide to continue the procedure, begin with the skeletonization of the duodenal bulb or with cutting the ileum. We prefer to create the duodenoileal anastomosis by hand sewing in a mini-laparotomy.

Step 2 – Cutting the Ileum

- Move the patient from the anti-Trendelenburg position into the Trendelenburg position for this step. Remove all instruments from the abdomen beforehand to avoid accidental injury of the liver. This includes the liver retractor, which must also be removed or at least loosened and placed between

the left hepatic lobe and the diaphragm, and the calibration tube from the gastric sleeve.
- Move to the patient's left side; the assistant with the camera will be standing next to you, cranially.
- Identify the cecum first.

> Some authors perform an appendectomy as a prophylactic measure, so that later possible pain in the right lower abdomen caused by a malfunctioning enteroenteral anastomosis cannot be confused with appendicitis. We omit this step.

- Next measure the complete small intestine (how to do so see p. 55). Mark the point for the future enteroenteral anastomosis (70–100 cm proximal from the ileocecal valve) with a suture or a clip.
- Continue measuring up to Treitz's arch. Go back from there to find the transsection point for the small intestine. The Roux loop should be 2–3 m long.

> Tension is never a problem for the duodenoileal anastomosis, even with a short and fatty mesentery.

- Tilt the table to the right a little before you cut the ileum.
- Remove the camera from the supraumbilical trocar and place it into the left working trocar or the left additional trocar, depending on the situation.
- Grasp the small intestine (atraumatic grasper, suprapubic trocar) and hold it close to the ventral abdominal wall in the right middle abdomen.
- The first assistant holds the small intestine with another grasper (right working trocar) about 10 cm from your grasper; the segment is thereby tensed between the two instruments.
- Cut a small opening into the mesentery. Extensive dissection is not necessary here; it should be just large enough for the jaw of the Endo-GIA to fit through.

> To avoid hemorrhage from the fatty mesentery, we do not begin dissection with ultrasound scissors, but with a monopolar hook. After opening the anterior mesenterial layer, we continue bluntly, with dissector or a coagulation suction tube until the posterior mesenterial layer is reached.

- Cut the intestine with a linear stapler.
- Then continue cutting the mesentery with ultrasound scissors, if necessary, usually about half way down.

> A long distance transsection of the mesentery is not necessary in BPD-DS, because the Roux loop does not have to be pulled all the way up to the proximal end of the stomach, but is connected to the duodenal bulb.

Step 3 – Creating the Enteroenteral Anastomosis

- Stay on the patient's left side with the assistant for the creation of the enteroenteral anastomosis. The patient remains in the Trendelenburg position, but the table is tilted a little to the left now.
- The camera is returned to the supraumbilical trocar. Insert an additional 12-mm trocar left to the umbilicus and a 5-mm trocar on the right side, both of them a little lateral to the medioclavicular line.
- Find the end of the biliopancreatic segment.
- The first assistant grasps the end of the biliopancreatic segment (atraumatic grasper, right working trocar) and pulls it caudally toward the ileocecal valve. He places it isoperistaltically parallel to the ileum next to the point marked beforehand for anastomosis. Place a stay suture (we prefer vicryl 2-0) between the two segments and tie the knot. This suture marks the middle of the future enteroanastomosis; it is placed opposite to the mesentery of both segments.
- After tying the knot, cut one side and let the other half long. The first assistant holds the suture with a grasper (right working trocar) and pulls it toward the anterior wall of the right lower abdomen.
- Next create small openings in the intestine on both sides opposite to the mesentery with ultrasound scissors; the stay suture remains in the middle of the two jaws of the stapler.
- Insert the jaws of the stapler through the newly positioned 12-mm trocar in the right middle abdomen. We use a 45-mm stapler with a blue cartridge. Grasp one of the segments (new 5 mm trocar, left middle abdomen) and pull slightly to facilitate the entrance of the jaws. The second assistant does the same with the other segment (atraumatic grasper, right additional trocar). Both jaws must be inserted completely into the lumen. Only then the stapler is closed and fired.

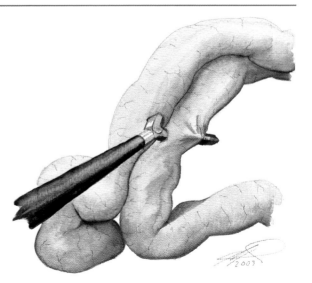

Fig. 5.2 Small bowel perforation by tangential insert a stapler

> *Attention*: Going parallel to the run of the intestine, it must be possible to insert the jaws into the lumen without any resistance at all. Touching the wall can easily result in a perforation (Fig. 5.2). The direction of the jaws must then be adjusted to match the course of the intestine. Sometimes it helps to open the stay suture and to insert the two jaws separately. The assistant must take care to hold the segment with an atraumatic grasper in a way that prevents the jaw from sliding out again.

- After firing the stapler close the enterotomy. We perform this step with two running sutures, vicryl 2-0. Place the suture line parallel to the run of the intestine. The upper suture is begun at the cranial end of the opening and tied. Then continue with a running suture, going through serosa, then mucosa, mucosa and again serosa. The first assistant constantly holds the suture under tension with a grasper (left working trocar).
- Continue sewing up to the middle of the opening. The assistant should now hold the suture under slight tension until it is tied together with the other suture.
- Begin this second suture at the caudal end and continue toward the middle in the same fashion. Knot both sutures together, but make sure to pull them tight enough to prevent leakage.

Step 4 – Cutting the Greater Omentum (Not Mandatory)

A fatty greater omentum may result in a certain tension around the duodenoileal anastomosis, if the antecolic pathway was chosen. Here it is necessary to transsect the greater omentum. In gastric bypass surgery only the pars libera is cut; in the duodenal switch however, the gastrocolic ligament is cut also, all the way to the stomach wall. Transsection is not performed through the middle, but more to the right, leaving two thirds to the left.

Step 5 – Removing the Gall Bladder (Not Mandatory)

In BPD, we perform a cholecystectomy only, if the patient has gall stones; it is done before the duodenoileal anastomosis is performed.

Step 6 – Dissecting and Cutting the Duodenal Bulb

This step is elaborate and technically demanding and therefore especially prone to complications. The duodenal bulb is cut about 3–4 cm distal to the pylorus. The proximal part must be well prepared for anastomosis, i.e., be well mobilized and well supplied with blood at the same time.

- The patient is tilted back into the anti-Trendelenburg position, you stand between the legs.
- Reinsert the liver retractor and review the operative findings.
- The first assistant takes hold of the gastric sleeve below the beginning of the stapler seam in the antrum with a babcock forceps (left additional trocar) and pulls craniad so that the duodenal bulb and the gastric sleeve are in one line.
- The omental bursa has already been opened during sleeve gastrectomy, just as the gastroepiploic arcade has already been cut.
- As soon as the hepatoduodenal ligament has been identified, begin dissection at the upper edge of the duodenal bulb.
- Cut into the upper layer of the hepatoduodenal ligament close to the duodenal wall and the pylorus with a monopolar hook (left working trocar). You are now between the gastroduodenal artery and the right gastric artery. As there are many small blood vessels in this area (pyloric and duodenal branches), cut the tissue only in very small bits at a time to avoid hemorrhage. We therefore

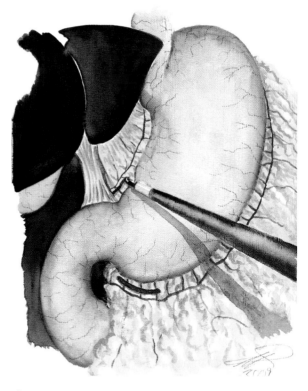

Fig. 5.3 Opening the hepatoduodenal ligament close to the duodenal wall and the pylorus

consider a hook with monopolar electricity to be the most suitable instrument for this part of the procedure (Fig. 5.3).
- Insert an atraumatic grasper into the right working trocar. Use it to tense the operation field by pulling either the duodenum or the lateral edge of the hepatoduodenal ligament.

Dissection can also be started in the pars flaccida of the lesser omentum near the pylorus.

- After opening the pars flaccida or the outer layer of the hepatoduodenal ligament about 2 cm, the assistant will flip the gastric sleeve upward with the babcock forceps to show the backside. This enables the surgeon to cut the right gastroepiploic artery. It is best done next to the middle of the backside of the duodenum, because the fatty strand with the artery inside is clearly visible there if the stomach is pulled up and tensed.

- Grasp the strand with an atraumatic grasper (right working trocar). Pull it caudally with a babcock forceps (left additional trocar) into the opposite direction.
- Preparate the strand from the duodenal wall first through blunt dissection. We use a monopolar hook and a bent dissector (left working trocar).
- After preparing the right gastroepiploic artery from the duodenal wall, cut it with ultrasound scissors.
- Create a channel behind the duodenal bulb next with a coagulation suction tube (left working trocar). The end of the tube should appear at the upper edge of the duodenal bulb, which has already been dissected.

> Pulling the gastric sleeve toward the spleen with a babcock forceps (left additional trocar) after placing the coagulation suction tube next to the distal end of the pylorus facilitates the dissection of the retroduodenal channel.

- Then insert a 60-mm linear stapler with a blue cartridge into the abdomen (left working trocar) and cut the duodenum about 3 cm from the pylorus. There must be only duodenum between the jaws of the stapler, but no fat tissue.
- Inspect both stapler sutures. Stop an eventual hemorrhage with electricity or sutures.
- Now inspect the proximal segment of the duodenum to determine its suitability for the creation of a duodenoileal anastomosis. If the anastomosis is to be created with circular stapler, no further dissection is required. For a hand-sewing anastomosis however, you will almost always have to continue dissection, including transsection of the right gastric artery.

Step 7 – Creating the Duodenoileal Anastomosis

The creation of the duodenoileal anastomosis is the most challenging step of the procedure. There are several ways to proceed:

- Endoscopic end-to-side anastomosis with a circular stapler
- Endoscopic end-to-end anastomosis by hand
- Conventional end-to-side anastomosis with a circular stapler
- Conventional end-to-end anastomosis by hand.

In order to minimize the risk of stenosis, a 25-mm circular stapler is desirable. However, this can be quite difficult at times, because the ileum has a smaller diameter than the jejunum and is less elastic. In case of an especially small ileum, the insertion of a 25-mm stapler can be very difficult.

The Roux segment can be pulled up following the antecolic or the retrocolic pathway. When operating endoscopically, the antecolic pathway is easier to perform. For the retrocolic pathway an opening must be created on the right side of the middle colic artery, which is technically demanding in laparoscopy. We guide the segment up the retrocolic pathway to create the duodenoileal anastomosis in a minilaparotomy.

Anastomosis with the circular stapler is as difficult as the hand sewn suture in laparoscopy, which is why this step of the procedure shows the highest risk of postoperative complications. We have not reached a satisfying level of skill in laparoscopy here so far, so we perform a mini-laparotomy (BPD-DS hybrid technique) check online. The cut is about 10-cm long and goes upward in the middle line, beginning directly above the umbilicus. We never cut horizontally, because the vertical cut facilitates interventional measures in case of complications.

- After opening the abdomen, remove the stomach specimen and also the appendix and the gall bladder, if necessary.
- The decision whether to create the anastomosis per hand or with the circular stapler is made during the procedure. If the ileum is very narrow ("spastic"), perform a double end-to-end anastomosis by hand. Use a 4-0 absorbable running suture for the inner seam and absorbable single sutures (2-0) for the outer row and the opening in the duodenal bulb.
- If the anatomy of the ileum permits it, use the circular stapler. Cut 1.5 cm (the stapler suture) from the lower edge of the duodenum and place a purse string suture there with nonabsorbable 2-0 monofilament.
- Then insert the anvil of the circular stapler into the duodenum and close the purse string suture.
- Now remove the stapler suture from the Roux segment and insert the stapler into the ileum.
- Create an end-to-side duodenoileal anastomosis and remove the "blind loop" with a linear stapler.
- After testing for tightness with methylene blue, add a row of single hand sutures (2-0), even if no leakage was detected.
- Close all openings in the mesentery.
- Insert a drainage tube next to the anastomosis; the procedure is now completed.

Difficult Situations and Intraoperative Complications

Difficult situations during sleeve gastrectomy are described in Chap. 4, other difficulties are listed here.

Measuring the Intestine Reveals That Several Segments Are Stuck in the Lower Abdomen Through Adhesions

Prevention: Measure the small intestine before you cut the stomach. Only if the surgeon is convinced that the Roux segment can be pulled upward without tension, he may proceed to sleeve resection.

Management: Try to estimate the extent of the adhesions and to decide, whether to continue laparoscopic or to switch to an open approach. Slight adhesions with only one or two attached segments can be taken care of without switching. Severe long-distance adhesions with tightly attached segments in very obese patients however produce a very confusing situation. There is a very high risk of injuries to the intestine that even may remain unnoticed, to make things worse. In this case you have the following options:

- Finish the procedure as sleeve gastrectomy. A second procedure will follow 4–6 months after weight loss.
- Switch to a conventional approach.
- Change strategy and perform a gastric bypass with only one anastomosis (only if the first 2 m of the intestine are free from adhesions). The segment is connected about 2 m from Treitz's arch with the gastric sleeve with a side-to-side anastomosis. Do not create a Braun's anastomosis. If sleeve gastrectomy has already been performed, this procedure is modified slightly (for a description of the original technique see p. 103–107, Garcia-Caballero).

Gastric Bypass with One Anastomosis
Step 1 – Cutting the Gastric Sleeve and Creating a Gastric Pouch

- Move the patient into an anti-Trendelenburg position. The surgical team stands as for sleeve gastrectomy.
- Cut the gastric sleeve distally between antrum and corpus. To stay away from the antrum, position the linear stapler (45 or 60 mm, green cartridge) about 1 cm above the beginning of the stapler suture, coming from the side of the stapler suture (left working trocar).

> You can also begin dissection below the stapler suture. In this case however, the cutting line will go through the antrum, where the stomach wall is thickest due to marked muscular layers. There is higher risk of hemorrhage from the stapler suture or a breakdown of the suture.

- Place the first linear stapler perpendicular to the vertical axis of the gastric sleeve. Stretch the stomach between two atraumatic graspers (right working trocar and left additional trocar).
- The stapler is then pointed cranially, in a 45° angle to the vertical axis of the gastric sleeve and fired.
- Before positioning the second stapler, remove the fat tissue and the branches of the right and left gastric arteries from the lesser curvature. If the gastric sleeve is cut together with the fat tissue, a quite massive diffuse hemorrhage will occur and quickly lead to hematoma. On the other hand you should avoid extensive devascularization to not compromise the blood supply of the pouch. The opening must be wide enough for the jaw of the stapler.
- Begin dissection close to the lesser curvature. The gastric sleeve is grasped with a babcock forceps (left additional trocar) and pulled to the left toward the spleen.
- Open the lower part of the pars flaccida. Grasp the fat tissue alongside the lesser curvature with an atraumatic grasper (right working trocar) and pull to the right toward the liver. The front layer of the lesser omentum is best opened with a monopolar hook. Continue with blunt dissection to expose a segment of the backside of the stomach. A slight diffuse hemorrhage here usually stops spontaneously.
- The gastric sleeve must be pulled toward the spleen continuously (babcock forceps, left additional trocar), so that the backside of the stomach is visible.
- Now create a channel with a blunt instrument (e.g., a coagulation suction tube) beginning with the front opening in the lesser omentum.
- Now insert the linear stapler into the prepared channel and cut the gastric sleeve.

Step 2 – Identifying and Fastening the Segment for the Pouch

- Move the patient back to a Trendelenburg position.
- Move to the patient's left side to stand next to the first assistant.
- Measure 2 m of small intestine, beginning at Treitz's arch. Adhesions are usually rare here; the chosen segment can easily be pulled up to the stomach pouch following the antecolic pathway.

> If massive adhesions are found around the proximal part of the small intestine, refrain from performing a gastric bypass with one anastomosis. Before you choose this procedure, make sure the proximal segments are free of adhesions.

- Fasten the segment to the pouch with two stay sutures (distal part of the pouch, close to the stapler suture after sleeve gastrectomy). Place the afferent loop above the efferent loop. Do not cut the lower stay suture.

Step 3 – Creating the Gastroenteral Anastomosis with the Linear Stapler

- Grasp the long suture with a grasper and pull in cranial direction. Cut small openings into the front side of the stomach and into the small intestine opposite to the mesentery with the ultrasound scissors. Insert a linear stapler with a 60-mm (blue) cartridge into both openings (left working trocar). Close and fire.
- Close the front part of the anastomosis by hand. Begin with placing two single sutures into the corners. Hold on to these sutures with graspers (endodissector, left additional trocar) and pull the upper one in cranial, the lower one in caudal direction. The suture line follows the vertical axis of the gastric sleeve. The grasper for the lower suture can also be inserted through the additional trocar in the right middle abdomen, instead of the liver retractor. If the left hepatic lobe still needs to be held, an additional 5-mm trocar in the right upper or middle abdomen is helpful.
- Insert a gastric tube through the pouch into the intestinal segment. Tense the opening between two graspers and close it with two absorbable running sutures (2-0). Use the outside-inside-inside-outside-

technique and tie the sutures together in the middle of the opening.
- Close the lumen of the efferent loop below the tip of the gastric tube with an atraumatic forceps and inject 50 mL methylene blue through the gastric tube. If no leak is visible, the creation of the gastro-enteral anastomosis is completed.

Step 4 – Creating Sero-Serosal Sutures Between the Afferent Loop and the Gastric Pouch

Sero-serosal sutures are placed between the afferent loop and the gastric pouch as a prophylactic measure against biliary reflux. The aim is to create anatomical conditions that facilitate the flow of bile and pancreatic juices from the efferent loop into the afferent loop, passing the gastric pouch by. This way a reflux of bile into the esophagus is avoided.

- Place —four to six single sutures (absorbable material, 2-0) between the afferent loop opposite to the mesentery and the stapler suture of the gastric pouch. As the anastomosis is quite far distal, there should be no tension between the intestine and the pouch.
- After placing sero-serosal sutures, remove the stomach specimen through the widened opening for the left working trocar.
- The procedure is completed after positioning a drainage tube.

Perforation of the Small Intestine While Positioning the Linear Stapler for the Enteroenteral Anastomosis

Predisposing factors: This complication is rare, but can happen nevertheless. Predisposing factors are massive intraabdominal fat tissue and anatomic particularities of the ileum. The wall of the ileum can be very thin and rigid in some obese patients; a stapler jaw touching it can lead to perforation, even if it is handled with care.

Prevention: The jaws of the stapler must be inserted parallel to the run of the intestine and remain so without manipulating the wall too roughly. Surgeon and first assistant must work together well. Inserting the thicker jaw of the stapler into the biliopancreatic loop and the thinner one into to the Roux loop works best. Create a slightly larger opening into the wall of the biliopancreatic loop for this reason. Surgeon and first assistant must both show and fix the two segments while inserting the stapler to keep it straight and from touching the walls.

Management: This complication is easy to detect during the procedure. It is nevertheless advisable to inspect both the front and the back wall of the future anastomosis carefully after inserting the jaws and closing the stapler, but before firing. Do not fire before you have made sure that both jaws are positioned correctly inside the intestine. If a wall was perforated, proceed as following: Identify the perforated segment.

- *Perforation of the biliopancreatic loop* is easy to manage; the perforated segment is simply removed with a linear stapler and ultrasound scissors.
- *Perforation of the Roux loop* is much more difficult to handle. Exact localization and extent of the damage are crucial to further proceedings. If the perforation is on the fat-free side of the intestine, suture it and insert the stapler through another opening in the segment in the other direction. The segment has to be turned for this purpose. If the perforation is close to the mesentery or is too large to be closed with a suture, the segment needs to be removed altogether. In this situation do not hesitate to switch to the conventional surgical approach to be able to perform the necessary steps under better conditions.

"Blue" Duodenoileal Anastomosis

Predisposing factors: Visible impaired blood supply is most often found around the anastomosis on the duodenal side. Reasons are an overly extensive skeletonization of the pylorus and/or anatomical particularities of the intramural blood vessels. Impaired blood supply on the ileal side is very rare and usually caused by tension because of a short and fatty mesentery.

Prevention: Try to spare the right gastric artery. It should be the last structure to be approached while mobilizing the pylorus. In many cases the artery can remain untouched and at the same time good conditions for the creation of the duodenoileal anastomosis can be produced.

Management: The breakdown of the duodenoileal anastomosis is a serious complication with a high potential mortality, so a "compromise" is no option. If impaired blood supply is suspected, open the anastomosis and remove the distal part of the gastric sleeve. Follow your preferred technique for a new ileogastral anastomosis.

Revision Procedures

Revision procedures after BPD with duodenal switch can be divided into the following categories:
- Revision procedures because of surgical (technical) problems
- Revision procedures because of negative effects due to the changes of the anatomy of the gastrointestinal tract
- Revision procedures because of no or insufficient weight loss

Revision Procedures Because of Surgical Problems

These are:
- Complications after sleeve gastrectomy
- Breakdown of the duodenoileal anastomosis
- Stenosis of the duodenoileal anastomosis
- Duodenal stump leakage
- Breakdown of the ileoileal anastomosis
- Ileus of the small intestine

Revision procedures because of surgical problems are emergency procedures; their outcome is therefore worst. A broken duodenoileal anastomosis and a duodenal stump blow-out are feared most. Therapy is individually adapted to the patient's situation.

Drainage of Bile Within the First Ten Days After Surgery

Additional diagnostic measures: None.

Diagnosis: Duodenal stump leakage or a breakdown of the ileoileal anastomosis.

Therapy: In these cases an emergency laparoscopy or laparotomy must be performed to close the broken suture. If a breakdown of the ileoileal anastomosis is found, it is safest to remove it and create a new one.

Duodenal stump leakage is more difficult to manage. It is often hardly possible to create a stable suture in highly infiltrated and fragile tissue. As duodenal stump leakage is an extremely rare complication, make sure to inspect the entire biliopancreatic segment carefully to exclude a mechanical obstruction as the cause for the breakdown.

Any obstructions must be eliminated first. Straighten kinked segments of the intestine. If an inflammation has caused a stenosis of the ileoileal anastomosis, the latter must be removed and recreated as wide as possible. Only then the duodenal stump is closed. The procedure is completed if this is possible with single sutures or a U-shaped running suture. If the sutures tear out of the tissue, an omental patch is used to close the broken segment. If this also fails, insert a Foley catheter into the stump and fasten it with single sutures. Create a new opening in the abdominal wall for the catheter.

Drainage of Putrid or Turbid Discharge and Fever and Raised Inflammatory Parameters Within the First Ten Days After Surgery

Additional diagnostic measures: CT of the abdomen with water-soluble contrast swallow, scanning for a breakdown of the duodenoileal anastomosis and an intraabdominal abscess.

Diagnosis No 1: Breakdown of the duodenoileal anastomosis

Therapy: Depending on the extent of the findings and the patient's overall condition there are different therapeutic options. Conservative therapy consists of a stent through the broken suture with or without drainage of the abscess. Surgical therapy can either be suturing the broken suture line or removing the distal end of the gastric sleeve (including the broken duodenoileal anastomosis) and creating an ileogastral anastomosis.

Diagnosis No 2: Intraabdominal abscess without signs of a broken anastomosis.

Therapy: Interventional drainage of the abscess. If this fails, a surgical procedure (either laparoscopy or laparotomy) to remove the abscess is necessary.

Intense Abdominal Cramps and Nausea

Additional diagnostic measures: X-ray of the abdomen with water-soluble contrast swallow; scanning for stenosis of the duodenoileal anastomosis and/or small bowel obstruction.

Diagnosis No 1: Stenosis of the duodenoileal anastomosis

Prevention: We recommend a 25-mm circular stapler for the anastomosis. If the ileum is too small, we create the anastomosis by hand. Others use 21-mm circular staplers (i.e., Gagner and Topart, see p. 151 and 157). We insert a soft gastric tube for 3 days and believe it functions as a splint to reduce the risk of stenosis.

Therapy: If the x-ray reveals that stenosis at the duodenoileal anastomosis is not complete, we begin with conservative measures to relieve the strain on the

gastric sleeve, such as a gastric tube, parenteral feeding, and in some cases hydrocortisone. In case of a complete obstruction at the distal end of the stomach gastroscopy is performed. If a small opening is visible, a guidewire is inserted with fluoroscopy. If this maneuver is successful, dilatation of the stenosis is possible. If not, a surgical procedure is performed – removal of the distal end of the gastric sleeve and the anastomosis and creation of an ileogastral anastomosis.

Diagnosis No 2: Small bowel obstruction

Prevention: All openings in the mesentery and below the Roux loop must be closed to avoid herniation, which happens frequently after weight loss. Take care not to twist the intestine while creating the enteroenteral anastomosis.

Therapy: Small bowel obstruction after duodenal switch is usually located in the Roux segment. An obstruction of the common channel is rare. The most frequent causes are interior herniation after weight loss or adhesions. A twist of the alimentary loop or the ileoileal anastomosis is less common. All these cases require immediate surgical therapy to get rid the ileus. It can be done laparoscopic or with laparotomy; we prefer the latter.

Persistent Abdominal Pain and Bloating Without Nausea or Constipation

Additional diagnostic measures: CT of the abdomen with water-soluble contrast swallow, scanning for change of caliber, obstruction, and dilatation of the duodenum.

Diagnosis: Dilatation of the duodenum.

Causes: Obstruction of the biliopancreatic loop due to adhesions, a twist of the segment, interior herniation or stenosis of the ileoileal anastomosis.

Prevention: Avoid twisting the intestine while creating an enteroenteral anastomosis. It also must be wide enough, use at least a 45 mm or two 30 mm staplers. All openings in the mesentery and below the Roux segment must be closed to avoid herniation, which happens frequently after weight loss.

Therapy: An obstruction of the biliopancreatic loop must also be treated surgically. The procedure can be performed selectively at an earlier point. Identify the exact location of the obstruction (in the alimentary or the biliopancreatic loop or in both) first, then determine the extent of the procedure.

Revision Procedures Because of Negative Effects of the Anatomical Changes in the Digestive System

The most frequent reasons for revision procedures in this category are a therapy-resistant malabsorption syndrome and uncontrollable weight loss; most of these patients have both. The decision for the procedure should be made within an interdisciplinary team; all conservative opportunities by endocrinologists, nutritionists, gastroenterologists, and psychologists must be explored first.

The aim of a surgical procedure is to lengthen the common channel by creating a new enteroenteral anastomosis about 100 cm proximal to the old one ("Kissing-X anastomosis").

Revision Procedures Because of Missing or Inadequate Weight Loss

These procedures are rare after biliopancreatic diversion surgery, but can be necessary. The common channel is shortened to about 50 cm by creating a new ileoileal anastomosis. If the gastric sleeve is dilated, a repeated sleeve gastrectomy can be discussed individually.

5.1 Surgical Technique by Laurent Biertho (Canada) and Rudolf Steffen (Switzerland)

Laurent Biertho and Rudolf Steffen

Introduction

Biliopancreatic diversion was first described by Dr Scopinaro in the mid-1970s. In the early 1980s, Drs Marceau and Hess exchanged the conventional 2/3 gastrectomy for a sleeve gastrectomy, retaining the pylorus yet excluding the duodenum (duodenal switch). The procedure has been adapted for laparoscopy by Dr Gagner in the early 1990s and is considered by many as one of the most technically demanding of all laparoscopic operations.

Biliopancreatic diversion with duodenal switch (BPD-DS) is one of the procedures endorsed by the American Society for Metabolic and Bariatric Surgery for the surgical treatment of obesity. Surgical indications follow the current National Institute of Health guidelines.

During the learning curve of the laparoscopic approach, patients' selection is key to minimize operative risks and decrease operative time. Female patients with a BMI under 50 kg/m^2 and minimal previous abdominal surgery are ideal candidates. Surgeons should also be familiar with the open BPD-DS before trying a laparoscopic approach. Working with someone experienced in laparoscopy will also decrease operative time and frustration.

Preparation

Setting, Positioning, and the Surgical Team

- Good laparoscopic instruments are essential for all advanced laparoscopic procedures. A bariatric surgery set should further include extra-long instruments (bowel grasper, clip applier), 15-mm trocars, and bariatric endoscopic staplers. In this technique, we also use an endoscopic 21-mm circular stapler to create the duodenoileal anastomosis. A 30° camera and a high flow insufflator are also required. Most of the dissection is performed using a Harmonic Ace scalpel (Ethicon Endo-Surgery, Johnson and Johnson). A "snake" 5-mm liver retractor with table-mounted holding device is usually sufficient to provide a good exposure.
- Thrombo- and antibio-prophylaxis are given 2 h prior surgery (Heparin 5,000–10,000 Units s/c and Cefazolin 1–2 g for patients below and above 150 kg, respectively).
- The patient is placed in a split-leg position with both arms opened.
- A monitor is placed on each side of the patient.
- Intermittent pneumatic leg compression devices are routinely placed.
- The surgeon stands between the legs of the patient, the cameraman on the right and the second assistant with the scrub nurse and tables on the left of the patient at the beginning of the procedure. The surgeon moves to the left of the patient for the ileoileal anastomosis.
- A long Veress needle (15 cm) is introduced in the left upper quadrant to create a 15 mmHg pneumoperitoneum.

- A 12-mm optical trocar (Xcell trocar, Ethicon Endo-Surgery, Johnson and Johnson) is used to enter the abdominal cavity, 15 cm below the xiphoid and slightly off-midline to the left, to avoid the hepatic ligament.
- Two 12-mm trocars are then placed in the left flank and left subcostal area (both on the left mid-clavicular line).
- A 15-mm trocar is placed in the right flank (right mid-clavicular line) at the level of the optic port. The 15-mm incision is used for the introduction of the circular stapler and the extraction of the gastric specimen and the gallbladder.
- Finally, three 5-mm ports are placed in the left flank, epigastria (liver retractor), and right subcostal area.

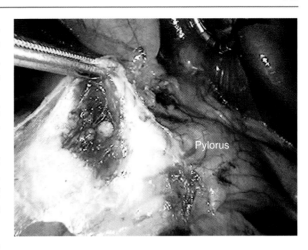

Fig. 5.4 Duodenal dissection

Surgical Technique

Gastric Mobilization

- The patient is placed in a steep reverse Trendelenburg position. The surgeon stands between the legs of the patient.
- The second assistant retracts the omentum laterally with two bowel graspers while the surgeon retracts the stomach medially.
- Dissection begins along the gastric body (where the lesser omental cavity is easily entered) by dividing with the Ultracision the branches of the gastroepiploic artery, near the gastric wall.
- Dissection progresses toward the angle of His and the short gastric vessels. The first short gastric vessels are usually controlled with large clips.
- Posterior adhesions to the pancreas are frequent and have to be released to have a good mobilization of the stomach.
- A good exposure of the upper part of the fundus is critical. The patient is placed in a maximum reverse Trendelenburg position, with the 30° camera looking slightly to the left.
- The second assistant retracts the posterior fundus toward the right iliac fossa (left subcostal port) and the omentum laterally (left flank port).
- The surgeon retracts the fundus medially (right flank port) and divides the gastro-splenic ligament with a combination of clips and Ultracision. Dissection is carried up to the left diaphragmatic crus.

- The remainder of the greater curvature is then released distally to about 10 cm proximal to the pylorus, down to where adhesions between the pre-pyloric region and the retroperitoneum begin.

Duodenal Dissection

- The liver retractor is now placed to expose the duodenum and pylorus. The pylorus is identified using palpation and the pyloric vessels as a landmark (Mayo's vein).
- The second assistant (on the left side) now holds the camera with his left hand and retracts the pre-pyloric region to the left with his right hand (left subcostal port). The assistant to the right of the patient retracts the gastro-colic ligament caudally (right subcostal port).
- The peritoneum above and below the first duodenum is first opened. The choledochus is usually easily identified and represents a good landmark for dissection.
- First the duodenum is lifted up by the surgeon's left hand and a retro-duodenal window is created with the ultracision (Fig. 5.4). That window starts about 3–5 cm distal to the pylorus (between the second and third vessels to the inferior part of the duodenum) and ends up just lateral and above the choledochus. That window should be done in an avascular plane, with blunt dissection.
- A 15-cm Penrose drain is then passed into that window to retract the duodenum (surgeon's left hand). That window is slightly enlarged to accommodate the jaw of a linear stapler.

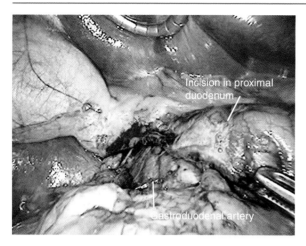

Fig. 5.5 Mobilization of the duodenal stump

- A 3.5-mm linear stapler (Echelon, Ethicon Endo-Surgery, Johnson and Johnson, 60-mm length) is then introduced into the retro-duodenal window (through the left flank port) and the duodenum is stapled-cut.
- The posterior attachments of the proximal duodenal stump are released on a few centimeters to obtain a good mobilization of the duodenum (Fig. 5.5).
- A gastrotomy is then created on the greater curvature of the stomach, to accommodate a 21-mm anvil. The anvil of a 21-mm circular stapler is connected to an 18 Fr Foley catheter, cut to 15 cm. The anvil is then introduced into the abdomen through the 15-mm incision in the right flank.
- A small opening is then created on the inferior aspect of the duodenal stump, just above the staple line, using the hot blade of the Ultracision (through the right subcostal port).
- A Maryland grasper is introduced into the duodenum and through the gastrotomy in a retrograde fashion (through the right subcostal port). That grasper is used to pull the Foley catheter connected to the 21-mm circular anvil into the duodenum.

> Buscopan or glucagon is routinely used to relax the pylorus and allow the passage of the anvil.

- The duodenal stump is inspected to ensure that the opening is tight around the shaft of the anvil.

Sleeve Gastrectomy

- A sleeve gastrectomy is then performed using a 4.8-mm Echelon stapler (60-mm length). The first stapling is done at the level of the crow's foot, about 7 cm proximal to the pylorus; through the right flank port to avoid any stenosis at the level of the incisura.
- The subsequent staplings are usually done through the left flank trocar with the same staple length (the gastrotomy on the greater curvature is resected at the same time).
- Gastrectomy is done along the lesser curvature of the stomach, to create an estimated 60-Fr gastric remnant. An esophageal bougie is used only when there is no duodenal switch added to the sleeve gastrectomy. It is however important to remove the whole fundus to avoid long-term dilatation at that level.
- The staple line is checked for hemostasis and clips are applied if required.

> We do not routinely oversew the staple line or use buttressing material.

- The specimen is then introduced into a large plastic bag and extracted through the 15-mm incision in the right flank.

Alimentary Limb

- The patient is positioned in a head-down position with a slight tilt to the patient's left.
- The surgeon and first assistant now stand on the patient's left side, and the second assistant is between the patient's legs.
- The camera is introduced through the left subcostal port and the surgeon uses the 5 and 12-mm ports in the patient's left flank.
- The cecum and the ileocecal junction are identified first. The ileum is then measured with small bowel graspers (the length of the metallic part of the bowel graspers being 5 cm).
- The ileum at 100 cm from the ileocecal valve is marked using a clip on each side of the mesentery.
- The small bowel is then run another 150 cm, to create a 250-cm alimentary limb.
- A mesenteric window is then created at that level and the small bowel is stapled using a 2.5-mm Echelon stapler. The distal end of the ileum (going

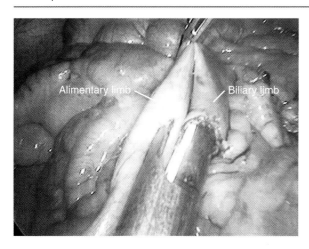

Fig. 5.6 Ileoileal anastomosis

to the duodenum) is directly identified with a clip on the staple line.

- The mesentery is then opened on a few centimeters to avoid any tension on the duodenal anastomosis.

Ileoileal Anastomosis

- A side-to-side anti-peristaltic anastomosis will be created at 100 cm from the ileocecal valve. The alimentary limb runs from its proximal end to the cecum.
- The clips previously placed at 100 cm are identified.
- The alimentary limb is positioned on the patient's right side with the biliary limb placed medially.
- The patient is positioned to obtain a good exposure (head and right side downward slightly). The biliary limb is held close to the ileum at 100 cm above the ileocecal valve.
- The two limbs are stitched together using 3/0 vicryl. That stitch is used to hold the bowel into place (supra-umbilical port).
- Two small enterotomies are done on each limb, to allow the introduction of 2.5-mm Echelon stapler (60-mm length).
- The anastomosis is then created (Fig. 5.6).
- The remaining enterotomy is closed using a running suture of 3/0 vicryl.
- Finally, the mesenteric window is closed using a running suture of 3/0 silk.

Duodenoileal Anastomosis

- The patient is now placed in a slight reverse Trendelenburg position.
- The surgeon stands between the legs of the patient with one assistant on each side.

- The distal end of the alimentary limb (previously identified with a clip on the staple line) is opened along the staple line. The Foley catheter is disconnected from the circular anvil in the duodenal stump.
- A 21-mm endoscopic circular stapler is then introduced through the 15-mm incision in the right flank.
- The camera is moved to the left flank port and the surgeon now uses the supra-umbilical port for his right hand.
- The circular stapler is then introduced into the alimentary limb, and advanced about 5 cm into the small bowel lumen, where the spike of the stapler is pushed through the anti-mesenteric bowel wall.
- It is then connected to the anvil. The stapler is closed progressively, to ensure that there is no fat coming into the stapler and to avoid any rotation of the duodenum or ileum.
- The duodenoileal anastomosis is created and the stapler is extracted from the small bowel.

There should be no tension on the duodenal anastomosis. If this is not the case, the small bowel mesentery can be opened further, the attachments on the upper part of the duodenal stump can be released, and sutures can be placed to reinforce the duodenoileal anastomosis.

- The camera is then moved back to the supra-umbilical port. The mesentery of the small bowel is released a few centimeters along the ileal stump to allow its closure.
- A 2.5-mm stapler is introduced through the right flank port and the ileum is transected 2–3 cm away from the duodenoileal anastomosis (Fig. 5.7).
- The anterior and posterior walls of the anastomosis are checked for leaks.

The anastomosis is not routinely tested with methylene blue. If there is any concern about the integrity of the duodenal anastomosis or gastric stapling, an intraoperative gastroscopy is performed. This allows to rule out any bleeding or bubbling on the staple-lines and to inspect the anastomosis for a leak or a stenosis.

- The mesenteric defect is then closed using 3.0 silk and a routine cholecystectomy is performed.

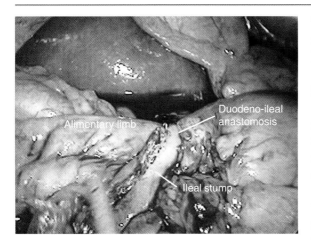

Fig. 5.7 Duodenoileal anastomosis

A closed suction drain is placed in Morisson's space in selected cases.

- The 12 and 15-mm ports are closed using 0 vicryl with a fascia closure device.

Conclusion

With an operative time around 3 h, a partial gastrectomy, two small bowel anastomoses, and a surgery involving three different quadrants of the abdomen, laparoscopic biliopancreatic diversion with duodenal switch remains a technically challenging procedure. The benefits for the patient include a shorter hospital stay, quicker postoperative recovery, and a decrease in abdominal wall complications. A good selection of the patients is however crucial to avoid any increase in operative complications during the learning curve of the procedure.

5.2 Surgical Technique by Michael Gagner (USA)

Michael Gagner and Nelson Trelles

Introduction

In 1988, Hess and Hess (USA) [1] first added the sleeve gastrectomy (SG), and simultaneously the duodenal switch (DS), as a modification to the biliopancreatic diversion (BPD) to improve clinical outcomes.

This procedure was called BPD with DS and combines malabsorption with restriction to optimize and ensure long-term weight loss.

The laparoscopic approach of the BPD with DS, first performed by Gagner in 1999 [2, 3], has demonstrated to be safe and effective for the treatment of morbid obesity [4, 5] with comparable morbidity and mortality to the open approach [6]. However, the initial reports on BPD with DS showed an increased rate of complications and deaths among males and super-super-obese patients (BMI > 60 kg/m^2) [4, 6]. Thus, in 2000, Gagner and co-workers [7] suggested that separating the restrictive and malabsorptive components of the BPD with DS into two operative stages would reduce morbidity and mortality. Both short-term and long-term weight loss exceed that of the any other procedure including that of the gastric bypass [8, 9].

We prefer to start with the SG rather than the distal ileoileostomy because occasionally patients cannot tolerate pneumoperitonium and may require a shortened procedure. Other factors for considering the two-stage approach include extensive intraabdominal adhesions or reduced working space despite higher pneumoperitoneum pressures. The SG alone (first stage) will effectively achieve significant weight loss without major complications, thus the patient can return some months later for the second stage or completion of the BPD with DS.

Two different techniques have been described to perform the SG. The first starts with the stapling of the stomach as soon as the surgeon accesses to the lesser sac, then the greater curvature devascularization is performed after completion of the gastric transection. We advocate the second technique in which the stapling is performed after complete devascularization of the greater curvature [10] because we find it easier and more logical to perform gastric division after devascularization to prevent bleeding from the staple line. By doing so we can also avoid injuries to the pancreas and the splenic artery because once the greater curvature dissection is complete, the lesser sac is best exposed and all posterior attachments to the pancreas can easily be divided. Otherwise these attachments may tear during stapling and cause bleeding (Fig. 5.8).

Surgical Technique

- A total of seven trocars are used, extra-long trocars may be required (Fig. 5.9).

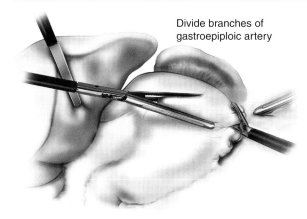

Divide branches of
gastroepiploic artery

Fig. 5.8 Dissection of the greater curvature

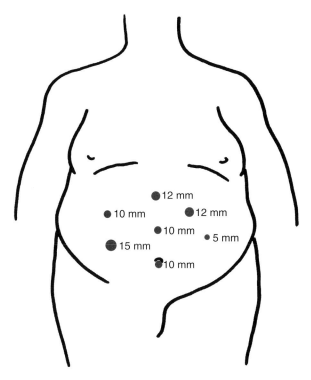

12 mm
10 mm   12 mm
10 mm
5 mm
15 mm
10 mm

Fig. 5.9 Trocar placement

We perform an open technique at the top of the umbilicus to enter the peritoneal cavity. This trocar arrangement facilitates exposure and dissection of the stomach and the small bowel, allowing the surgeon to perform smooth maneuvers of the instruments while he operates in-between the legs and from the left side of the patient, avoiding continuous position changes.

SG and Duodenal Transection

- The most critical step is the dissection of the angle of His, which must be completely freed from the left crus to facilitate subsequent stapling.
- The anterior perigastric fat just to the left of the gastroesophageal junction must be cleared to minimize tissue thickness during stapling.
- However, avoid dissecting to the right of the gastroesophageal junction because of the risk of injury to the vagus nerve. Careful attention must also be taken due to the risk of esophageal injury that could lead to leaks.
- If a significant hiatal hernia is found, it should be reduced and repaired to prevent or improved postoperative reflux symptoms and because failure to recognize or repair a herniated fundus may lead to inadequate weight loss.
- Once the greater curvature dissection is complete, the first 2–5 cm of duodenum are dissected free circumferentially with the ultrasonic scalpel. We prefer the reusable 5 mm Sonosurg device (Olympus; Orangeburg, NY, USA). The supraduodenal window created should be small and medial to the common bile duct and lateral to the hepatic artery.
- The gastroduodenal artery, which lies posteriorly between the first and second portion of the duodenum, marks the distal aspect of the dissection. It is usually not necessary to perform a Kocher maneuver. Meticulous attention to the pancreas and the gastroepiploic and pyloric vessels is needed to avoid injuries or bleeding.
- The duodenum is transected at this point with a 60-mm/3.5-mm Endo-GIA linear stapler (Tyco Healthcare, Norwalk, Conn, USA) buttressed with bioabsorbable material (Seamguard W.L. Gore & Associates, Inc, Flagstaff, AZ, USA), leaving a 2–5 cm duodenal cuff.

Another issue of concern during SG is the antrum preservation. As Weiner in Germany, but in contrast to Baltasar in Spain, we advocate preservation of the antrum to ensure adequate postoperative gastric emptying. Thus, at approximately 6–8 cm proximal to the pylorus the SG begins with sequential firings of 60-mm/4.8-mm linear staplers reinforced with Seamguard, with the stomach retracted flat and laterally. The bioabsorbable buttressing material increases costs, however it reduces staple-line hemorrhage, possibly leakage rate [11–15] and operative time [16].

Two important reasons to preserve the antrum:

- The reservoir volume of the antrum is very low, therefore the capacity of the stomach by resection of the antrum will not be markedly decreased.
- The accelerated pump function of the antrum after SG may contribute to achieve weight loss [17].

• After the second firing, a 60-Fr bougie is inserted transorally and carefully positioned under laparoscopic vision. Inserting the bougie after the first two stapler firings helps align the bougie along the lesser curvature into the duodenum.

> For all BPD with DS cases, we use the 60-Fr bougie to ensure enough gastric volume to permit adequate protein intake. Patients undergoing BPD with DS are more prone to protein deficiencies, so by leaving a larger reservoir we avoid nutritional deficiencies – in particular, protein malnutrition.

• The remainder of the SG is completed by sequential firings of 3.5-mm or 4.8-mm linear staplers (depending on an assessment of the thickness of the stomach wall) along the bougie toward the angle of His. The anesthesiologist must prevent the bougie from retracting cephalad during stapling to avoid pexy of the bougie. At the gastroesophageal junction, the transection line deviates slightly from the bougie to avoid stenosis, but going further may lead to fundus dilatation and weight regain.

Missing the posterior folds of the fundus during transection could also lead to inadequate primary sleeve volume (too large) and then gastric dilatation. In case of sleeve dilatation, inadequate original gastric volume reduction or poor weight loss after SG (first stage) or BPD with DS, laparoscopic re-SG (LRSG) can be performed [18, 19].

The gastric pouch size usually varies from 150–200 mL. Consensus about the volume of the pouch, which is related to the bougie size, is still pending. However, surgeons advocate the construction of larger gastric pouches for BPD with DS than for independent SG.

During SG and duodenal transection, surgeons might encounter diverse intraoperative complications including:

• Leaks and bleeding from the staple line that can be treated by over-sewing if not prevented by Seamguard.

• Bleeding from the short gastric vessels that can be halted with the ultrasonic scalpel or in some cases with clipping.
• Splenic injuries during fundic dissection and bleeding due to a liver injury caused by the liver retractor, thus careful dissection and manipulation of organs are necessary.

Postoperative complications related to surgical technique include leaks and strictures. Temporary stenting is an effective and new strategy for the treatment of a gastric fistula, and may be performed safely in a patient with a leak of the staple line following SG or LRSG with or without BPD with DS [20, 21] Sleeve strictures mostly occur at the incisura and are likely related to suture reinforcement more than to bougie size [22]. For this reason, we avoid over-sewing of the whole staple line because this could contribute to stricture development. Instead, figure-of-eight/and 3-0 Maxon sutures (monofilament absorbable to preventing stricture) are placed at the apex of the SG (the area most prone to developing leak), at the intersections of the staple lines (also prone to suboptimal healing) and at the most distal end of the staple line (thickest part of the stomach). Moreover, the first two stapler firings are performed aiming approximately 2-cm away from the lesser curvature so we can prevent stenosis at this level.

Small Bowel Measurement

• The ileum is measured from the ileocecal valve using a 50-cm umbilical tape. Flat 5 mm forceps (Dorsey, Karl Storz; Tutlingen, Germany) are used to avoid serosal tears during measurements.
• Once the ileum is run, a 100-cm common channel is measured on the antimesenteric border.
• Several clips are placed in the mesentery to temporarily mark this spot.

> We prefer clips instead of a silk stitch because their use and retrieval are easier, thus we can spare time.

• An additional 150 cm are measured proximally from this mark to become the alimentary limb.
• At this point (250 cm from the ileocecal valve), the small bowel is transected using a 45- or 60-mm/2.5-mm linear stapler buttressed with Seamguard.
• The ultrasonic scalpel is used to transect 1–2 cm of mesentery between the two ends of the ileum.

Duodenoileal Anastomosis

The anvil of a 21-mm circular end-to-end stapler (CEEA 21, Tyco Healthcare, Norwalk, Conn, USA) is delivered transabdominally into the proximal duodenal stump where 1–2 cm of the duodenal staple line were removed using the ultrasonic scalpel.

> We prefer to use a circular stapler not only because it is time saving but also because it allows the surgeon to perform a more physiologic anastomosis.

- Once the base of the anvil is in place, it is secured with a 3-0 Prolene purse-string suture.
- The staples on the distal ileum are now removed.
- The 15-mm right port site is enlarged by 1–2 cm to permit the introduction of the CEEA 21 into the abdominal cavity, which is secured to a plastic camera drape for wound protection during removal of the contaminated device after completion of the anastomosis.
- The CEEA 21 is next inserted into the open distal ileum for approximately 6 cm where the spike perforates on the antimesenteric side under direct vision.
- The distal ileum is rotated cephalad in a clockwise manner to bring the alimentary limb up toward the anvil and then the stapler is attached to the anvil to create an antecolic end-to-side duodenoileal anastomosis with minimal or no tension (Fig. 5.10).

> It may be required to divide the omentum along its right lateral third to facilitate subsequent passage of the ileum toward the duodenum.

- It is also important that there is no tissue between the ileum and duodenum and that there is no pinching of the bowel wall (which can create an obstruction later).
- Then, the CEEA 21 is fired and removed from the abdominal cavity. The CEEA 21 is not a flipped-top and therefore – two to three rotations of the stapler are required in conjunction with counter-traction on the antrum in order to pull the CEEA through the anastomosis.
- The open ileum limb is inspected for bleeding at the anastomotic site. If bleeding is present, we can proceed to over-sewing (extraluminal), use of heat coagulation (intraluminal) or packing of the anastomosis with hemostatic agents (intraluminal).

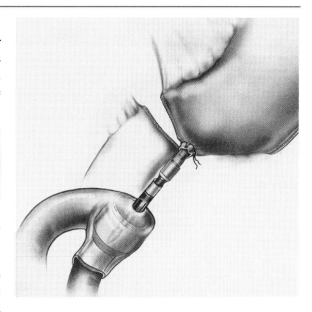

Fig. 5.10 Duodenoileal anastomosis with a circular stapler

- In the absence of bleeding, the opening in the ileum is closed with a 2.5-mm linear stapler buttressed with Seamguard, and a 3-0 Maxon running suture is carried across the musculoserosa of the anterior duodenoileostomy staple line to reinforce the anastomosis and relieve tension.

> We prefer absorbable sutures for this because non-absorbable sutures (e.g., silk sutures) have been associated with marginal ulcers and strictures.

- Then, methylene blue-tinted sterile saline is instilled under pressure, through an orogastric tube, with the distal ileum clamped to test the anastomosis and the SG for leaks. Over-sewing is used if leaks are identified.

> Note that the CEEA 25 stapler is too large for the distal ileum and frequently tears it during insertion. The delivery of the anvil 21 through the proximal duodenal stump can also be done transorally using the modified nasogastric tube-anvil apparatus (commonly used for gastric bypass) but it can be cumbersome because the anvil 21 does not flex and traverses the pylorus only with some difficulty. The passage of the anvil through a small hypopharynx can also be problematic.

Ileoileal Anastomosis

- We locate the marking clips at 100 cm from the ileocecal valve.

  We prefer the "M" triple-staple technique, a completely stapled anastomosis that provides a large patent anastomosis while avoiding the risk of narrowing the bowel lumen during closure of the enterotomy (Fig. 5.11).

- The clips on the ileal mesentery are removed.

- An enterotomy is made with the ultrasonic scalpel on the anti-mesenteric side of the marked ileum.
- Another enterotomy is made approximately 1–2 cm from the stapled end of the proximal ileum or biliopancreatic limb.

  Again, one must take care that there has been no twisting of the mesentery and that both staples are fired on the antimesenteric border to avoid ischemia.

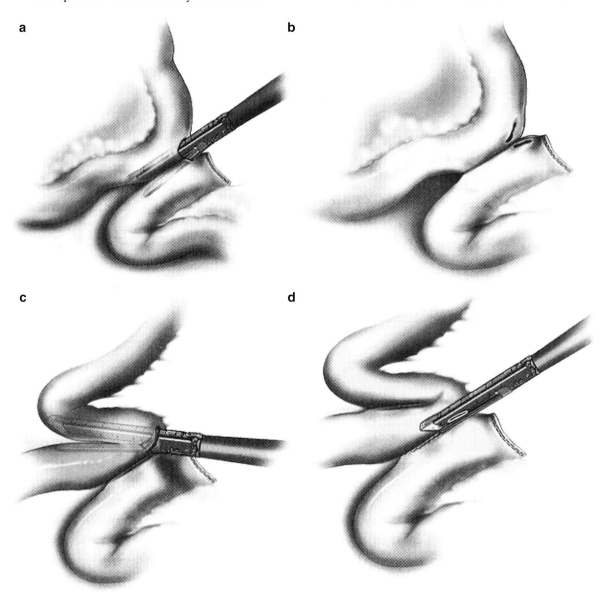

Fig. 5.11 Ileoileostomy with the "M" triple-staple technique

e

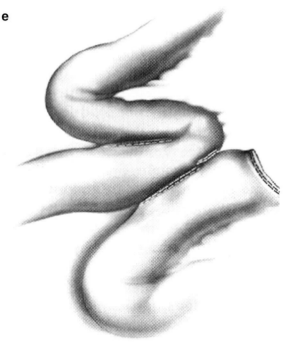

Fig. 5.11 (continued)

- The 60-mm/2.5-mm linear stapler is introduced, aiming toward the pelvis. It is best to insert the larger jaw of the stapler into the proximal ileum (larger diameter) and the smaller jaw into the distal ileum (narrower).
- A standard side-to-side anastomosis is created between the biliopancreatic limb and the last 100 cm of distal ileum to create the common channel.
- Through the same enterotomy, the 60-mm/2.5-mm linear stapler is fired between the alimentary limb and the common channel.
- A third firing of the linear stapler closes the enterotomy transversely.
- The specimen is removed without contaminating the wound.

> An alternate option for enterotomy closure is to carefully close the enterotomy with a running 2-0 silk suture, either in one or two layers.

Mesenteric Defects Repair
- The mesenteric defect at the ileoileostomy is repaired from right to left, in a transverse fashion using a running suture with 2-0 silk (24 cm length).

- Petersen's defect is also repaired using a running nonabsorbable suture.

> We prefer to close this from the patient's left side because there is a wider space on the left and because closure from the left side permits visualization of the ligament of Treitz and helps the surgeon avoid catching proximal jejunum in the closure.

- The omentum must be positioned superior to the transverse colon and must not be included in the closure. The repair must bring together the whole length of the transverse mesentery with mesentery of the ileum.

> We include in the suture the serosa of the transverse colon with the serosa of the ileum to bring more support to the repair because mesenteric fat closure alone may eventually (with significant weight loss) enlarge and lead to an internal hernia.

Inspection and Closure
- The SG staple line and both proximal and distal anastomoses are inspected for any evidence of bleeding or leaks. The biliopancreatic limb must be coming from the patient's left and the alimentary limb and common channel must be on the patient's right side.
- All fascial defects larger than 5 mm are closed using a suture-passer (Karl Storz, Tuttlingen, Germany) with 0 vicryl sutures. The umbilical wound is usually closed under direct vision with a #1 Prolene suture.

> We do not perform routine liver biopsy, appendectomy, or drainage. Cholecystectomy is performed for well-documented symptomatic cholelithiasis. Intraoperative ultrasonography may aid in diagnosis or confirmation.

5.3   Surgical Technique by Philippe Topart (France)

Philippe Topart and Guillaume Becouarn

Introduction

Based on the original Scopinaro procedure, today's BPD-DS was first used by Hess and first published by Marceau. The new gastrectomy was designed after the "Duodenal switch" operation for duodenogastric reflux as described by De Meester in 1985. Changes from the Scopinaro procedure include:

- A vertical "sleeve" gastrectomy removing approximately 50% of the stomach but retaining most of the antrum as well as the pylorus and the first 2–3 cm of duodenum.
- A longer (100 cm) common channel whereas the bowel length from the duodenoileal anastomosis to the ileocecal valve remains 250 cm.

Preparation

- The operation setup does not differ from other bariatric procedures. Six trocars (two 5 mm, two 10 mm, one 12 mm, and one 15 mm) are needed (Fig. 5.12).
- A nasogastric tube is positioned at the beginning of the procedure.

Surgical Technique

- The operation can start by performing the sleeve gastrectomy or by the measurement of the 250 cm of terminal ileum and the ileoileal anastomosis.

> I usually prefer to start with the first stage of the sleeve gastrectomy, freeing the greater curvature from 6–7 cm proximal to the pylorus. Care must be taken to extend dissection of the vessels to the right (toward the pylorus) in order to avoid injury of the vessels and bleeding when firing the first linear stapler shot coming from the right lower quadrant (RLQ) trocar and slightly angled.

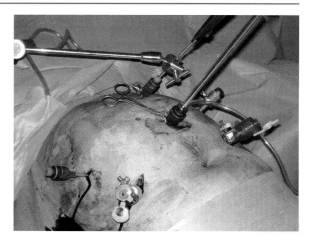

Fig. 5.12 Trocar placement

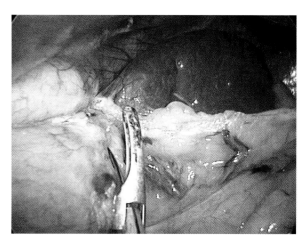

Fig. 5.13 Skeletonization of the greater curvature near the short gastric arteries with ultrasound scissors

- Up to the angle of His the stomach must be entirely mobilized including its posterior aspect with the left crus of the diaphragm exposed (Fig. 5.13).
- At this point the liver retractor usually needs to be repositioned under the right hepatic lobe to allow exposure of the gallbladder and duodenum (the liver retractor holding arm should be placed on the right side of the operating table to avoid too short a course).
- The duodenum is exposed first and the peritoneum is incised approximately 4–5 cm distal from the pylorus. In fact the true marker is the common bile duct (CBD) which is usually clearly visible.

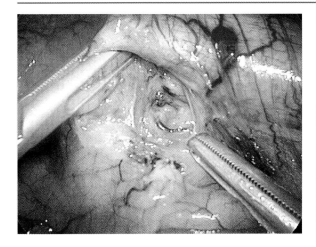

Fig. 5.14 Beginning dissection of the retroduodenal channel. The assistant's forceps holds the prepyloric stomach and maintains the duodenum stretched

- The duodenum should be divided approximately 2 cm to the right of the CBD. This avoids being too close to the duodenal papilla with the risk of injury. The peritoneum should be incised not only on the lower border of the duodenum but also and especially on the upper border. The assistant's forceps holds the prepyloric stomach and maintains the duodenum stretched (Fig. 5.14).
- Care must be taken to free the duodenum extensively on its posterior aspect as the duodenum does not lay in a sagittal plane but is inclined, with its posterior and superior aspect being deeper attached. Failure to perform extensive dissection at the upper border of the duodenum in the division area (2 cm wide is enough) will dramatically increase the risk of perforation of the posterior wall of the duodenum when the atraumatic forceps is inserted between the duodenum and the pancreatic head.
- Once the forceps has emerged at the superior border of the duodenum a tape can be passed around the duodenum allowing a gentle enlargement with the forceps.
- The 60 mm linear cutter/stapler is then inserted with anvil down preferably loaded with a vascular (white) cartridge (to minimize the risk of bleeding) or a blue one.
- At this time the nasogastric tube must be removed at least partially in case it has passed the pylorus to avoid the risk of an inadvertent section by the stapler.

- Once inserted into the space between the duodenum and the pancreas, the stapling device can be moved slightly downstream to keep as much duodenum length as possible in order to perform a safe and easy duodenoileal anastomosis later on.

Cholecystectomy can be recommended as a routine procedure in BPD-DS to avoid the increased risk of secondary cholecystitis which will develop in the area of the duodenoileal anastomosis. A cholangiogram does not appear to be mandatory if biliary structures are clearly identified. Cholecystectomy is best performed after dissection and division of the duodenum as local swelling may render this step more difficult.

- One way of doing the duodenoileal anastomosis is positioning the anvil of the 21 mm circular stapler in the proximal duodenum before performing the sleeve gastrectomy itself. The anvil is mounted on a 10–15 cm segment of a Foley catheter first.
- The anvil is then inserted in the peritoneal cavity after the LLQ trocar has been removed.
- A 2 cm gastrotomy is performed on the greater curvature; the sleeve gastrectomy includes removal of this area.
- A small opening is made 5 mm–1 cm proximal to the staple line on the proximal duodenum. Using an atraumatic forceps, the anvil of the circular stapler is brought through the gastrotomy and the pylorus in position into the proximal duodenum using a pull-through method (Fig. 5.15).

To facilitate the passage of the anvil through the duodenum, it is recommended to inject glucagon (1 mg) intravenously to allow smooth muscle (pylorus) relaxation.

- Always check for the "bump" when passing the anvil through the pylorus. To avoid any tearing and unwanted enlargement of the duodenal opening, the anvil is secured with a 3/0 purse-string suture which also allows removal of the Foley catheter "leading tube" (active blade of the Harmonic scalpel cuts rubber very easily) (Fig. 5.16).

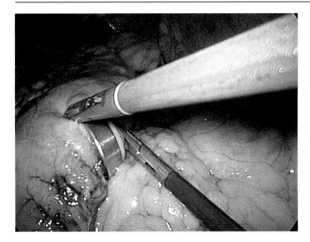

Fig. 5.15 Inserting the anvil through the gastrotomy close to the greater curvature. This section will be removed during the following sleeve gastrectomy

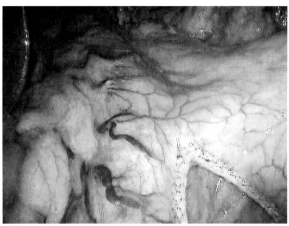

Fig. 5.17 In sleeve gastrectomy the stapler suture is placed beyond the gastric vessels entering the lesser curvature

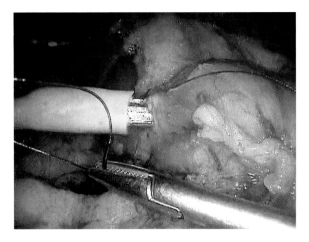

Fig. 5.16 The handle of the anvil is secured with a purse string suture

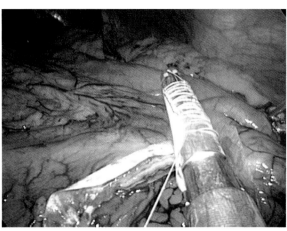

Fig. 5.18 Staple line reinforcement with bovine pericardium

Sleeve gastrectomy is now performed on a 50 Fr bougie. Care must be taken not to remove more than 50% of the stomach in order to avoid excessive restriction and prolonged postoperative hypoproteinemia.

- In this case the position of the stapler is beyond the penetration of the lesser curvature vessels into the gastric wall (Fig. 5.17).
- The 1st and 2nd stapler sutures are applied from the right lower quadrant trocar, the subsequent firings from the LLQ trocar. Absorbable staple line reinforcement (Fig. 5.18) can be used to minimize the risk of bleeding and leakage on gold and green cartridges only.

In case of revision surgery after primary sleeve, gastric banding or Mason procedure always use green cartridges to prevent staple line disruption. The use of staple line reinforcement is highly recommended. Reinforcement with a running suture is not advisable as it can promote ischemia. If staple line reinforcement is not available, hemostasis and securing the staple line junctions can be obtained with clips.

- Small bowel measurement is done with the surgeon standing on the left side of the patient. A 50-cm fabric surgical tape is used to measure the ileum from the ileocecal valve.

> It is essential to stretch the bowel to minimize the risk of excessive bowel limbs length.
>
> Stitches or clips on the mesentery can be used to mark the location of the future side to side ileoileal anastomosis 100 cm proximal to the ileocecal valve.

- The small bowel is then divided at a point located further proximally 250 cm from the ileocecal valve using a linear cutter/stapler (vascular white cartridge). This step can also be performed prior to the division of the duodenum to make sure the segment can be sutured to the duodenum without tension.

> This happens rarely, but can be expected in case of a very thick and short mesentery. Options include the division of the greater omentum (which is not performed routinely), extensive mobilization of the duodenum and pylorus or downsizing the procedure by performing a sleeve gastrectomy only.

- The duodenoileal anastomosis can be done either manually or using a circular stapler and in an antecolic fashion. The 21-mm circular stapler will allow a safe and large enough anastomosis.

> Always check if this is the correct bowel limb by confirming the location of the clips.

- The stapler is inserted through the slightly dilated RLQ trocar incision (a temporary 15 mm trocar which will be eventually necessary to remove the resected specimens can help to dilate this opening). In practice the opening must be about two fingers wide to allow an easy passage of the circular stapler. Care must be taken to avoid air leaks once the trocar is replaced. An end to side anastomosis is performed (Fig. 5.19).
- 3–4 stay 3/0 sutures reinforce the stapling and relieve tension on the anastomosis (Fig. 5.20).
- The ileal stump is closed with the linear stapler (white cartridge).

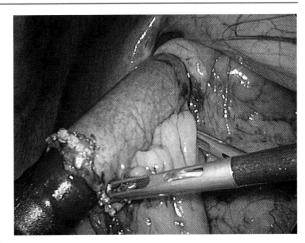

Fig. 5.19 The 21-mm circular stapler is inserted into the ileum and connected to the anvil in the duodenum

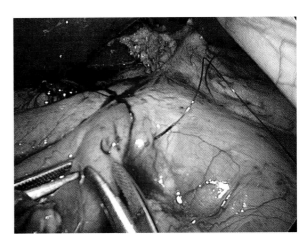

Fig. 5.20 3 to 4 stay 3/0 sutures reinforce the circular stapler suture and relieve tension on the anastomosis

- All resected specimens are placed in a plastic bag in the left upper quadrant.
- A methylene blue test is performed after the nasogastric tube is moved back down into the gastric sleeve.

> Additional sutures may be necessary in case of a leak as well as a manual anastomosis.

- Ileoileal anastomosis is performed side to side. The biliopancreatic limb is easily brought into an antiperistaltic position (staple line facing the head of the patient) and is located medially to the alimentary limb (Fig. 5.21). This setting avoids twisting.

> We do not perform any mesenteric defect closure.

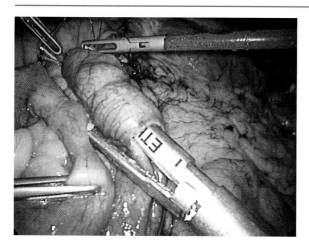

Fig. 5.21 Ileoileal anastomosis is performed side to side. The biliopancreatic limb is easily brought into an antiperistaltic position (staple line facing the head of the patient) and is located medially to the alimentary limb

- Openings are made with the harmonic scalpel on both limbs, the 60 mm linear stapler (white cartridge) is inserted and closure is performed with a running 3/0 suture.
- The nasogastric tube is removed at the end of the procedure; drainage is not routinely performed.
- Resected specimens are extracted through the RLQ trocar opening after replacing the 12-mm trocar by a 15-mm trocar. This incision is closed by a 0 suture on the aponeurosis.

Difficult Situations and Intraoperative Complications

Injury of the Duodenum
- In case of an injury of the duodenum always try to apply the stapler distally to the perforation. It is always preferable to have a safe closure of the duodenal stump.
- If closure or stapling of the proximal duodenum is not feasible, the perforation can be opened in order to place the anvil of the circular stapler for the duodenoileal anastomosis inside. It is secured by with a purse-string suture. Performing a manual duodenoileal anastomosis is also an option.
- If the proximal duodenum cannot be salvaged or is inadequate for a duodenoileal anastomosis, a distal gastrectomy with resection of the pylorus and 2–3 cm of proximal duodenum may be the only option; in this case a Scopinaro procedure will be performed.

- If an adequate closure of the (distal) duodenal stump is not possible or a manual suture fails, always try to not get too far distal and too close to the duodenal papilla in order to avoid injury/stricture. In this case a biliary T tube (KEHR drain) should be placed into the perforation/opening of the duodenal stump and secured with a purse-string suture.
- In case of a duodenal injury always try to drain the common bile duct (or the cystic duct) whenever possible to minimize the consequences of a duodenal stump leakage. Biologic glue can also be applied onto the repair suture.

Revision Procedures

Revision and reversal are rare after biliopancreatic diversion with duodenal switch. The global rate of revision accounts for 2–4.7% [1–3] of the procedures in largest series of up to 1,400 and 10 years follow-up. These revisions are usually indicated by hypoproteinemia or diarrhea and seem less frequent when a common channel of 100 cm is used instead of the "classic" 50 cm common channel of the original biliopancreatic diversion [2]. Most revision procedures can be safely performed laparoscopic, especially when the initial procedure was a laparoscopic DS or BPD.
- The patient is positioned on his back on the operating table.
- At least three trocars are needed: 1 umbilical and 1 working port on each side. Additional ports and/or different locations can be required according to the type of revision performed. In case of a redo sleeve gastrectomy a standard bariatric surgery installation is advised.
- In every situation it is recommended to clearly identify the alimentary and the biliopancreatic limbs and their anastomoses and the common channel. Visualization of the duodenoileal anastomosis is usually not required.

Both pioneers of the DS, Marceau, and Hess, recently reported less than 1% reversal rate which is indicated only in the most severe cases of hypoproteinemia or intractable diarrhea after failure of a previous revision. Although complete laparoscopic restoration of the digestive tract has been recently published 4, this challenging operation will be possible only in certain cases because it requires sufficient length of distal duodenum to re-create duodenal continuity. A much simpler and less dangerous alternative

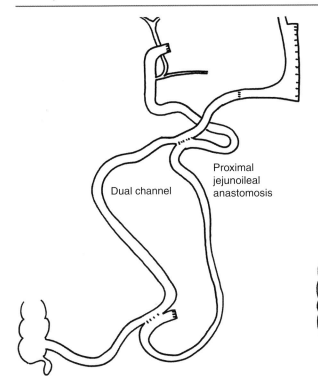

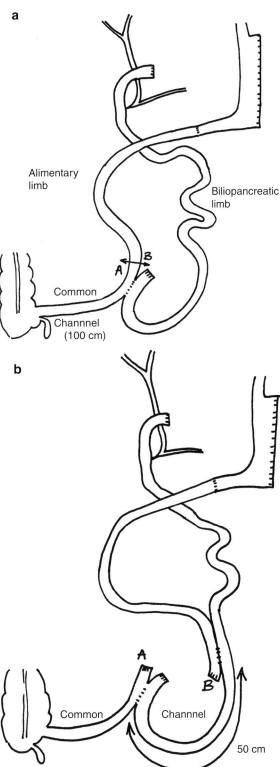

Fig. 5.22 Revision after duodenal switch. Proximal anastomosis between the alimentary and the biliopancreatic loop creating a dual channel in case of intractable malnutrition after a duodenal switch

is to perform a proximal anastomosis between the alimentary and the biliopancreatic limbs, thus creating a "dual channel" small bowel (Fig. 5.22). In this case all the consequences of the bariatric procedure (including weight loss) will disappear.

Excessive Weight Loss, Chronic and/or Severe Hypoalbuminemia, Diarrhea

These are the most frequent indications for revision after DS and require lengthening of the common channel. Lengthening is done using 50-cm increments and total added length varies according the severity of the problem and the initial common channel length. For this reason, it is necessary to measure preoperatively, using a 50 cm tape to determine the exact length of the alimentary and common channel. The alimentary limb is divided proximal to the anastomosis between the alimentary and the biliopancreatic limbs. A new anastomosis is performed 50 cm or more proximally along the biliopancreatic limb. Thus, not only the length of the common channel, but also the total length of the alimentary limb is augmented (Fig. 5.23a and b).

Fig. 5.23 (a, b) Lengthening the common channel

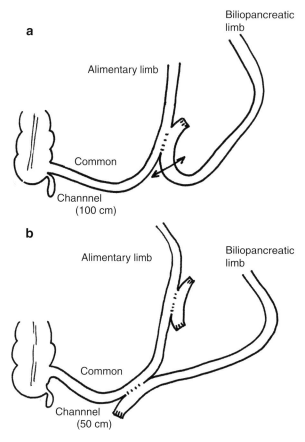

Fig. 5.24 (**a**, **b**) Shortening the common channel

Insufficient Weight Loss, Weight Regain

Shortening the common channel does not seem to lead to significant weight loss [5] but a 100 cm ("standard" DS length) can be shortened to 50 cm. Hess criteria 6 [common channel length 10% of the total small bowel length and alimentary limb (duodenoileal anastomosis to cecum) 40% of total small bowel length] can be applied in search of a more efficient procedure. However, no weight loss data support the use of these limb lengths criteria. In this case, the total length of the alimentary limb remains unchanged (250 cm) but the common channel length is reduced from the usual 100–50 cm. To perform this length reduction, the biliopancreatic limb is divided proximal to the junction with the alimentary limb and a new anastomosis is done on the alimentary limb 50 cm downstream (Fig. 5.24a and b).

Besides shortening the common channel, gastric pouch size reduction "redo sleeve gastrectomy" in case of an enlarged gastric remnant seems to lead to a significant weight loss after revision [5, 7]; sleeve gastrectomy is done in a similar fashion as during the initial procedure with stapling along a 50–60 Fr bougie [5]. Care must be taken not to add too much restriction as the malabsorptive component is the prime mechanism of weight loss in DS. This surgery is similar to the primary sleeve gastrectomy, epiploic adhesions along the already stapled stomach must be freed but this is usually bloodless. However because of the thickened stomach wall the use of Seamguard staple line reinforcement on green cartridges is highly recommended to minimize the risk of staple line disruption.

5.4 Surgical Technique by Ernesto Di Betta (Italy)

Ernesto Di Betta and Francesco Mittempergher

Introduction

Biliopancreatic diversion represents the only bariatric procedure able to reach two gold standards in obese patients: to reduce the Body Mass Index (BMI), with a percentage of Excess Weight Loss (EWL%) of about 70% after 2 years (stable over time), and to improve comorbidities such as diabetes, hypertension, dislipidemia, and obstructive sleep apnoea.

There are some alternative techniques to perform a biliopancreatic diversion. The different techniques regard the length of common ileal tract and mostly the management of the stomach. The most popular BPD was introduced in 1979 by Scopinaro N. et al. [1]; it includes a partial gastrectomy. Hess DS. et al. in 1998 [2] reported a large series of obese patients in which sleeve gastrectomy was combined with a duodenal switch.

DS-TVG is a hybrid procedure of transitory restriction and malabsorption (Fig. 5.25), first described in 1997 by Vassallo C. et al. [3] The early good weight control is due to the vertical gastroplasty, which is able to reduce the food intake and to provide an early sense of satiety when eating. After about 6–8 months the resorbable band reduces its effect and the patient can eat without any restrictive limit. Therefore all patients can have a complete meal as before the operation, but the malabsorbitive procedure allows to control the

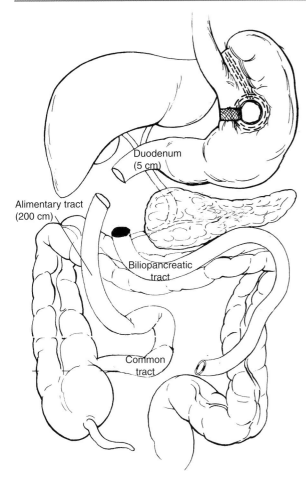

Fig. 5.25 Diagram of the duodenal switch procedure with transitory vertical gastroplasty

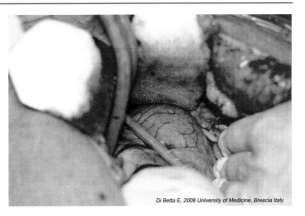

Fig. 5.26 Measuring the spot for the transgastral opening, 7 cm from the angle of His

Identification of the Lower Esophagogastric Sphincter (LES)

- The right index finger is used in the angle of His to blindly dissect a retrogastric tunnel from the greater curvature side to and through the peritoneum of the lesser curvature.
- When the tunnel is created, the Nelaton tube is passed through it.

> In case it is difficult to find the retrogastric space, a gastric tube 40 CH, introduced orally, may be useful to identify the posterior wall of the esophagus. The passage of the Nelaton tube has to be performed very carefully to avoid esophagus or gastric perforation.

caloric intake. The downside of this procedure is the risk of malnutrition due to the malabsorption of calcium, iron, protein, and vitamins, if supplementation is not correct.

DS-TVG is a safe and effective surgical option in super-super obese patients [4].

Partitioning the Stomach

- A nasogastric tube 40 CH is introduced orally and positioned through the lesser curvature, held down between the surgeon's left thumb and forefinger.
- The first step to partition the stomach is to create a circular hole in the stomach wall. The distance between the angle of His and the circular hole should be 7 cm (Fig. 5.26).

Surgical Technique: Transitory Vertical Gastroplasty

The first step of this operation is similar to a Vertical Banded Gastroplasty as described by Mason EE et al. [5] with the only difference regarding the absorbable banding in PDS instead of nonabsorbable material used in the original technique.

> A circular stapler (Ethicon Endosurgery 21 mm) is used to create a circular hole through the anterior and posterior walls of the stomach along the side of the nasogastric tube (Fig. 5.27a and b).

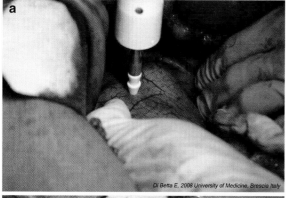

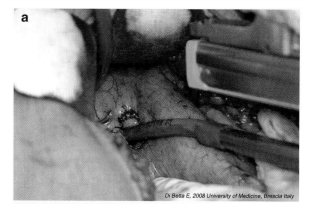

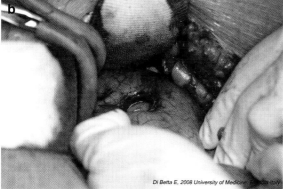

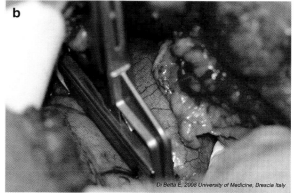

Fig. 5.27 (**a**) Creating the transgastral opening. The handle of the circular stapler is pushed through the stomach wall. (**b**) Completed circular transgastral opening

- The surgeon should gently fold the lesser curvature of the stomach around the nasogastric tube and then he should put the circular stapler far enough away from the lesser curvature so when it is closed there is no tension on that portion of the wall between the nasogastric tube and the circular stapler.
- A linear stapling device (TA 90) is then placed through the circular opening, parallel and next to the nasogastric tube pointing toward the left crus, using the Nelaton tube as guide for the stapler TA 90 (Fig. 5.28a–c).
- When the operation is completed, a collar of polydioxanone (PDS) is used to encircle the stomach wall (Fig. 5.29a and b). It is important to suture the ends of the PDS banding together to secure the circumference and to determine the outlet of the pouch.

Difficult Situations and Intraoperative Complications

The volume of the pouch does not depend on how close the window is to the lesser curvature but it is determined by the position of the linear stapler suture.

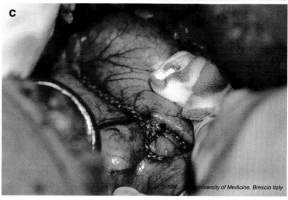

Fig. 5.28 (**a**) The TA 90 stapler is guided through the transgastral window toward the angle of His with a Nelaton tube. (**b**) Position of the TA 90 stapler before firing. (**c**) A vertical gastric pouch has been created

A shorter pouch facilitates the creation of a small volume and a cylindrical shape. A small pouch causes less disrupting force on the staple lines, because, according to Laplace's law, the distending tension on the wall is related to the radius of the lumen. When filled, a small pouch is also less likely to force the esophagogastric junction to open and to cause reflux.

Disruption of the staple line is infrequent with this technique, in particular with a small pouch and using the four-row stapler.

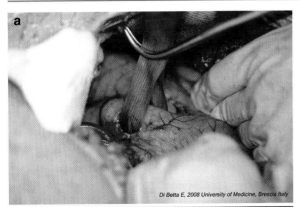

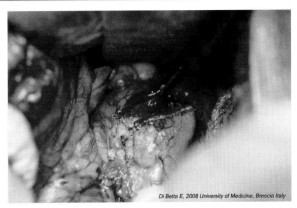

Fig. 5.30 The duodenum is cut 4–5 cm distal from the pylorus with a 60-mm linear stapler

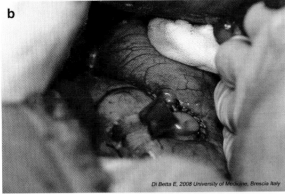

Fig. 5.29 (**a**) A slowly absorbable PDS band is used to reinforce the exit of the pouch. (**b**) View of a completed transitory vertical gastroplasty

Migration of the PDS mesh into the lumen has been never reported in literature, due to its absorbable feature.

Internal calibration using the nasogastric tube 40 CH provides a more accurate internal diameter than an external calibration with a standard pre-measured PDS mesh. The PDS collar has to be sutured leaving at least 2–3 mm of space between the mesh and the gastric wall (a forceps should stay in between).

If the pouch distends, the distal stomach wall can be pulled into the pouch if the PDS band is not adhered to the gastric serosa. The stomach wall that herniates into the pouch from below may stretch and form a diverticulum just above the ring, which may obstruct the outlet.

Surgical Technique: The Duodenal Switch

Dividing the Duodenum

The duodenal switch is performed by dividing the duodenum 3–4 cm distal to the pylorus.

- A small window is opened in the superior border of the proximal duodenum.

This is a critical step and dissection of the distal part of the duodenum has to be stopped where the anterior pancreatic tissue joins the duodenal wall. The superior arterial arcade is preserved in order to prevent severe ischemia of the duodenopyloric area.

- Another small window is opened in the inferior border of the proximal duodenum and a retroduodenal plane is developed. A 60-mm blue cartridge linear stapler (Tyco Healthcare, Norwalk) is used to transect the duodenum (Fig. 5.30).

Preparation of the Alimentary Limb, the Biliopancreatic Limb, and the Common Tract

- Using a previously measured 250-cm tape, the ileum is measured 50 cm proximally and marked with a suture on the antimesenteric border.
- An additional 200 cm are measured and the bowel is divided with a 60-mm blue cartridge linear stapler.
- The mesenteric fat of the transected ileum is partially divided between vessels.
- A running suture with silk or vicryl 3/0 is performed on both ileal stumps. The alimentary limb is followed to the marking suture, which was previously placed.
- The transected proximal ileum can be easily located by following the mesentery.
- A side-to-side or end-to-side ileoileostomy is then performed manually or with a 60-mm white cartridge linear stapler (Tyco Healthcare, Norwalk).

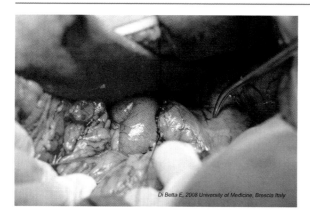

Fig. 5.31 Hand-made end-to-end duodenoileal anastomosis

- The enterotomy is then closed with a running 3/0 silk or vicryl sero-muscolar suture. The mesenteric defect next to the ileoileostomy is closed with a running 3/0 vicryl suture.

Duodenoileal Anastomosis
- The distal end of the ileal limb is brought through a hole in the mesocolic transversum next to the second portion of the duodenum, in an avascular section.
- A small incision is created on the proximal duodenum, next to the staple line, and on the lateral ileal stump.
- An end to side sero-muscolar anastomosis is then performed manually, using 2/0 single silk or vicryl stitches. The first stitch between the superior duodenal border and the ileum is performed using a 0 silk or vicryl suture (Fig. 5.31).
- The anastomosis is tested by injection of methylene blue diluted with saline through a nasogastric tube, with occlusion of bowel distal to the anastomosis.

Revision Procedures

When undertaking a revisional procedure, the bariatric surgeon has to take in consideration the increased risks and benefits of revisional bariatric surgery. In particular the surgeon should consider certain technical details to minimize the risk of further adverse outcome.

After DS-TVG causes of failure could be:
- Complications of the stomach
- Complications of the duodenoileal anastomosis
- Leakage of duodenal stump

- Internal hernia
- Excessive diarrhea and/or malabsorptive syndrome

Complications of the Stomach
Stenosis
We have never reported gastric stenosis. In a few cases we have observed patients with symptoms of vomiting, rapid satiety, and esophageal reflux. This functional obstruction may be related to the lack of propulsive contractile activity in the proximal stomach or a tilting of the external band thereby narrowing the functional luminal diameter of the stoma. This was not readily apparent endoscopically but could be documented by a radiographic contrast examination with gastrografin. In all cases we observed a resolution of symptoms after a mean of 6 months of PPI therapy.

Band Erosion
Erosion of the band can result in bleeding, ulceration, mechanical obstruction and, rarely, perforation. Endoscopic removal of eroded ring should be the treatment of choice when the band is completely migrated inside the stomach and a scar is formed in the serosa layer.

Leakage
Another possible complication could be a fistula in the stapler line. In that case a conservative treatment or a re-operation could be considered depending on the leakage volume. We have never observed this complication.

Complications of the Duodenoileal Anastomosis
Stenosis
This complication could be due to a marginal ulcer or a fibrotic stenosis. In the first case a PPI therapy and a correct diet are enough to resolve the problem. In the other case an endoscopic dilatation should be considered.

Leakage
In this case a conservative treatment or a re-operation are feasible options. In our experience we observed a case of high volume duodenoileal leakage treated successfully by draining the anastomotic fistula, excluding the antrum by a stapler line and performing a gastric-ileal anastomosis on the alimentary limb and an ileoileal anastomosis within the alimentary limb (Fig. 5.32).

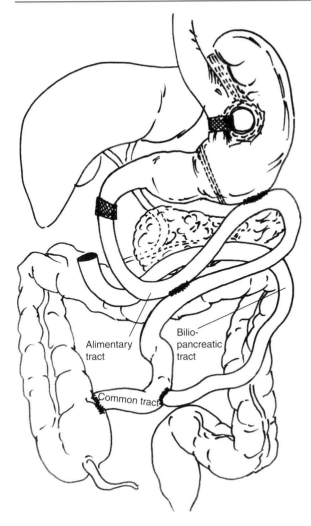

Fig. 5.32 Treatment of a breakdown of the duodenoileal anastomosis by closing the antrum with a stapler suture and creating an ileogastral anastomosis

(Labels in figure: Alimentary tract; Bilio-pancreatic tract; Common tract)

Leakage of Duodenal Stump

This is a rare complication. A conservative treatment draining the fistula or a re-suture of the duodenal stump adding fibrin glue are valid options, depending on the volume of leakage. In our experience we never reported any case of leakage of duodenal stump.

Internal Hernia

Internal hernias may occur at one of the different openings created by the passage of the alimentary limb behind the transverse mesocolon for retrocolic placement or at the mesenteric defect at the enteroenterostomy. Conservative management, with placement of a nasogastric (NG) tube, intravenous fluids, and obser-

vation could be the treatment of choice at the beginning. There is the possibility to inject water-soluble contrast Gastrografin as a therapeutic agent through the NG tube to stimulate the intestine and to help clear the bowel obstruction.

In case of a surgical approach, the proximal biliary limb and the distal common limb have to be identified by following the bowel proximately to the ligament of Treitz and distally to the cecum. The segments are inspected to rule out any dilatation in their entire length. Afterward, the remaining two defects in the transverse mesocolic space and the one associated with the enteroenterostomy should be inspected. If some space is open, it should be approximated with a permanent running suture, even if no bowel is apparent in the defect during the procedure.

Excessive Diarrhea and/or Malabsorbitive Syndrome

Occasionally patients will develop diarrhea which can be associated with severe protein/calorie/fat/vitamin malabsorption. These patients should be fed up nutritionally first, their mineral and vitamin deficiencies should be sought and normalized and their electrolyte abnormalities corrected; this usually requires a period of parenteral nutrition. Operative procedures then follow to lengthen the ileal common channel. In our experience we observed only one case (0.5%) with severe malnutrition who underwent a side-to-side enteroenterostomy 100 cm before the anastomosis between the biliopancreatic limb and the common channel. With a new common channel of 150 cm we observed a reduction of the diarrhea and resolution of the malabsorbitive syndrome.

References

5.2 Surgical Technique

1. Hess DS, Hess DW (1998) Biliopancreatic diversion with a duodenal switch. Obes Surg 8(3):267–282
2. de Csepel J, Burpee S, Jossart G et al (2001) Laparoscopic biliopancreatic diversion with a duodenal switch for morbid obesity: a feasibility study in pigs. J Laparoendosc Adv Surg Tech A 11(2):79–83
3. Gagner M, Patterson E (2000) Laparoscopic biliopancreatic diversion with duodenal switch. Dig Surg 17:547–566
4. Ren CJ, Patterson E, Gagner M (2000) Early results of laparoscopic biliopancreatic diversion with duodenal switch: a case series of 40 consecutive patients. Obes Surg 10(6):514–524

5. Baltasar A, Bou R, Miro J et al (2002) Laparoscopic biliopancreatic diversion with duodenal switch: technique and initial experience. Obes Surg 12(2):245–248
6. Kim WW, Gagner M, Kini S et al (2003) Laparoscopic vs. open biliopancreatic diversion with duodenal switch: a comparative study. J Gastrointest Surg 7(4):552–557
7. Regan JP, Inabnet WB, Gagner M, Pomp A (2003) Early experience with two-stage laparoscopic Roux-en-Y gastric bypass as an alternative in the super-super obese patient. Obes Surg 13(6):861–864
8. Prachand VN, Davee RT, Alverdy JC (2006) Duodenal switch provides superior weight loss in the super-obese (BMI > or = 50 kg/m²) compared with gastric bypass. Ann Surg 244(4):611–619
9. Strain GW, Gagner M, Inabnet WB et al (2007) Comparison of effects of gastric bypass and biliopancreatic diversion with duodenal switch on weight loss and body composition 1–2 years after surgery. Surg Obes Relat Dis 3(1):31–36
10. Trelles N, Gagner M. Sleeve gastrectomy. In: Koltun WA (Hrsg.) Operatives techniques in general surgery. Elsevier, Hershey (September 2007); 9(3):123–131
11. Consten EC, Gagner M (2004) Staple-line reinforcement techniques with different buttressing materials used for laparoscopic gastrointestinal surgery: a new strategy to diminish perioperative complications. Surg Technol Int 13:59–63
12. Yo LS, Consten EC, Quarles van Ufford HM et al (2006) Buttressing of the staple line in gastrointestinal anastomoses: overview of new technology designed to reduce perioperative complications. Dig Surg 23(5–6):283–291
13. Nguyen NT, Longoria M, Chalifoux S et al (2005) Bioabsorbable staple line reinforcement for laparoscopic gastrointestinal surgery. Surg technol Int 14:107–111
14. Consten EC, Gagner M, Pomp A et al (2004) Decreased bleeding after laparoscopic sleeve gastrectomy with or without duodenal switch for morbid obesity using a stapled buttressed absorbable polymer membrane. Obes Surg 14(10):1360–1366
15. Nguyen NT, Longoria M, Welbourne S et al (2005) Glycolide copolymer staple-line reinforcement reduces staple site bleeding during laparoscopic gastric bypass. A prospective randomized trial. Arch Surg 140:773–778
16. Weiner RA, Weiner S, Pomhoff I, Jacobi C, Makarewicz W, Weigand G (2007) Laparoscopic sleeve gastrectomy-influence of sleeve size and resected gastric volume. Obes Surg 17:1297–1305
17. Melissas J, Koukouraki S, Askoxylakis J et al (2007) Sleeve gastrectomy: a restrictive procedure? Obes Surg 17(1):57–62
18. Gagner M, Rogula T (2003) Laparoscopic reoperative sleeve gastrectomy for poor weight loss after biliopancreatic diversion with duodenal switch. Obes Surg 13(4):649–654
19. Baltasar A, Serra C, Pérez N, Bou R, Bengochea M (2006) Re-sleeve gastrectomy. Obes Surg 16(11):1535–1538
20. Serra C, Baltasar A, Andreo L et al (2007) Treatment of gastric leaks with coated self-expanding stents after sleeve gastrectomy. Obes Surg 17(7):866–872
21. Eisendrath P, Cremer M, Himpens J, Cadière GB, Le Moine O, Devière J (2007) Endotherapy including temporary stenting of fistulas of the upper gastrointestinal tract after laparoscopic bariatric surgery. Endoscopy 39(7):625–630
22. Lalor PF, Tucker ON, Szomstein S, Rosenthal RJ (2008) Complications after laparoscopic sleeve gastrectomy. Surg Obes Relat Dis 4:33–38

5.3 Surgical Technique

1. Hess DS (2005) Biliopancreatic diversion with duodenal switch. Surg Obes Relat Dis 1:329–333
2. Marceau P, Biron S, Hould FS et al (2008) Duodenal switch improved standard biliopancreatic diversion. Surg Obes Relat Dis 5(1):43–47
3. Hamoui N, Chock B, Anthone GJ, Crookes PF (2007) Revision of the duodenal switch: indications, technique, and outcomes. J Am Coll Surg 204:603–608
4. Dapri G, Cadiere GB, Himpens J (2008) Laparoscopic restoration of gastrointestinal continuity after duodenal switch. Surg Obes Relat Dis 4:451–454
5. Gagner M, Rogula T (2003) laparoscopic reoperative sleeve gastrectomy for weight loss after biliopancreatic diversion with duodenal switch. Obes Surg 13:649–654
6. Hess DS, Hess DW (1998) Biliopancreatic diversion with a duodenal switch. Obes Surg 8:267–282
7. Serra C, Baltasar A, Perez N, Bou R, Bengochea M (2007) Laparoscopic reoperative sleeve gastrectomy. Cir Esp 82: 37–40
8. Baltasar A, Bou R, Miro J, Bengochea M, Serra C, Perez N (2002) Laparoscopic biliopancreatic diversion with duodenal switch: technique and initial experience Obes Surg 12: 245–248
9. Consten EC, Gagner M, Pomp A, Inabnet WB (2004) Decreased bleeding after laparoscopic sleeve gastrectomy with or without duodenal switch for morbid obesity using a stapled buttressed absorbable polymer membrane. Obes Surg 14:1360–1366
10. Gagner M, Matteotti R (2005) laparoscopic biliopancreatic diversion with duodenal switch Surg Clin North Am 85: 141–149, x–xi
11. Hinder RA (1992) Duodenal switch: a new form of pancreatobiliary diversion. Surg Clin North Am 72:487–499
12. Marceau P, Biron S, Bourque RA, Potvin M, Hould FS, Simard S (1993) Biliopancreatic diversion with a new type of gastrectomy. Obes Surg 3:29–35
13. Rabkin RA, Rabkin JM, Metcalf B, Lazo M, Rossi M, Lehmanbecker LB (2003) Laparoscopic technique for performing duodenal switch with gastric reduction. Obes Surg 13:263–268
14. Weiner RA, Blanco-Engert R, Weiner S, Pomhoff I, Schramm M (2004) Laparoscopic biliopancreatic diversion with duodenal switch: three different dudeno-ileal anastomotic techniques and initial experience. Obes Surg 14:334–340

5.4 Surgical Technique

1. Scopinaro N, Giannetta E, Civalleri B et al (1979) Biliopamcreatic by-pass for obesity. II. Initial experience in man. Br J Surg 66:619–623
2. Hess DS, Hess DW (1998) Biliopancreatic diversion with duodenal switch. Obes Surg 8(3):267–282
3. Vassallo C, Negri L, Della Valle A et al (1997) Biliopancreatic diversion with transitory gastroplasty preserving duodenal bulb: 3 years experience. Obes Surg 7:30–33
4. Di Betta E, Mittempergher F, Nascimbeni R et al (2008) Outcome of duodenal switch with a transitory vertical gas-

troplasty, in super-super-obese patients in an 8-year series. Obes Surg 18(2):182–186

5. Mason EE (1982) Vertical banded gastroplasty for morbid obesity. Arch Surg 117:701–709

Further Reading

5   Biliopancreatic Diversion with Duodenal Switch

Cossu ML, Meloni GB, Alagna S, Tilocca PL, Pilo L, Profili S, Noya G (2007) Emergency surgical conditions after biliopancreatic diversion. Obes Surg 17:637–641

Dapri G, Cadiere GB, Himpens J (2008) Laparoscopic restauration of gastrointestinal continuity after duodenal switch. Surg Obes Relat Dis 4(3):451–454

Gracia JA, Martinez M, Elia M, Aguilella V, Royo P, Jimenez A, Bielsa MA, Arribas D (2008) Obesity surgery results depending on technique performed: long-term outcome. Obes Surg 19(4):432–438. Epub 2008 Nov 12

Gracia JA, Martinez M, Elia M, Aguilella V, Royo P (2007) Postoperative morbidity of biliopancreatic diversion depending on common limb length. Obes Surg 17(10):1306–1311

Hamoui N, Chock B, Anthone GJ, Crookes PF (2007) Revision of the duodenal switch: Indications, technique, and outcome. J Am Coll Surg 204:603–608

Korenkov M, Sauerland S (2007) Clinical update: bariatric surgery. Lancet 370(9604):1988–1990

Lee CW, Kelly JJ, Wassef WY (2007) Complications of bariatric surgery. Curr Opin Gastroenterol 23(6):636–643

Marceau P, Biron S, Hould FS, Lebel S, Marceau S, Lescelleur O, Biertho L, Simard S (2007) Duodenal switch: long-term results. Obes Surg 17(11):1421–1430

Serra C, Baltasar A, Perez N, Bou R, Bengochea M (2006) Total gastrectomy for complications of the duodenal switch, with reversal. Obes Surg 16:1082–1086

Shikora SA, Kim JJ, Tarnoff ME (2007) Nutrition and gastrointestinal complications of bariatric surgery. Nutr Clin Pract 22(1):29–40

Silecchia G, Rizzello M, Casella G, Fioriti M, Soricelli E, Basso N (2008) Two-stage laparoscopic biliopancreatic diversion with duodenal switch as treatment of high-risk super-obese patients: analysis of complications. Surg Endosc 23(5):1032–1037. Epub 2008 Sep 24

Spyropoulos C, Bakellas G, Skroubis G, Kehagias I, Mead N, Vagenas K, Kalfarentzos F (2008) A prospective evaluation of a variant of biliopankreatic diversion with Roux-en-Y reconstruction in mega-obese patients (BMI > or = 70 kg/m²). Obes Surg 18(7):803–809

The Magenstrasse and Mill Procedure

6

Michael Korenkov, Paolo Millo, Rosaldo Allieta, and Mario Nardi Jun

The Magenstrasse and Mill procedure (M&M procedure) was first performed in 1987 by David Johnston. The slightly unusual name of the procedure goes back to the anatomic and physiological peculiarities of the stomach. Back in 1908, Waldeyer named the lengthwise folds within the lesser curvature that carry liquid and food from the cardia down to the pylorus very quickly, "Magenstrasse" or gastric canal. Aschoff identified the magenstrasse as a preferred location for gastric ulcers. Studies later proved that orally ingested food and drink moves along the magenstrasse down to the pylorus first. The rest of the stomach is filled only after that (Fig. 6.1).

The function of the antrum is referred to as the antral mill; grinding and propelling solid food through the pylorus into the duodenum takes place here. In this procedure a magenstrasse is created by cutting the stomach alongside the lesser curvature from the antrum to the angle of His. The milling function of the antrum remains unaltered, which facilitates the emptying of the stomach in portions at a time. This helps prevent the dumping syndrome.

The magenstrasse and mill operation is a purely restrictive procedure, but in contrast to gastric banding and vertical gastroplasty no foreign material is implanted. Surgical technique is quite similar to gastroplasty.

According to Johnston the following steps are performed:

- Create an opening into the antrum wall at the angular notch with the circular stapler, 5–6 cm away from the pylorus.
- A sufficiently large lumen must remain between the lower edge of the opening and the greater curvature, so that secretions from the bypassed fundus and the corpus can flow freely into the antrum.

M. Korenkov (✉)
Abteilung für Allgemein- und Visceralchirurgie, Klinikum Werra-Meissner, Akademisches Lehrkrankenhaus der Universität Göttingen, Elsa-Brendström-Straße 1, 37269 Eschwege, Germany
e-mail: michael.korenkov@klinikum-wm.de

P. Millo • R. Allieta • M.N. Jun
Department of General Surgery, Regional Hospital "Umberto Parini", Center of Excellence in Bariatric Surgery, Viale Ginevra 3, 11100 Aosta, Italy
e-mail: paolomillo@yahoo.com, www.chirurgia-aosta.org

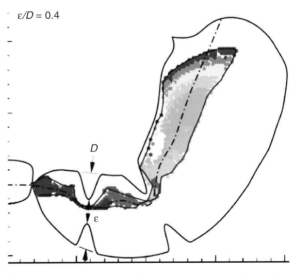

$\varepsilon/D = 0.4$

Fig. 6.1 Geometric model of the Magenstrasse (A. Pal et al.)

M. Korenkov (ed.), *Bariatric Surgery*,
DOI 10.1007/978-3-642-16245-9_6, © Springer-Verlag Berlin Heidelberg 2012

- The branches of Latarjet's nerve that lead to the antrum must be spared carefully to maintain undisturbed function of the antrum.
- Transect the stomach from the circular opening up to the angle of His, following the lesser curvature. Insert a large calibration tube as a splint while doing so. Johnston used a 40-fr tube at first, but switched to a 32-fr tube because of insufficient weight loss.

Johnston performed the M&M-procedure conventionally and recommended this for patients with a BMI between 35 and 45. Later other authors performed it endoscopically (hand-assisted or completely laparoscopic). Authors who favor this procedure argue as follows:

- Comparatively easy technique, as far as the stomach is concerned
- No need to implant foreign bodies
- In case of no or inadequate weight loss distal gastric bypass surgery can be performed later

There are also technical modifications of this procedure:

- *"Classical" M&M procedure*: A circular opening is created in the stomach about 5–6 cm from the pylorus away (original procedure by Johnston)
- *Super-magenstrasse with pyloroplasty*: To improve weight loss after the classic M&M procedure, an Italian team headed by Vassallo suggested to lengthen the magenstrasse and partially cut the antrum, too. The procedure begins just like the classic method with the creation of a circular opening in the stomach 5–6 cm from the pylorus away; the stomach is also cut alongside the lesser curvature toward the angle of His. But then the antrum is cut with a linear stapler, beginning at the circular opening and going parallel to the lesser curvature toward the pylorus. The distal end of the stapler suture is about 3–4 cm from the pylorus. To reduce the risk of gastric voiding disorder the authors performed a digitoclastic pyloroplasty – by crushing the pylorus between thumb and forefinger.

As in any other procedure with staplers involved, there is a risk of hemorrhage from the suture line or a breakdown, as the supporters of this technique report. The place value of this procedure is not yet clarified. Studies to compare the M&M procedure with other restrictive techniques, such as gastric banding or sleeve gastrectomy, have not been carried out so far. Further developments in bariatric surgery will show if it will prevail among the standard procedures or rather be abandoned in the future.

6.1 Surgical Technique by Paolo Millo (Italy)

Paolo Millo, Rosaldo Allieta, and Mario Nardi Jun

Introduction

In the first two cases, we used a very similar technique to the one described by Johnston (Fig.6.2a and b). But in order to make the procedure more simple, reproducible, and safe with the laparoscopic approach, we then modified the technique.

Preparation

Setting, Positioning, and the Surgical Team

- General anaesthesia with endo-tracheal intubation is used.
- The patient is placed in lithotomy position with a steep reverse Trendelenburg tilt.
- Abdominal insufflation, up to 14 mmHg, is achieved with a Veress needle inserted on the left subcostal margin. A 30° angled telescope is used.

Surgical Technique: Original Technique

- We use six trocars (four of 5–12 mm and two of 5–15 mm); the first is always an optic trocar (T1) placed just to the left of the middle third-upper third of the xyphoumbilical line.
- Two other trocars (T5 and T3 of 5–15 mm) are placed in the left subcostal region near the midclavicular line and on the right side near the umbilicus, respectively.
- For the hepatic retractor T2 is inserted on the left side on the anterior axillary line.
- A fifth trocar (T6) for the assistant is placed on the left side on the anterior axillary line.
- One 5–12 mm trocar is placed in the right hypochondrium (T4) for the surgeon's left hand (Fig. 6.6a).
- After a general inspection of the abdominal cavity we proceed by measuring 6 cm from the pylorus (Fig. 6.3).
- After creation of an access to the lesser sac by a window in the gastro-colic omentum vessels with the LigaSure Vessel Sealing device, a circular 21 mm stapling device is inserted by a minilaparotomy

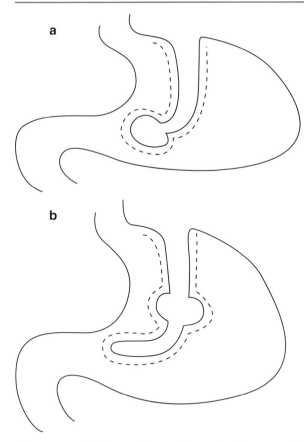

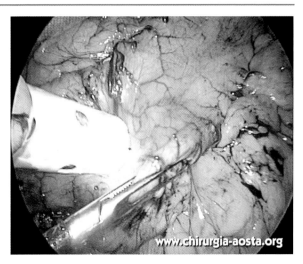

Fig. 6.4 A 21-mm circular stapler is used to create a transgastral window

Fig. 6.2 (a) Original M&M technique by Johnston. (b) Modification

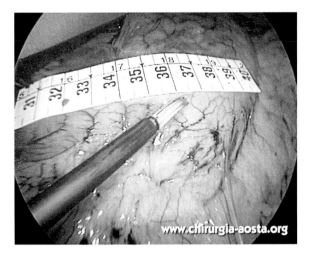

Fig. 6.3 Measuring the spot for the creation of a circular transgastral window (6 cm from the pylorus)

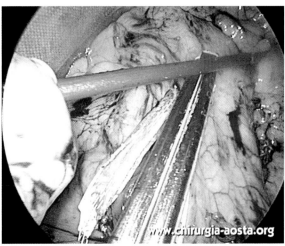

Fig. 6.5 The stomach is cut through the transgastral window toward the angle of His with a 60-mm linear stapler

- A 36-Fr bougie is inserted into the stomach close to lesser curvature down to the pylorus to calibrate the resection.
- The 60-mm linear stapler (green cartridge) is inserted through T3, the stomach is divided close to the tube, up to the angle of His with sequential firings of the linear roticulator stapler (Fig. 6.5).
- During this step the tube prevents any accidental stenosis or cardio-oesophageal junction transection and is used to realise a standard sized gastric pouch (~150 ml).

in the side of T4. It is used to create a defect in the gastric antrum, just beyond the incisura angularis, 6 cm from the pylorus (Fig. 6.4).

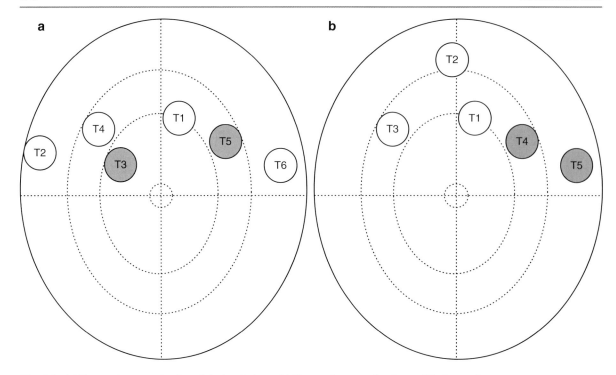

Fig. 6.6 (**a**) Trocar placement for the original technique. (**b**) Trocar placement for the modified procedure

- A running suture is placed over the staple line for haemostatis and leaks prevention. Alternatively it is possible to reinforce the staple line with Seamguard which we use routinely.
- A methylene blue test is performed to check the presence of fistula. A drain is left along the section line and a NG tube is inserted into the stomach by the anaesthesist.

Surgical Technique: Modified Technique

The creation of the gastro-gastric window is the most difficult part of the procedure for the following reasons:
- The difficulty to perform traction between the antrum and the circular stapler
- The danger of injuries of the aortic vessel in this region by the shaft during perforation of the gastric wall
- The possibility of perforation of the pancreas
- The lack of a good control of the instruments in this zone because of the size of the hepatic ligament.

For these reasons we modified this technique as follows.
- We use five trocars (three of 5–12 mm and two of 5–15 mm).The first is always an optic trocar (T1) placed just to the left of the middle third-upper third of the xyphoumbilical line. We maintained the same disposition for the other trocars, except for the hepatic retractor T2, which is inserted subxiphoidally (Fig. 6.6b) and a 15-mm trocar on the left side.
- The intended site for placement of the endoscopic circular stapler, more than 6 cm down from the gastroesophageal (GE) junction near the lesser curvature is determined.
- We open the pars flaccida of the little epiploon to have access to the lesser sac and to check for adhesions (Fig. 6.7).
- Calibration of the gastric tube is determined by positioning a 36-French tube along the lesser curvature which is blocked by a babcock forceps inserted in T4 (Fig. 6.8).
- Perforation of the stomach is performed by the 21-mm circular stapler inserted through the right flank into the lesser sac. The anvil is secured and

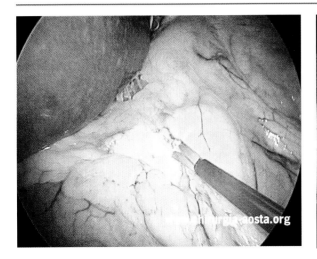

Fig. 6.7   Entering the omental bursa through the pars flaccida

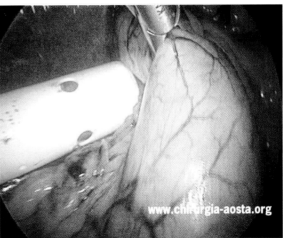

Fig. 6.9 The handle of the 21-mm circular stapler is inserted through the marked spot

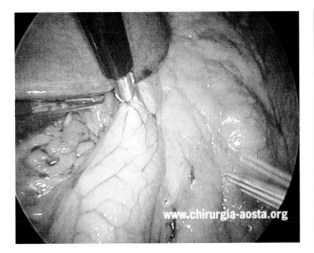

Fig. 6.8 Preparing the creation of a transgastral window. The stomach with the calibration tube is held with a babcock forceps close to the lesser curvature

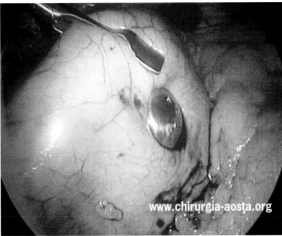

Fig. 6.10 The 21-mm circular stapler is connected to the anvil and screwed together

the device is closed and fired, producing a transgastric circular defect like in the VBG technique (Figs. 6.9–6.11).

- After dissection of the posterior surface of the stomach until the angle of His, the endoscopic 60-mm linear cutting stapler (green cartridge) with Seamguard is advanced into the peritoneal cavity though T3. It is placed in the circular stapled ring to divide the stomach toward the angle of His (Figs. 6.12 and 6.13).
- We complete the procedure with the insertion of the endoscopic linear stapler through T6 and by using the stapler again but directed to the antrum to reach 7 cm from the pylorus.

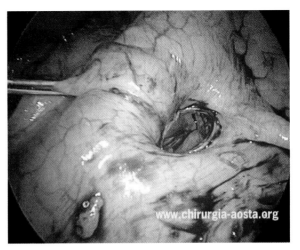

Fig. 6.11 Completed circular transgastral window

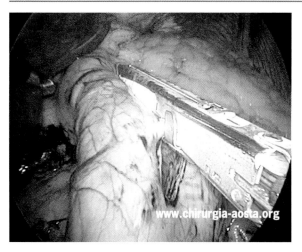

Fig. 6.12 The stomach is cut through the transgastral window toward the angle of His with linear stapler

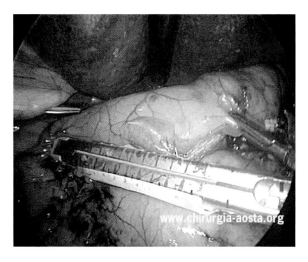

Fig. 6.13 After cutting the stomach in cranial direction, the antrum is cut through the transgastral window toward the pylorus with a linear stapler

Further Reading

Carmichael AR, Tate G, King RFG, Sue-Ling HM, Johnston D (2002) Effects of the Magenstrasse and Mill operation for obesity on plasma plasminogen activator inhibitor type 1, tissue plasminogen activator, fibrinogen and insulin. Pathophysiol Haemost Thromb 32:40–43

Johnston D, Dachtler J, Sue-Ling HM, King RF, Martin G (2003) The Magenstraße and Mill operation for morbid obesity. Obes Surg 13(1):10–6

Lossen H (1927) Über Magenstraße und Magenisthmus. Klinische Wochenschrift 26:1217–1218

Pal A, Brasseur JG, Abrahamsson B (2007) A stomach road or "Magenstrasse" for gastric emptying. J Biomech 40:1202–1210

Robinson J, Sue-Ling H, Johnston D (2006) The Magenstraße and Mill procedure can be combined with a Roux-en-Y gastric bypass to produce greater and sustained weight loss. Obes Surg 16(7):891–896

Vassallo C, Berbiglia G, Pessina A, Carena M, Firullo A, Griziotti A, Ramajoli F, Palamarciuc E, Fariseo M (2007) The Super-Magenstrasse and Mill operation with pyloroplasty: preliminary results. Obes Surg 17(8):1080–1083

Waldeyer W (1908) Die Magenstraße. Sitzungsberichte der König. Akademie der Wiss., Preuss, June 1908

Gastric Pacing

7

Michael Korenkov, Arthur Bohdjalian,
Gerhard Prager, and Stefanie Wolf

Introduction

The aim of the procedure is to reach a feeling of satiety quickly by stimulating the stomach wall with an electric pacer. This method is neither restrictive nor malabsorptive nor combined; it opens a new chapter in bariatric surgery: gastric pacing (Fig. 7.1).

This very interesting and promising new therapy is so far merely performed experimentally within studies.

Gastric pacing was developed in the 1990s by Cigaina and colleagues to treat gastroparesis. In animal experiments they produced peristalsis going forward and backward by stimulating the gastric wall. The test animals also changed their eating habits; they ate less. These experiments formed the prerequisite for clinical testing of the method.

M. Korenkov (✉)
Abteilung für Allgemein- und Visceralchirurgie,
Klinikum Werra-Meissner, Akademisches
Lehrkrankenhaus der Universität Göttingen,
Elsa-Brendström-Straße 1, 37269 Eschwege, Germany
e-mail: michael.korenkov@klinikum-wm.de

A. Bohdjalian • G. Prager
Department of Surgery, Medical University of Vienna,
Waehringer Guertel 18-20, A-1090 Wien, Austria
e-mail: arthur.bohdjalian@meduniwien.ac.at

S. Wolf
Klinik für Allgemein-Visceral- und Gefäßchirurgie,
Otto-von-Guericke Universität Magdeburg, Leipziger Str. 44,
39120 Magdeburg, Germany
e-mail: stefanie.wolff@med.ovgu.de

Electrical Stimulation of the Stomach Wall

The human stomach wall has its own intrinsic myoelectric activity, the so-called slow waves. They arise continuously three times per minute from the pacemaker area between fundus and corpus close to

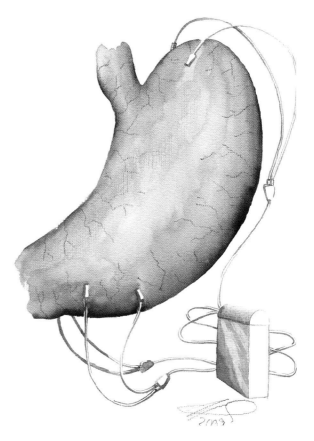

Fig. 7.1 Gastric pacing

M. Korenkov (ed.), *Bariatric Surgery*,
DOI 10.1007/978-3-642-16245-9_7, © Springer-Verlag Berlin Heidelberg 2012

the greater curvature. From there they move toward the pylorus. The activity of the stomach muscles is not generated by these slow waves, however, but by the so-called spike potentials. These spike potentials are produced sychronously with the slow waves after depolarization of the membrane of the smooth muscle cells [2, 3].

Pathophysiology of gastric pacing is closely related to the anatomical structures of motility. These are the smooth muscles of the gastric wall, the neuronal network, made up of interstitial Cajal calls and enteric neurons (for motory, sensory, and integratory signal procession), and the afferent and efferent nerve fibres that are connected to the CNS. Electrical stimulation of these structures affects their activity and changes their function. This effect depends on the excitability of the structures and the nature of the stimulus. Stimulation can be continuous or sequenced.

A specialized software changes the following parameters from the outside: amplitude of the impulse, length and frequency of the stimulation, and duration of the pacing process.

The amplitude of the impulse characterizes the electrical intensity of the impulse; for gastric pacing an amplitude between 2 and 10 mA is used.

The length of the individual impulse is measured in μs. About 30–500 μs is a common time in gastric pacing.

Frequency is the number of stimulating impulses per second, usually between 3 and 50 Hz.

Frequency is the most important parameter in stimulation. Different effects can be achieved, depending on the frequency:

- Frequencies in the sub-Hertz-range activate the interstitial Cajal cells and/or the cells of the smooth muscles, but not the intramural cholinergic nerves.
- Fast pacing (up to 1,200 Hz) cannot induce propulsive slow waves, but probably effects the CNS directly [4].
- A frequency between 5 and 10 Hz stimulates smooth muscles by releasing acetylcholine from the nerve endings.

Bortolotti defines three methods of gastric pacing: Gastric Electrical Stimulation (GEP), fast gastric pacing, and neural electric gastric pacing [1].

Gastric electrical stimulation is induced by permanent stimulation of the stomach wall with extra-slow waves of about 30–500 μs. These waves spread in oral and aboral direction, depending on the location of the stimulation. If the area between the antrum and the corpus is stimulated, the waves spread in both directions, to the fundus and the pylorus. If however a spot between fundus and corpus (pacemaker area) is stimulated, the impulse spreads distally toward the pylorus. If the antrum is stimulated, the waves spread in the opposite direction toward the fundus. For this kind of stimulation impulses from the sub-Hertz-range are used. The artificial slow waves can only develop if the frequency of the impulses is slightly higher than the intrinsic frequency. This stimulation is called gastric electrical pacing, because the stomach is not only stimulated to move by its own slow waves, but also by the extrinsic impulses. The formation of a spike wave however cannot be guaranteed.

Fast gastric pacing uses frequencies that are 4–40 times faster than the intrinsic impulses. The body's own slow waves will continue to arise, only slightly modified.

For neural electrical stimulation, impulses have frequencies over 10 Hz. Now the stomach wall does not move propulsively, but contracts concentrically.

Systems for Gastric Pacing

The idea of gastric pacing sparked the interest of various companies; different systems were developed. There are two systems available today: The ISG-system (Implantable Gastrostimulator by Medtronic, MN, USA) and the Tantalus-system (by MetaCure). As all pacemakers do, they consist of the pacemaker unit and the electrodes for stimulation, either mono- or bipolar.

Preparation

- Positioning of the patient and the surgical team as well as the creation of the pneumoperitoneum are similar to gastric banding.
- Usually four trocars are inserted; some authors use only three, depending on the operation site.

Surgical Technique

This procedure is technically rather simple; there are hardly any risks for serious intraoperative complications. The IGS-system is easier to implant than

Tantalus, because the backside of the stomach does not have to be dissected. For a detailed description of technical details and difficult situations see the articles by S. Wolf (p. 181–184) and A. Bohdjalian (p. 177–181). Two aspects need to be considered: There are no long-term evaluation results available so far concerning the technical aspects of the procedure and there are the following difficulties concerning the construction of the pacemaker and the surgical principle to pay attention to:

- Intraoperative intragastral placement of the electrode
- Postoperative intragastral dislocation of the electrode
- Intraoperative damage to the electrode due to surgical manipulation or postoperatively through shearing forces
- Symptoms linked to the pacemaker:
  - Pain around the pacemaker
  - Difficulties with coding a pacemaker that is implanted too deep within the abdomen
  - Inflammation

7.1 Surgical Technique by Arthur Bohdjalian (Austria)

Arthur Bohdjalian and Gerhard Prager

Introduction

The Tantalus system was developed to treat type II diabetes in obese patients [1]. The mechanism of action is thought to be an interaction with afferent vagal signals to the hypothalamus, which causes a feeling of satiety. In some studies, however, a reduction of the HbA1c was shown even without weight loss [2, 3]. For this reason other mechanisms of action are suspected, which are examined in studies worldwide at the time.

This chapter gives an overview of the surgical technique needed to implant the Tantalus system.

Preparation

Setting, Positioning, and the Surgical Team
- The Tantalus system consists of implantable and non implantable parts. The implantable parts are the pulse generator (IPG), the Ultraflex electrodes (UF), and the charging coil (CC) (Fig. 7.2a–d and Table 7.1).

- Mark the positions for the IPG and the CC on the patient's skin with a pen immediately before the procedure, to prevent postoperative motion-dependent discomfort. The IPG is implanted below the left costal arch, anterior to the straight abdominal muscle. The CC is placed right on top of the costal arch about 4 cm from the IPG away (Fig. 7.3).

> Avoid the bra line in female patients.

- Administer an i.v. antibiotic prophylaxis 30 min before the procedure is begun.
- Insert five trocars, including the camera trocar (Fig. 7.4).
  1. Working trocar right hand (10–12 mm) for the electrodes and the clip applicator
  2. Working trocar left hand (5 mm)
  3. Connector trocar (5 mm)
  4. Liver retractor (5 mm)
  5. Camera trocar (10 mm)
- To prepare the UltraFlex electrodes for implantation, attach the stay sutures for later beforehand. We recommend a braided 2/0 suture (such as Ethibond). Place the suture into the dent of the eyelet. Leave about 7 cm of suture between the needle and the knot. Do not leave the other end for the intracorporal knot too long (Fig. 7.5).

Surgical Technique

Electrode Positioning
Figure 7.6 shows a diagram of the electrodes connected to the stomach.

The electrodes at the antrum (front and back wall) record electric gastric activity, but are also used for stimulating the stomach. The electrodes at the fundus record the extension of the fundus and contribute to the recognition of food intake, together with the measured electric gastric activity [4].

Mobilization of the Stomach
- Open the hepatocolic ligament with ultrasound scissors and mobilize the greater curvature, proceeding from the middle toward the pylorus. Be very careful not to injure the gastroepiloic vessels.

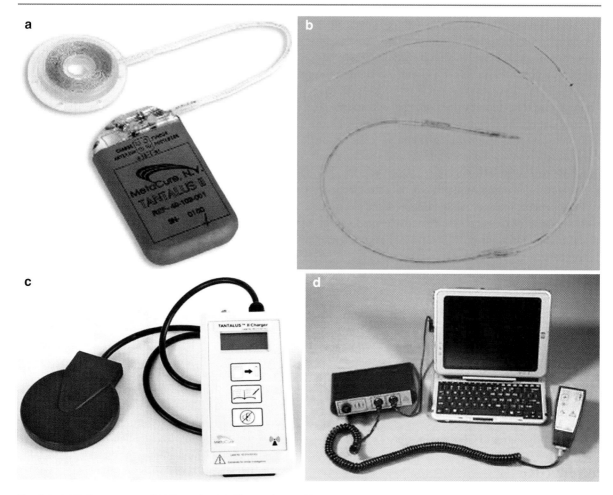

Fig. 7.2 (**a**) Pulse generator. (**b**) Electrodes. (**c**) Charger for weekly recharging of the battery. (**d**) Program unit to adjust the device individually according to the patient's needs. The IPG and the electrodes are implanted laparoscopic

Table 7.1 Recommended endoscopic instruments and equipment

Laparoscopy stack
30°/0° camera
Needle holder
Grasper
Ultracision
Electrocautery unit
Liver retractor/probe
5 mm trocars (3)
12 mm trocars (2)
Clips (i.e., EthiconLigaclip 10 M/L)
2/0 Ethibond suture
DVD/Video recording system

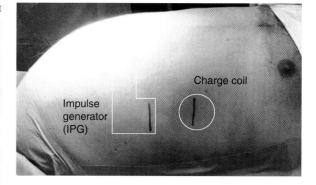

Fig. 7.3 Preoperative marking of the position of the IPG and the CC

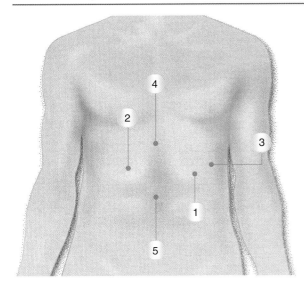

Fig. 7.4 Trocar placement

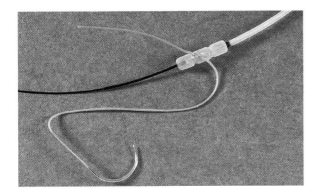

Fig. 7.5 Fastening suture. The knot is placed into the dent of the eyelet. The black ring marks this electrode for posterior application

- Remove retrogastric adhesions from the distal stomach and the pylorus with the ultrasound cutter or scissors.
- After completing mobilization, insert the electrodes one by one into the abdomen. They are either inserted through a 10/12 mm trocar with a grasper or pushed through the trocar and then pulled from within with the grasper.
- Tense the stomach wall with the stay suture to facilitate placement of the electrodes in the subserosa.

Fundus Electrodes
- Place the electrodes 2-cm below the lower esophageal sphincter, 2-cm apart from each other.
- Tense the stomach between the stay suture and a grasper (Fig. 7.7).
- Insert the UF needle parallel to the tension line right above the stay suture, directing toward the grasper. Make sure the electrode is positioned subserosally.
- Secure the wire close to the electrode with two titanium clips and cut the needle off.
- Fasten the fixtures of the electrodes to the stomach with the prepared suture.
- Perform gastroscopy to rule out a perforation of electrodes into the stomach.

Antrum Backside Electrodes
- After displaying the pylorus, place the electrode into the subserosa with the help of the UF-needle and the stay suture (Fig. 7.8).
- Insert the UF needle from the greater curvature toward the lesser curvature. The stay suture (not depicted) keeps the greater curvature under

Fig. 7.6 Electrode positioning. The distal antrum electrodes are placed 2 cm above the pylorus, the proximal antrum electrodes 4 cm above the distal electrodes (i.e., 6 cm above the pylorus). This is repeated on the backside. The fundus electrodes are placed 2 cm below the esophageal sphincter 2 cm apart from each other

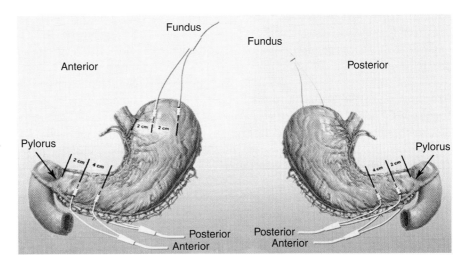

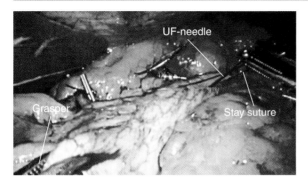

Fig. 7.7 Inserting the UF needle into the subserosa; the stay suture is also depicted

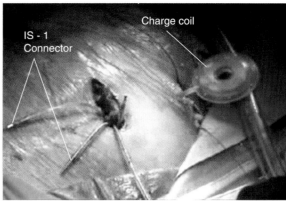

Fig. 7.9 Incision for the IPG below the left costal arch with the electrodes coming out of the abdomen and the incision for the CC

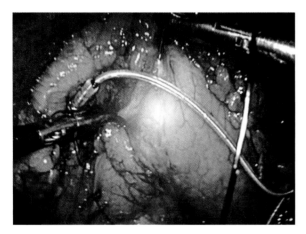

Fig. 7.8 Antrum backside electrode

tension. The already implanted distal electrode with its two titanium clips is seen on the lower left side (Fig. 7.8).

Antrum Frontside Electrode

This one is usually the easiest to place. It belongs opposite to the backside electrodes, i.e., 2 and 6 cm above the pylorus.

Preparation of the Subcutaneous Pocket for the IPG

- Usually the channel for the right trocar is turned into the IPG pocket. Create space for the IPG through blunt dissection with your finger.

To prevent rotation/migration, make sure the pocket is not too large.

Preparation of the Subcutaneous Pocket for the CC

- Create the incision on the beforehand marked lines near the left costal arch about 4 cm cranial to the IPG.
- After dissecting the subcutis, prepare three to four non absorbable sutures. The coil should not be positioned more than 1.5 cm below the skin to not impair charging.
- Pull the charging electrode of the coil through to the IPG subcutaneously with a clamp.
- After successful test charging, fasten the coil to the fascia (Fig. 7.9).
- Connect the plug to the IPG very carefully, so as not to harm the spring (Fig. 7.10).
- Before you connect the plugs with the IPG, clean the ends with saline or alcohol and dry them. Three clicking sounds are supposed to be heard in the process.
- Now place the IPG into the subcutaneous pocket.
- Move the long electrodes back into the abdomen with a grasper.
- Close both pockets with subcutaneous and skin sutures.
- Prepare sutures for the fascia, remove the trocars under visual control and close the sutures of the fascia. Finish the procedure with skin sutures.

Postoperative Recommendations

Have the patient wear an abdominal bandage until the stitches are removed.

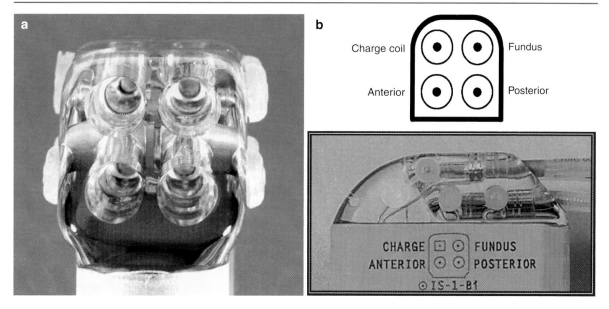

Fig. 7.10 IPG plugs. On the left upper hand is the plug for the CC electrode, the other plugs are for the IPG electrodes. The plugs must be connected by hand under visual control and fastened with a screwdriver

7.2   Surgical Technique by Stefanie Wolf (Germany)

Stefanie Wolf

Introduction

Gastric pacers are implanted for two reasons today: gastroparesis and severe obesity.

Gastroparesis has various causes, first of all diabetes. It can also be induced by other diseases, such as chronic pseudo-obstruction, connective tissue diseases, or anorexia nervosa. Pharmaceutical causes must also be considered as a differential diagnosis, before a gastroparesis can be named idiopathic. It presents with a feeling of fullness or of having a rock inside the stomach and sometimes vomiting.

This reduces the quality of life and in an advanced stage impairs food intake, but therapeutical options are scarce. New treatment ideas are looked for.

First results of a multicenter gastroparesis study showed only an insignificant improvement of nausea and vomiting and gastric emptying after 1 year. Average weight gain was 5.5%.

The gastric pacer was approved by the FDA for chronic gastroparesis refractory to pharmaceutical treatment with nausea and vomiting in cases of diabetes or idiopathic in 2000.

Based on results by Cigaina et al. [1], the working mechanism of the gastric pacer for the *treatment of obesity* was investigated. First implantations in humans were performed in 1995, the first pilot study was begun in 1998 [2]. Cigaina et al. just recently published their data concerning patient safety and effectiveness from a long-term follow-up of 8 years and 65 patients [3].

The first European multicenter studies reported an average loss of excess body weight of 23% in 12 months [4]. A group in France even reached 30% by applying higher stimulation amplitudes [5].

Multicenter studies from the USA (U.S.O-01 Trial, Digest Trial) prove the safety of the procedure, but excess weight fell only by 20% in 29 months in the O-01 trial and by 23% after 16 months in the Digest Trial [6]. In summary, all trials concerning gastric pacers have well proved the safety of the procedure, but so far a proof of efficiency has not been given in larger groups of patients.

Implantation of a gastric pacer to lose weight should therefore only be performed in specialized centers or in trials. Indications are the same as for established bariatric procedures.

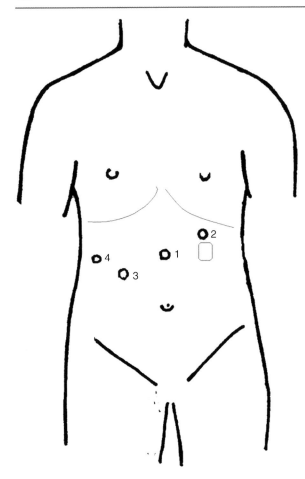

Fig. 7.11 Trocar placement: 1 Camera trocar; 2,3 working trocars, 4 trocar for liver retractor

Preparation

Setting, Positioning, and the Surgical Team

- All patients receive antithrombotic and antibiotic prophylaxis perioperatively. The procedure is performed laparoscopic [7].
- Bring the patient into an anti-Trendelenburg position with spread arms and legs.
- You as the surgeon stand between the patient's legs, the assistant on the right side.
- Four trocars are needed for the procedure (Fig. 7.11). We insert a Visiport first; it is positioned on the middle line between the umbilicus and the xiphoid.
- After inserting the optic trocar and inspecting the upper abdomen, add two to three more working trocars (12 mm) under visual control. They are placed next to the middle line on the right side and at the left and right (liver retractor) costal arch.

Surgical Technique

- Begin with removing any adhesions, until you can see the anterior side of the stomach completely. A liver retractor is usually necessary (right costal arch). Only if the left hepatic lobe is very small, you can omit the retractor and thus the fourth trocar.
- Insert the electrode into the abdominal cave through the working trocar in the left upper abdomen. The electrode comes with an application needle fastened to it.
- Grasp the needle and implant the electrode 6-cm away from the pylorus intramurally at the lesser curvature. The exact localization varies in the different trials. In gastroparesis, the electrodes were implanted at the greater curvature, in obesity at the lesser curvature. You could also implant two electrodes (antrum and cardia), depending on the design of the trial (Fig. 7.12a and b).
- Perform gastroscopy to confirm the intramural position of the electrode.

  If gastroscopy reveals an injury of the mucosa, remove the needle. As insertion is performed tangentially and the needle is fairly thin, there is no need to suture the puncture site. The needle is inserted and controlled again. If another injury is ruled out, push the needle into its final position.

- Cut off the needle. Placing a titanium clip over the end of the electrode and suturing the electrode to the stomach will keep it from slipping out of the gastric wall.
- Pull the other end of the electrode out of the abdomen and remove the trocars under visual control.
- Drainage tubes are usually not necessary.
- Connect the electrode with the pacemaker.
- After checking the function of the device, fasten it with sutures within a subcutaneous pocket over the fascia in the left upper abdomen.

Postoperative Proceedings

- Perform a water-soluble contrast swallow to document the correct position of the electrodes.
- Patients can begin to eat the next day.
- They are usually discharged on day 2.

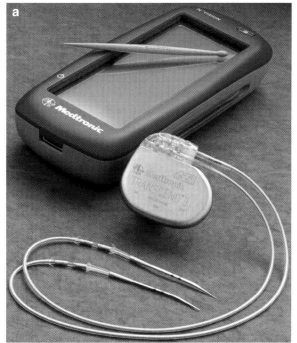

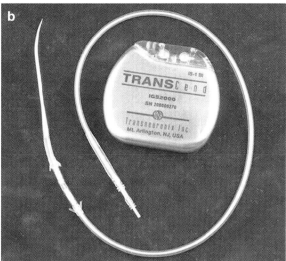

Fig. 7.12 (**a**) Pacemaker with double electrode. (**b**) Single electrode

- The pacemaker is switched on 2–4 weeks after implantation on an outpatient basis.
- From then on, the patient returns every 2–3 months to have weight loss and wounds checked. Sometimes an individual adjustment of the stimulation parameters is necessary. Therapy time (24 h or interval therapy) can also be varied.
- Regular gastroscopies are strongly recommended, even in symptom-free patients.

- Battery replacement can be performed within a small procedure, just as with a cardiac pacemaker.

> **Particularities of patients with a gastric pacemaker**
> They carry a *pacemaker ID*. Regarding possible diagnostic measures and treatments, they are to be treated just like carriers of cardiac pacemakers.
> *MRI scans* are only to be performed in life-threatening emergencies to save the IPG from harm. Avoid diathermy (short wave, micro wave, and ultrashort wave treatments) as the tip off the electrode might heat up.
>   Due to limited experience, refrain from treating women who are *planning a pregnancy* or are *pregnant* already. If the device has been implanted before, it should be switched off or even removed altogether. If it remains implanted during a pregnancy, make sure the electrodes have not dislocated before treatment is restarted.

Difficult situations and Intraoperative Complications

We have encountered three typical kinds of complications in the last 7 years: electrode dislocation, penetration into the stomach, and inflammation of the IPG pocket.

Electrode Dislocation

Electrode dislocation from the stomach was quite frequent in the beginning, when ways of attaching the electrode to the stomach wall were not perfected yet. Surgical technique was improved; the electrodes are now fastened with clips and additional sutures. Electrode dislocation has become a rare event.

Symptoms: Sometimes abdominal pain is present. As energy is still delivered through the tip of the electrode, misguided contractions of the abdominal wall can be painful. Localization of pain depends on the position of the lose end of the electrode.

Diagnosis: We recommend an ultrasound scan and an X-ray (Fig. 7.13). A water-soluble contrast swallow can facilitate localization; fluoroscopy shows, if the electrode moves with the stomach or not.

The pacemaker is switched off by placing a magnet on the IPG. Acute pain will resolve quickly, although

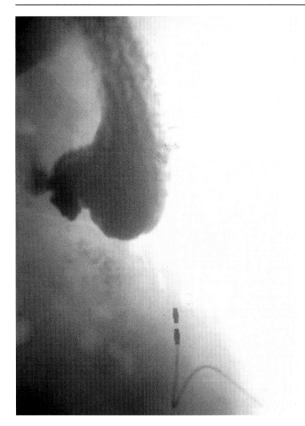

Fig. 7.13 Electrode dislocation

the affected abdominal muscles might remain sore for a while.

Now the system is either removed or the electrode is repositioned; both procedures are performed laparoscopic.

Penetration into the Stomach

In more than 400 obese patients with a gastric pacer, this complication has occurred three times. We have only observed one case so far. The patient participated in a double blind placebo-controlled trial and belonged to the placebo group, i.e., he received no stimulation for 6 months. A routine gastroscopy revealed penetration of the electrode into the stomach. The patient had no symptoms whatsoever. The device was removed laparoscopic; the electrode was covered with serosa along the entire length. A single suture was placed on the stomach wall after removal of the electrode.

Symptoms: Penetration of the electrode can provoke symptoms or not (as in the case mentioned above). Asymptomatic penetration is usually detected through routine follow-up examinations and is usually the result of chronic migration of the electrode through the stomach wall. Reasons could be continuous mechanical irritation due to the contractions of the stomach wall or a microperforation that was overlooked during implantation. Penetration of foreign bodies into the stomach has been reported before, i.e., with gastric bands.

Diagnosis: We recommend the same measures as with suspected electrode dislocation, gastroscopy being the key examination. Treatment is removal of the device.

Inflammation of the IPG Pocket

This complication usually requires removal of the entire system.

Summary

Gastric pacing in bariatric surgery is performed since 2000. In contrast to the other established techniques, such as gastric bypass, gastric banding, sleeve gastrectomy, and BPD, the effect is neither restrictive nor malabsorptive, but is based on the electrical stimulation of the gastric wall. The exact mechanism that provokes the feeling of satiety remains unknown, possibly a change in the distension capacity of the stomach wall.

Surgical technique is safe and easy to master by surgeons with laparoscopic experience.

Problematic is the rather modest effectiveness of the procedure. With an Excess Weight Loss (EWL) of only about 20% it lags behind the other bariatric techniques.

Indication in cases of gastroparesis must be considered individually.

Generally spoken, this procedure should only be performed within controlled trials, independent of the indication.

References

7   Gastric Pacing

1. Bortolotti M (2002) The electrical way "to cure gastroparesis. Am J Gastroenterol 97(8):1874–1883
2. Kwong NK, Brown BH, Whittaker GE, Duthie HL (1970) Electrical activity of the gastric antrum in man. Br J Surg 57:913–916

3. Monges H, Salducci H (1970) A method of recording the gastric electrical activity in man. Dig Dis 15:271–276
4. Tack J, Coulie B, Van Cutsem E, Ryden J, Janssens J (1999) The influence of gastric electrical stimulation on proximal gastric motor and sensory function in severe idiopathic gastroparesis (abstract). Gastroenterology 116:A1090

7.1   Surgical technique

1. Bohdjalian A, Prager G, Aviv R, Policker S, Schindler K, Kretschmer S, Riener R, Zacherl J, Ludvik B (2006) One-year experience with Tantalus: a new surgical approach to treat morbid obesity. Obes Surg 5:627–634
2. Peles S, Petersen J, Aviv R, Policker S, Abu-Hatoum O, Ben-Haim SA, Gutterman DD, Sengupta JN (2003) Enhancement of antral contractions and vagal afferent signaling with synchronized electrical stimulation. Am J Physiol Gastrointest Liver Physiol 285(3):G577–G585
3. Bohdjalian A, Ludvik B, Guerci B, Bresler L, Renard E, Nocca D, Karnieli E, Assalia A, Prager R, Prager G (2009) Improvement in glycemic control by gastric electrical stimulation: TANTALUS(TM)) in overweight subjects with type 2 diabetes. Surg Endosc 3(4):964–970
4. Policker S, Lu H, Haddad W, Aviv R, Kliger A, Glasberg O, Goode P (2008) Electrical stimulation of the gut for the treatment of type 2 diabetes: the role of automatic eating detection. Diabetes Sci Technol 2(5):906–912

7.2   Surgical technique

1. Cigaina V, Saggioro A (1996) The long-term effects of gastric pacing on an obese young woman. Obes Surg 6:312, A 41
2. Cigaina V, Saggioro A, Gracco L, Pivotto L, Tamburrano G (2001) Gastric pacemaker to treat morbid obesity – five year experience. Obes Surg 11:171, A P8
3. Cigaina V (2004) Long-term follow-up of gastric stimulation for obesity: the Mestre 8 year experience. Obes Surg 14:S14–S22
4. Cigaina V, Dargen J, Belachew M, Melissas J, Miller K, Favretti F, Dietl KH, Horber F (2002) Treatment of obesity with the transcend implantable gastric stimulator: multi-center open label study.Obes Surg 12:194, A6
5. D'Argent J (2002) Gastric electrical stimulation as therapy of morbid obesity: preliminary results from the French study. Obes Surg 12:21S–25S
6. Shikora SA (2004) What are the Yanks doing? The US experience with implantable gastric stimulation (IGS) for the treatment of obesity – update on the ongoing clinical trials. Obes Surg 14:S40–S48
7. Wolff S, Pross M, Knippig C, Malfertheiner P, Lippert H (2002) Gastric pacing. A new method in obesity surgery. Chirurg 73(7):700–703

Gastric Balloon

8

Michael Korenkov, Richard Merkle,
and Sybille Abegg-Zips

Introduction

Gastric balloons are implanted and filled to achieve a temporary restriction of stomach size. The balloons are supposed to remain in the stomach for 6 months; patients will learn to modify their eating habits by then.

The implantation of an intragastric balloon is not a surgical procedure. The first balloon, the so-called GEB (Garren-Edwards bubble by American Edward Lab., Inc., Santa Ana, CA, USA), was developed in the USA in 1984. This balloon was made of polyurethane and was filled with up to 220 mL of air (Fig. 8.1).

The concept of the balloon is based on the idea of reducing the volume of the stomach by placing something large inside. This was supposed to produce a faster feeling of satiety, which was to result in a lower calorie intake and consequent weight loss.

The gastric balloon was soon established as the initial procedure in complex bariatric treatments. After having lost weight as desired and the removal of the balloon, patients were to receive further therapy (nutrition (800–1,200 kcal/day), exercise, and behavioral therapy).

The principle of gastric balloon therapy as an adjuvant treatment for obesity was presented first at the International Conference at Tarpon Springs, FA, in 1987 [12]. But low quality of the material lead to various negative events, such as broken balloons, stomach ulcers, stomach perforations, and obstructions, which resulted in a poor acceptance of the technique [1].

The shortcomings of the GEB were overcome by other manufacturers. In contrast to the sharp-edged GEB with its rough surface, the BIB (Bioenterics Intragastric Balloon, Inamed Corporation, Santa Barbara, CA, USA) is an elastic, soft spheric silicone balloon that is filled with saline. Using the BIB reduced the number of complications noticeably [11].

Implantation Technique

- The BIB system has a soft and smooth silicone balloon that can be inserted into the stomach through gastroscopy, while it is empty and folded (Fig. 8.2).
- After inserting the balloon into the stomach, fill it over a thin catheter that is connected to the balloon with 600–700 mL of sterile saline.
- Add methylene blue to the saline. If the balloon breaks, blue saline will leak. The patient will notice blue stool or urine and is warned of a leak in the balloon.

M. Korenkov (✉)
Abteilung für Allgemein- und Visceralchirurgie,
Klinikum Werra-Meissner, Akademisches Lehrkrankenhaus der
Universität Göttingen, Elsa-Brendström-Straße 1,
37269 Eschwege, Germany
e-mail: michael.korenkov@klinikum-wm.de

R. Merkle • S. Abegg-Zips
Leiter der Viszeralchirurgischen Sektion des
Medizinischen Competenz Centrum München GmbH,
Taulerstr. 14, 81739 München, Germany
e-mail: richard.merkle@mnet-online.de

Fig. 8.1 Garren-Edwards bubble

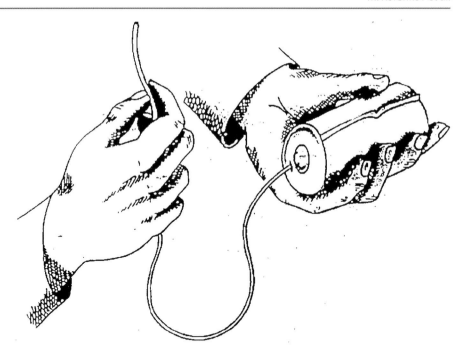

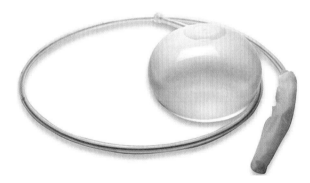

Fig. 8.2 BIB gastric balloon

- After filling the balloon, disconnect the catheter from the balloon by pulling and remove it. The balloon is equipped with a self-closing valve and will float freely inside the stomach.
- Six months later the balloon is removed during another gastroscopy.

Difficult Situations, Complications, and Adverse Events

In contrast to surgical bariatric procedures and conservative methods with valid long-term studies to confirm their effectiveness and safety, therapy with the gastric balloon has little scientific evidence to support it. Data from the Cochrane Database of Systematic Reviews show that the longest follow-up studies do not reach further back than 2 years [5]. Weight loss after 6 months of therapy with an IGB averages 25–40% of the excess weight [5, 8]. There are no long-term studies available.

Analysis of morbidity and mortality shows that serious complications, such as perforations of the stomach and the esophagus, bowel obstruction and massive hemorrhage from the stomach (Mallory-Weiss syndrome) are extremely rare [7, 10]. Lethality rates are around 0–0.2% [5].

There is however a characteristic morbidity associated with IGB-therapy, the *adjustment phase*. Patients almost always suffer from severe spasmodic pain in the upper abdomen, combined with massive heartburn and nausea after implantation of the balloon. In spite of mandatory therapy with proton pump inhibitors, spasmolytics, analgetics, and antiemetics these symptoms can last for weeks. Two to 8% of the patients need to have the balloon removed early because of intolerance [3, 4]. Some patients need to be admitted to hospital to treat dehydration and electrolyte imbalance. The intensity of the symptoms can be reduced by replacing liquids or by reducing the size of the balloon endoscopically. It is however quite difficult to assess the correct amount of fluids [2, 6]; too much will hinder weight loss, too little will not alleviate the symptoms. There are no evident data available.

Adapting the size of the IGB is elaborate and technically difficult and often results in irreversible damage of the balloon.

An effective solution of the problems associated with IGB has therefore not been found.

Assuming that some of the problems of the adjustment phase are caused by the comparatively large weight of the saline-filled balloon (depending on the amount of saline), the idea of the air-filled balloon resurfaced. The French company Héliofrance developed an air-filled gastric balloon in 2005. It weighs about 30 g and is far better designed than the Garren-Edward bubble. A first study by Mion et al. shows acceptable results of the therapy with the Hélioscope balloon [9], but evident data comparing air- and saline-filled balloons are not yet available.

Another important negative effect of the balloon is the *chronic pangastritis* as a reaction to the foreign body.

Today IGB are used in the following cases:
- *I* Overweight patients with a BMI under 35 as part of a conservative therapy regimen; implantation can be repeated.
- *II* Morbidly obese patients; the IGB is used to assess the indication for restrictive bariatric procedures.
- *III* Overweight patients planning other surgery (heart, orthopedic surgery) to optimize their overall condition.
- *IV* Extremely obese patients (BMI over 60), preparing for surgical bariatric procedures.

> *Attention*: Surgery should take place approximately 2 weeks after removal of the balloon, otherwise the rate of complications is too high due to the massive swelling of the stomach wall.

Contraindication for an IGB is stomach surgery in the past; there is a high risk of stomach perforation.

Summarizing it can be said that the status of the IGB is not yet settled conclusively. This method is very successful for patients from the groups III and IV. The therapeutic effect for patients of group No. I is uncertain.

Long-term studies need to be conducted. The therapeutic effects for patients in group No. II are just as uncertain; available data are insufficient and in part contradictory.

Therapy with the IGB has low mortality and morbidity, but problems during the adjustment phase have not yet been solved satisfactorily.

In some countries therapy with the IGB is not covered by the health insurance companies.

Difficult Situations During and After Implantation of the Balloon

Implantation and removal of the IGB are performed throughout gastroscopy, which is why the potential for complications is rather low. But even here complications and difficult situations may arise.

Hematemesis and Later Melaena After Implantation of an IGB; Emergency Gastroscopy Reveals a Mallory-Weiss Syndrome

Predisposing factors: A Mallory-Weiss syndrome after implantation of an IGB is caused by repeated nausea. The reason is a too large volume of the balloon and insufficient education of the patient about this therapy.

Prevention: We fill the balloon with 500–600 mL liquid in patients with a BMI between 30 and 35. Each patient must be informed about the entire procedure. Massive nausea can occur in the first few days after implantation. In this case we recommend to admit the patient to hospital immediately and to treat with antiemetics, spasmolytics, analgetics, and infusion therapy.

Management: Hemorrhage in Mallory-Weiss syndrome is usually treated by injections during an emergency gastroscopy. We know a case from an expertise, in which a surgical procedure (laparotomy, gastrotomy, and suture of the torn mucosa) was necessary.

Sudden Change of Sensation in the Upper Abdomen Without Tightness, Large Amounts of Food Can Be Eaten Again; An Emergency Gastroscopy Reveals a Perforated Balloon Inside the Stomach

Predisposing factors: Sharp edged or pointed parts of food, such as fish bones can perforate the gastric balloon.

Prevention: Detailed information on what food to avoid during therapy with an IGB is mandatory.

Management: The balloon needs to be removed immediately to keep it from migrating into the intestine and causing an ileus. The use of blue saline for the filling is recommended to detect perforation of the balloon early.

> We fill our balloons with clear liquid, because we often encountered the following situation: a patient reports blue urine, but emergency gastroscopy revealed that the balloon is intact. To avoid these confusions, we stopped using tinted saline years ago and so far have not found a reason to revise our concept.

Sudden Abdominal Cramps and Nausea Long After the Adjustment Phase; X-Ray of the Abdomen Shows an Ileus; a CT Scan of the Abdomen Reveals Obstruction of the Small Intestine with a Foreign Body; the Balloon Is no Longer Inside the Stomach

Predisposing factors: This situation arises when a balloon perforates unnoticed and passes through the pylorus into the ileum.

Prevention: Early recognition of a perforation (s.a.)

Management: An ileus of the small intestine due to a broken balloon must be treated surgically with an emergency enterotomy, laparoscopically, or conventionally. Note that an ileus caused by a migrating balloon is a very rare event. Most of the broken balloons migrating into the intestine leave the body the natural way.

8.1   Implantation Technique by Richard Merkle (Germany)

Richard Merkle and Sybille Abegg-Zips

Introduction

Obesity, a complex disease pattern, affects all sectors of the population and all ages. The WHO reports 300 Mio obese people worldwide. This problem is not only prevalent in industrialized countries, but is also beginning to affect threshold countries. Latest studies show that 37 Mio adults and 2 Mio children in Germany are overweight or obese.

If conservative treatment, such as diets, increased physical activity, or pharmaceutical treatment alone does not result in long-term weight loss, the gastric balloon as an active therapy is a suitable treatment (Fig. 8.3 and Table 8.1). This is a restrictive technique, i.e., food intake is limited.

The gastric balloon helps build strategies to modify behavior without a surgical procedure. Patient motivation is crucial for success. The therapeutical concept includes the balloon, nutritional counseling, and behavior modification. Changing habits concerning physical activity and nutrition improves the chances for keeping the weight down after removal of the balloon. Nutritional counseling is strongly recommended, as a sensible use of food and not sacrifice is the goal.

In the first months weight loss is achieved without hunger due to the permanent partial filling of the stomach. A feeling of satiety is reached much earlier so that food intake can be reduced substantially.

The gastric balloon is a soft elastic silicone balloon.

After gastroscopy to rule out any pathology, the balloon is inserted into the stomach through the esophagus. Then it is filled with about 600 ml of sterile blue saline through a tube (Fig. 8.4), which is then removed. The balloon is now too large to migrate into the intestine and floats freely inside the stomach.

Insertion takes 15–20 min and can be performed on an outpatient basis.

The balloon should not remain in the stomach longer than 6 months. It must be removed after this period, because aggressive gastric juices will erode the balloon and cause leakage. It could be replaced by a new balloon immediately, although we recommend a break of 4–6 weeks.

The saline is tinted blue to serve as an indicator for leakage. If saline leaks from the balloon, the patient will notice blue urine. The balloon should then be removed as quickly as possible.

If large amounts of saline leak out and the balloon is propulsed into the intestine, an ileus might occur in rare cases in spite of laxative measures.

Preparation

Setting, Positioning, and the Surgical Team
- The patient should not eat in the last 6 h before the procedure.
- Anticoagulant medication must be stopped in time.

Fig. 8.3 Indications for the implantation of a gastric balloon depending on the BMI

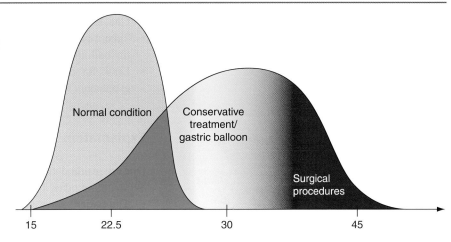

Table 8.1 Indications and contraindications for a gastric balloon

Indications

Patients with a BMI between 28 and 40, who have failed to achieve long-term weight loss with conservative weight loss programs

Weight loss in severe obesity (BMI over 55) before a bariatric procedure to reduce risks associated with the excess weight

Test before implantation of a gastric band: The willingness of the patient to change eating habits is tested. If patients "cheat" the balloon, similar unsuitable eating habits must be suspected after implantation of a band as well

Contraindications

Eating disorders, especially "sweet eaters," who can cheat the balloon with their choice and preparation of food

Abdominal surgery and bariatric procedures in the patient's history

Large hiatal hernia

Severe esophagitis

Peptic ulcers

Unsatisfactory compliance

- Patients with a BMI of up to 45 can be sedated, heavier patients receive intubation anesthesia. Expect chronic impaired nasal breathing and a tight pharynx in these cases.
- We recommend administering Pantozol and Zofran intravenously as an antiemetic prophylaxis.
- Perform gastroscopy beforehand to rule out ulcers, inflammation, tumors, large hernias, etc., and test for *Helicobacter pylori*.

Preparation for Intubation

- If intubation is necessary, place the tube on the side of the mouthpiece and fasten it carefully.
- Position the endoscopy stack next to the patient's head.

Implantation Technique

- The patient is lying on his left side.
- Insert the folded balloon through the large middle opening of the mouthpiece (in this case without intubation).
- Move the balloon down into the proximal esophagus like a gastric tube (Fig. 8.5). It is helpful to place your finger on the base of the tongue as a splint (Fig. 8.6) to prevent the balloon from unfolding in the throat.
- Place the folded balloon into the stomach.
- Position the gastroscope into the cardia and fill the balloon with 500–700 mL of blue saline.
- Disrupt the tube.
- After removal of the implantation devices, the balloon should be in the fundus, while the patient is lying on his left side (Fig. 8.7).

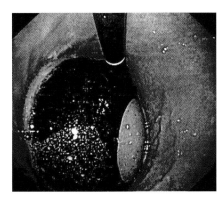

Fig. 8.4 Filled gastric balloon

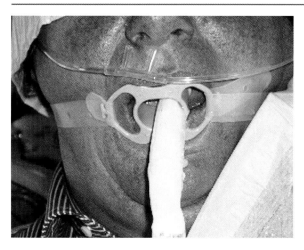

Fig. 8.5 The balloon is moved down into the proximal esophagus like a gastric tube

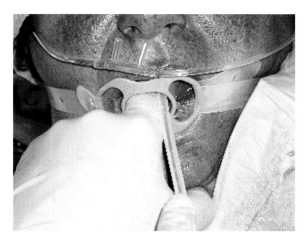

Fig. 8.6 It is helpful to place your finger on the base of the tongue as a splint

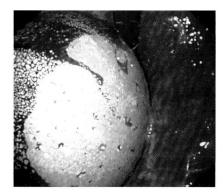

Fig. 8.7 Filled gastric balloon after removal of the implantation devices

- Check for free passage of the pylorus.
- Take a photograph to prove the correct position of the balloon in the fundus.
- Look for possible injuries of the stomach or the esophagus while retracting the gastroscope.

Explantation

Due to residual food and/or a thinned balloon wall, explantation takes a little longer than implantation.
- The patient should not eat in the last 12 h and not drink in the last 6 h before the procedure.
- Anticoagulant medication must be stopped in time.
- Because of the danger of aspirating residual food, we always perform this procedure in intubation anesthesia.
- Puncture the balloon under visual control (Fig. 8.8) with the endoscopic needle.
- Insert the catheter into the balloon and aspirate the tinted saline.
- Remove the empty balloon under visual control with a grasper.

> If there is no endoscopic needle at hand, you could also open the balloon with scissors.

- Aspirate the blue saline (Fig. 8.9) and remove the balloon with a grasper afterward.

> In some cases the balloon can be entered with the endoscope; the valve can then be grasped with a polypectomy snare and removed.

- Observe the patient for another 1 or 2 h, before he is discharged in company.

Compliance

The patient's compliance is of utmost importance for gastric balloon therapy. Patients will experience nausea and intense foreign body sensation for the first 1–3 days. This must be explained very clearly in the information beforehand to avoid having the first dropouts early (Table 8.2).

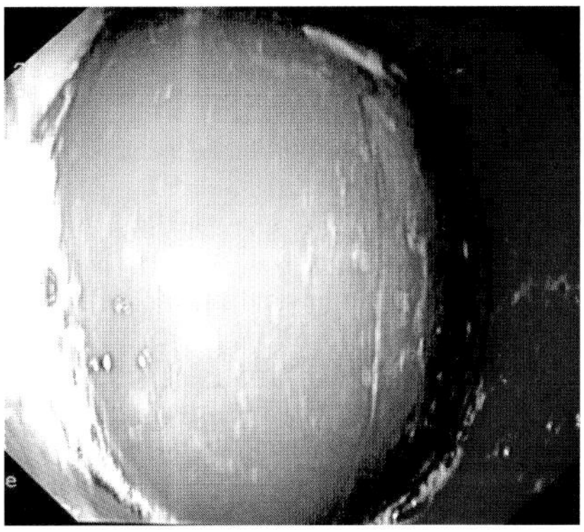

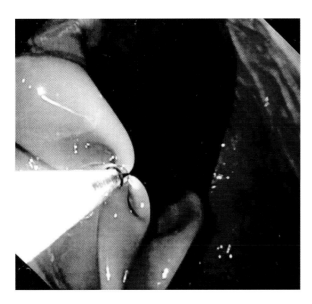

Fig. 8.8   Puncture the balloon under visual control for explantation

Table 8.2   Feeding and co-medication after implantation of the gastric balloon

Day 0	A little water or tea
Days 1 and 2	Tea
	If no nausea occurs, liquids or mashed food
From day 3 on	Light food
Nutrition counseling	
Antiemetic and analgetic medication	Dimenhydrinate 3 × 1 supp.
	Butylscopolamine 3 × 1 supp.
	Clorazepate dipotassium 2 × 10 mg p.o.
	Novaminsulfon 3 × 30 drops
Long-term medication	Omeprazole 1 × 40 mg p.o.

After this phase, frequent aftercare and careful instructions concerning nutrition and physical activity are mandatory. Until the balloon is removed, patients must be able to continue their new regimen without feeling deprived.

A major part of success is the aftercare after removal, including nutritional advice and other talks.

The more invasive a procedure is, the less compliance is asked from the patient, or to put it more positively, the less invasive a procedure is, the more it depends on the patient's compliance and his willingness to cooperate and change his eating habits (Fig. 8.10).

Success Rates and Complications

Evaluation of our patient data shows a female to male ratio of 3:1 (Tables 8.3–8.5). Average weight loss was 19 kg.

Absolute weight loss increases with the BMI, relative excess weight loss (EWL) however, decreases.

Fig. 8.9   The emptied balloon is held with a grasper and removed

Fig. 8.10   Patients' compliance depending on the bariatric procedure

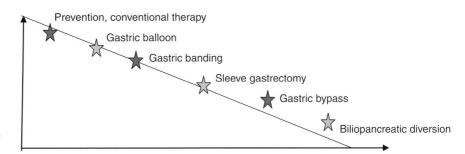

Table 8.3 Patient population

Time period: 11/1/2006–11/30/2008

Number of patients: $n = 227$

Balloon was not tolerated: $n = 6$

Non-compliance: $n = 17$

Complications:

1 × pneumonia due to aspiration

1 × gastric ulcer

Table 8.4 BMI reduction in men with the gastric balloon

Men	BMI	Body weight in kg	Excess weight loss in kg	Excess weight loss in %	BMI reduction
A1 $n = 17$	32, 3	101	16	52	5, 2
A2 $n = 18$	37, 8	118	19	39	6, 2
A3 $n = 18$	46, 2	145	26	35	8, 2
SO $n = 9$	60, 9	191	38	31	12, 1

Table 8.5 BMI reduction in women with the gastric balloon

Men	BMI	Body weight in kg	Excess weight loss in kg	Excess weight loss in %	BMI reduction
Excess weight $n = 23$	27, 4	77	14	73	5, 1
A1 $n = 52$	32, 6	92	15	44	5, 3
A2 $n = 49$	37, 3	105	17	36	6, 2
A3 $n = 33$	46, 1	130	21	29	7, 5
SO $n = 8$	57	161	27	26	9, 6

We saw one case of aspiration pneumonia and one patient with gastric ulcer. The patient with pneumonia spent several weeks in intensive care, but was discharged completely healthy. The gastric ulcer healed with high dose PPI therapy, the balloon was not removed.

References

1. Benjamin SB, Maher KA, Cattau EL, Jr., Collen MJ, et al. (1988) Double-blind controlled trial of the Garren-Edwards gastric bubble: an adjunctive treatment for exogenous obesity. Gastroenterology 95:581
2. De Waele B, Reynaert H, Van Nieuwen hove Y, Urbain D (2001) Endoscopic volume adjustment of intragastric balloons for intolerance. Obes Surg 11:223
3. Doldi SB, Micheletto G, Perrini MN, Librenti MC, Rella S (2002) Treatment of morbid obesity with intragastric balloon in association with diet. Obes Surg 12:583
4. Evans JD, Scott MH (2001) Intragastric balloon in the treatment of patients with morbid obesity. Br J Surg 88:1245
5. Fernandes M, Atallah AN, Soares BG, Humberto S, et al. (2007) Intragastric balloon for obesity. Cochrane Database Syst Rev CD004931
6. Ganesh R, Rao AD, Baladas HG, Leese T (2007) The Bioenteric Intragastric Balloon (BIB) as a treatment for obesity: poor results in Asian patients. Singapore Med J 48:227
7. Genco A, Bruni T, Doldi SB, Forestieri P, et al. (2005) BioEnterics intragastric balloon: the Italian experience with 2,515 patients. Obes Surg 15:1161
8. Herve J, Wahlen CH, Schaeken A, Dalle-magne B, et al. (2005) What becomes of patients one year after the intragastric balloon has been removed? Obes Surg 15:864
9. Mion F, Gincul R, Roman S, Beorchia S, et al. (2007) Tolerance and efficacy of an air-filled balloon in non-morbidly obese patients: results of a prospective multicenter study. Obes Surg 17:764
10. Nijhof HW, Steenvoorde P, Tollenaar RA (2006) Perforation of the esophagus caused by the insertion of an intragastric balloon for the treatment of obesity. Obes Surg 16:667
11. Sallet JA, Marchesini JB, Paiva DS, Komoto K, et al. (2004) Brazilian multicenter study of the intragastric balloon. Obes Surg 14:991
12. Schapiro M, Benjamin S, Blackburn G, Frank B, et al. (1987) Obesity and the gastric balloon: a comprehensive workshop. Tarpon Springs, Florida, March 19–21, 1987. Gastrointest Endosc 19–21;33:323

Plastic Surgical Corrections After Massive Weight Loss

Henrik Menke, Michael Ruggaber, and Nils-Kristian Dohse

Introduction

Plastic surgical corrections after weight loss have first been reported more than 75 years ago [4]. As obesity spreads, so does morbid obesity (BMI over 40 or 50 kg excess weight). More than 5% of adult Americans already are morbidly obese today, their number is increasing [3].

The development of modern methods in bariatric surgery has created new and increasingly popular dimensions of weight loss not possible before with conservative measures. Drastic weight loss has a marked health benefit, but the massive amounts of excess skin and remaining fat tissue cause considerable functional and aesthetic problems concerning hygiene, skin irritation, and pain. Abdomen, chest, thighs, buttocks, arms, and back are affected most.

Plastic surgical body lifts after bariatric procedures are therefore an important part of the treatment of morbid obesity and the only way to reduce large amounts of excess skin. These measures improve the patients' all over, sexual and physical self-confidence [8].

Patient Selection

Patients after massive weight loss have a number of various problems, such as comorbidities, preexisting scars, and nutritional effects. Strict criteria for the admission of patients to bariatric procedures are therefore recommended [13] and should be applied to subsequent procedures as well. In a group of body lift patients, the incidence of high blood pressure was 26%, gastroesophageal reflux 22%, hypothyroidism 11%, asthma 11%, diabetes 9%, and depression 22%; 43% had hernias that required surgical care [14]. These patients need specific surgical treatment.

The natural ability of the skin to retract is exhausted within the first few weeks and months after weight loss and depends on the age of the patient and amount and speed of weight loss. Further spontaneous regression of the skin is not probable after this period. Stabilization of body weight for at least 12 months is a prerequisite for plastic surgical procedures (Table 9.1). Massive weight loss affects the entire body from head to toe. Precise planning of the necessary procedures and their

Table 9.1 Basic principles for body shaping procedures after weight loss surgery

Confirm stable body weight for more than 12 months
Reduce preexisting risk factors (comorbidities, nutrition deficits)
Avoid surgery if the BMI is over 35
Plan all necessary procedures beforehand
Undermine the skin as little as possible
Suture superficial fascias
Minimize blood loss
Avoid extensive combined procedures
Mobilize the patient early

H. Menke (✉)
Chefarzt der Klinik für Plastische, Ästhetische und Handchirurgie, - Zentrum für Schwerbrandverletzte-Klinikum Offenbach, Starkenburgring 66, 63069, Offenbach, Germany

M. Ruggaber • N.-K. Dohse
Klinik für Plastische, Ästhetische, und Handchirurgie, - Zentrum für Schwerbrandverletzte- Klinikum Offenbach, Starkenburgring 66, 63069 Offenbach, Germany

M. Korenkov (ed.), *Bariatric Surgery*,
DOI 10.1007/978-3-642-16245-9_9, © Springer-Verlag Berlin Heidelberg 2012

sequence within the general concept is very important. Full body lifts after massive weight loss are nothing like usual aesthetic surgery procedures; there are special requirements for equipment and facilities due to the often still very high body weight (Fig. 9.1 a–c).

Patients must be informed in detail about the inevitable, usually quite extensive scars. Having scars instead of massive excess skin however is mostly met with a very high degree of acceptance. On a scale of evaluation ranging from 1 to 7 questioning criteria such as psychological situation, basic health, looks, self-confidence and vitality, ratings rose from 3.93 in average to 6.12 [11]. In some cases patients must be warned of unrealistic expectations concerning the effects of a body lift.

Corrections

> Standardized techniques have now superseded the rather eclectic incisions of the early years.
>
> (U. Kesselring)

Therapeutical goal is the enhancement of form and function by reducing excess skin and fat, placing the scars inconspicuously, reaching a lasting effect and closing muscular diastasis, especially in the front abdominal wall [9]. Lockwood recognized the major significance of superficial fascias for body shaping procedures; his work is the foundation of all skin reducing therapy [7]. Localized remnant fat deposits are minimalized by cautious liposuction.

The basic procedure is usually an abdominoplasty (Fig. 9.2a and b). Besides the classic inscision with a scar in the lower abdomen that is elongated to the flanks on the back, sometimes an additional vertical cut is required. This is located in the front middle line in patients with very extensive excess skin or preexisting scars.

In many cases even more skin needs to be removed at the flanks and on the back. This circular streamlining procedure is referred to as the body lift. In contrast to treating the abdomen alone, buttocks, lower back, and thighs can also be shaped (Fig. 9.3a–e).

Combining this with other procedures will lengthen the operation, aggravate blood loss, and extend recovery, but is not necessarily considered a risk factor [6]. Obesity definitely is a risk factor [5]. In many cases, especially in obese patients after multiple pregnancies, the aponeuroses and fascias of the front abdominal wall need to be streamlined, too, in order to achieve a good body contour. There are no negative effects concerning intraabdominal pressure or lung function [1].

Arm Lift

Interest in treatment of the upper arms after bariatric surgery has been increasing lately. Correction procedures require careful consideration of the technique, considering amount and localization of excess skin, softness of the skin and possible fat deposits [2]. Scars should be especially well hidden in this area. Remnant and redundant fat tissue is carefully removed by liposuction which spares the lymphatic system. Only skin is removed surgically; the incision can be elongated into the lateral axilla and the flanks, if needed.

Breast Lift

Massive weight loss often leads to a very slack and hypoplastic shape of the breasts due to a marked discrepancy between breast volume and the amount of skin. Reconstruction of an adequate shape is reached by shaping the mammary gland and removing excess skin (Fig. 9.4). If the size of the mammary gland is not sufficient, excess tissue from other parts of the body can be used and preferably so to heterologous material, such as breast implants. This method combines two advantages: reduction of excess tissue and more breast volume. Another possibility is the inverse tightening of the abdominal wall. Excess skin and fat tissue from the upper abdomen is moved cranially, de-epithelialized, parted with a t-shaped incision and used to augment breast volume. Transplanting a free muscle flap from the inside of the thigh (gracilis muscle) is an elegant microsurgical procedure, combining autologous breast augmentation and tightening of the thighs [12].

Complications

Complication rates after large body shaping procedures are comparatively high even among the many patients of specialized centers, up to 50% [10, 14, 15].

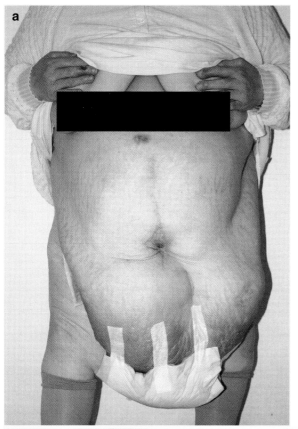

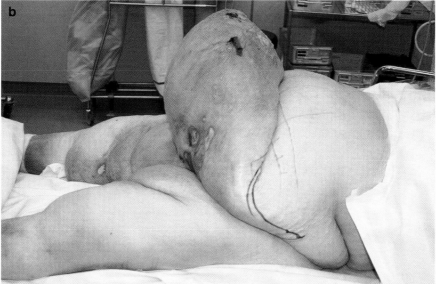

Fig. 9.1   (a–c) A massive fat paunch with severe intertriginous inflammation and ulcerations. (a) Before surgery. (b) During surgery; the fat paunch is lifted for autotransfusion. (c) Situation after removal of the fat paunch (14 kg)

Fig. 9.1 (continued)

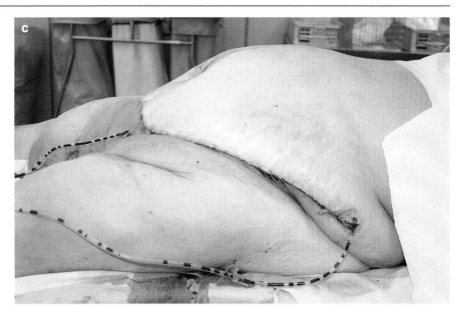

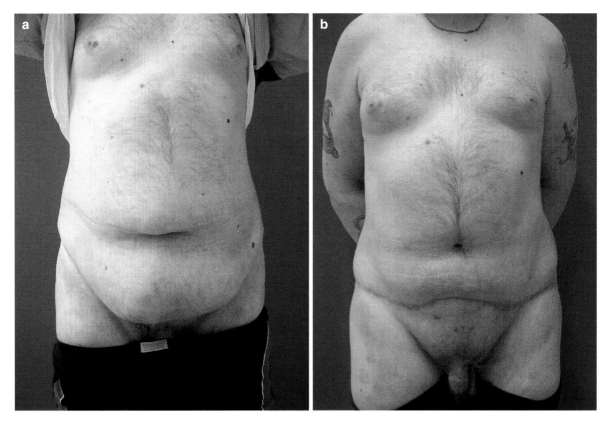

Fig. 9.2 A 36-year-old man after losing 45 kg. (**a**) Before and (**b**) 12 weeks after abdominoplasty

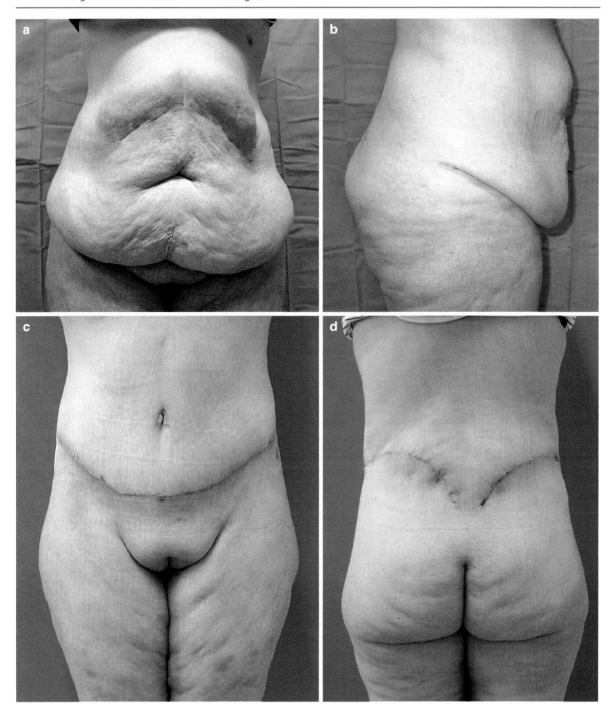

Fig. 9.3 (**a–e**) A 32-year-old woman 6 weeks after body lift; she had lost 55 kg after gastric banding. She gained 10 kg in the meantime.

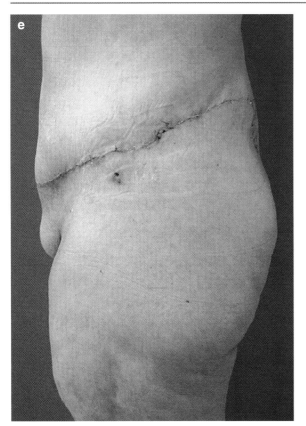

The most frequent complications are defective wound healing, such as wound dehiscence and seroma in up to 30% of all cases and skin necrosis in up to 10%. Extensive undermining of the skin must be avoided strictly during surgery. Inflammation and thromboembolism are rare and are seen only in 1–3% of all cases. Patients whose BMI is still over 35 should only be considered in exceptional cases.

Summary

Plastic surgical corrections after weight loss surgery with marked excess skin lead to a significant improvement of the quality of life. These patients with their complex problems require thorough interdisciplinary care by surgeons, internists, psychologists, and a personal trainer. Meticulous planning and perioperative care as well as experience with these extensive procedures are mandatory.

Fig. 9.3 (continued)

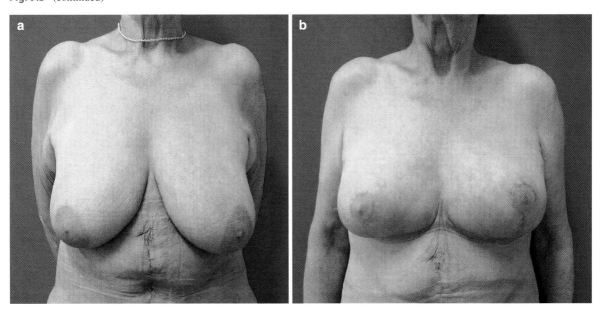

Fig. 9.4 A 58-year-old woman after losing 48 kg after gastroplasty and preexisting median laparotomy scar; stable weight for 5 years, 12 weeks after breast augmentation with inverse tightening of the abdominal wall

References

1. Al-Basti HB, El-Khatib HA, Taha A, Sattar HA, Bener A (2004) Intraabdominal pressure after full abdominoplasty in obese multiparous patients. Plast Reconstr Surg 113:2145–2150

2. Appelt EA, Janis JE, Rohrich RJ (2006) An algorithmic approach to upper arm contouring. Plast Reconstr Surg 118(1):237–246

3. Buchwald H (2002) Overview of bariatric surgery. J Am Coll Surg. 104:367

4. Felsch-Thebesius, Weinsheimer K (1931) Die Operation des Hängebauches. Chirurg 19:841–846

5. Gmur RU, Banic A, Erni D (2003) Is it safe to combine abdominoplasty with other dermolipectomy procedures to correct skin excess after weight loss? Ann Plast Surg 51:353–357

6. Hurwitz DJ, Holland SW (2006) The L brachioplasty: an innovative approach to correct excess tissue of the upper arm, axilla, and lateral chest. Plast Reconstr Surg 117(2):403–411; discussion 412–413

7. Lockwood TE (1991) Superficial fascial system (SFS) of the trunk and extremeties: A new concept. Plast Reconstr Surg 87:1009–1015

8. Menderes A, Baytekin C, Haciyanli M, Yilmaz M (2003) Dermalipectomy for body contouring after bariatric surgery in Aegean region of Turkey. Obes Surg 13:637–641

9. Menke H (2004) Atypische Straffungsoperationen nach massiven Gewichtsreduktionen. Panel Fettsucht "Morbide Adipositas". 35. Jahrestagung der Vereinigung der Deutschen Plastischen Chirurgen (VDPC). Düsseldorf 9:22–25

10. Nemerofsky RB, Oliak DA, Capella JF (2006) Body lift: an account of 200 consecutive cases in the massive weight loss patient. Plast Reconstr Surg 117(2):414–430

11. Romberg M, Piza-Kratzer H (2002) Plastisch-chirurgische Korrekturoperationen nach Gewichtsreduktion durch "gastric-banding". Chirurg 73:918–923

12. Schoeller T, Meirer R, Otto-Schoeller A, Wecheslberger G, Piza-Kratzer H (2002) Medial thigh lift free flap for autologous breast augmentation after bariatric surgery. Obes Surg 12:831–834

13. Schusdziarra V, Hausmann M, Erdmann J (2005) Bariatric surgery. Patient selection and indication][Adipositaschirurgie: Patientenselektion und Indikationsstellung]. Chirurg 76(7): 653–657

14. Shermak MA, Chang D, Magnuson TH, Schweitzer MA (2006) An outcomes analysis of patients undergoing body contouring surgery after massive weight loss. Plast Reconstr Surg 118(4):1026–1031

15. Strauch B, Herman C, Rohde C, Baum T (2006) Mid-body contouring in the post-ibariatric surgery patient. Plast Reconstr Surg 117(7):2200–2211

Anesthesiological Particularities in Bariatric Surgery

10

Hendrik W. Gervais, Annette Schmidt,
Matthias David, and Benno Wolcke

Introduction

Morbid obesity has become a global pandemic in recent years: 5% of the adult population of the USA are considered morbidly obese, i.e., have a BMI that exceeds 40. Every 90 seconds a US American dies of obesity and its consequences – making 1,000 people every day and 400,000 a year. This explains the dramatic rise of interest in bariatric procedures and with it in suitable anesthesiological methods.

Morbidly obese patients pose an anesthesiological challenge in many ways. To determine the best anesthesiological procedure for bariatric surgery, the following three issues must be considered:

- Lungs/ventilation
- Airway management
- Pharmacotherapy

Lungs/Ventilation

Lung volume, respiratory mechanics, and oxygenation are increasingly affected the higher the BMI rises. Functional residual capacity (FRC) and lung compliance decrease, resistance and breathing work increases. The result is a decline of oxygenation [38, 39].

This implies considerable consequences for anesthesia. The entire procedure in this extreme patient population, especially induction and termination of anesthesia, is balancing on a fine line separating two equally problematic situations. On one hand, a reliable and sufficient oxygen reserve must be created, on the other hand there is a risk of atelectasis and consecutive hypoxia due to pulmonal shunting, especially if inappropriately high concentrations of oxygen (FiO_2) are given; even more so here than in lean patients.

A conventional induction of anesthesia is considered unsafe in bariatric procedures, especially because one third of the patients suffer from gastroesophageal reflux [34].

Apart from difficulties with intubation (see below), a rapid sequence induction (RSI) without intermittent ventilation poses a great risk. It should be performed in theory, but obese patients fail to tolerate even very short phases of apnea. Even after optimal preoxygenation, reduced FRC and increased oxygen consumption lead to desaturation much faster than in lean patients [1, 21, 26]. Assuming an oxygen demand of 250 mL/h, lean patients can build an oxygen reserve of about 2,200 mL with optimal preoxygenation, which lasts for almost 10 min [48]. Morbidly obese patients however run into hypoxia after only 3 min [6, 27]. High inspiratory oxygen dosage stimulates the development of atelectasis from the induction of anesthesia on [35, 40]. Atelectasis that develops during anesthesia is not only dangerous perioperatively, but contributes significantly to postoperative complications, such as pneumonia [5, 18].

In lean patients, a reduction of the FiO_2 to 0.8 already lessens atelectasis, at the price of shortening apnea time without hypoxia (defined as the SaO_2 being 90% or more) by about 25% [18, 36]. In obese patients, however, apnea time without hypoxia is reduced even more if FiO_2 is below 1.0. A formation of atelectasis

H.W. Gervais (✉) • A. Schmidt • M. David • B. Wolcke
Klinik für Anästhesiologie, Universitätsmedizin der Johannes
Gutenberg-Universität Mainz, Mainz, Germany
e-mail: gervais@anaesthesie.klinik.uni-mainz.de

M. Korenkov (ed.), *Bariatric Surgery*,
DOI 10.1007/978-3-642-16245-9_10, © Springer-Verlag Berlin Heidelberg 2012

can be effectively avoided independently of patient's weight by applying CPAP during preoxygenation and PEEP (10 cm H_2O) immediately after intubation [12, 41]. This prolongs the duration of apnea without hypoxia in obese patients (average BMI 47) from 2 to 3 min [23]. The combination of CPAP during oxygenation (spontaneous breathing) with PEEP directly after intubation (ventilation) is crucial; CPAP during oxygenation without subsequent PEEP did not result in a longer apnea time without hypoxia [13].

The oxygen reserve can also be optimized by a special position during preoxygenation. Positioning the head upward (20°) elongated apnea time (until the SaO_2 dropped below 95%) from 283 s (Patient lying flat) to 186s in lean patients. This is similar with obese patients: positioning them head up (25°) during preoxygenation increases apnea (SaO_2 under 92%) time from 155 to 201 s, as compared to flat positioning. The tilt also increased PAO_2 from 360 to 442 mmHg [2, 7, 17].

Another effective measure to avoid hypoxia during apnea is to insufflate oxygen through a nasopharyngeal tube continuously between preoxygenation and endotracheal intubation. This way a SaO_2 of 100% could be kept up in almost all patients (average BMI 42) for a 4-min apnea [4]. For conventional orotracheal intubation, a modified RSI (rapid sequence induction) can be performed, analogous to the demands of pediatric anesthesiologists for RSI in children. In this modification, an intermittent ventilation with low pressure, represents a practical alternative, needs to be asserted in further studies [46].

Airway Management

The numerous alterations of the respiratory system in severely obese patients must also be taken into account for airway management. From an anesthesiological point of view, pulmonary risk combined with the high incidence of gastroesophageal reflux demands a primary fiber optic controlled intubation for the sake of safety of the morbidly obese. Reasoning that fiber optic intubation takes longer than conventional intubation is irrelevant, because a small gain in time should not be obtained at the expense of the patient's safety.

Another argument for fiber optic intubation is that difficulties in intubation are to be expected in extremely obese patients. There is a correlation between BMI and difficult intubation. The incidence of unexpectedly difficult intubations (conventional intubation) in morbidly obese patients is reported to be around 13% [9]. Circumference of the neck and a Mallampati score of III or IV correlate with a difficult intubation [20, 29, 30]. Still there is no defined maximum circumference of the neck up to which conventional intubation will probably be trouble free [8].

A BMI of 30 seems to be a kind of "cut-off" number; the incidence of difficult intubations rises threefold above this level [32, 42, 45].

When planning to perform conventional intubation, make sure to prepare alternative intubation methods beforehand. Intubating larynx masks (ILMA) and the ProSeal larynx mask have proved to be suitable in emergency situations for extremely obese patients, even if direct laryngoscopy reveals high Cormack and Lehane scores. Surprisingly, the ILMA can be placed even easier in obese patients. This is possibly due to the tighter placement of the mask within the more pronounced fat tissue in the lateral walls of the pharynx [11, 22, 31].

A further development of the ILMA is the so-called ILMA CTrach. This is an ILMA with an integrated fiber optic system, which combines visualization of larynx and vocal chords with administration of oxygen. First reports of the successful application of the device with patients with a BMI between 60 and 63 and expected difficult intubation (Mallampati score III and short thyromental distance) are available [47].

Dhonneur and colleagues recently described another technique that is supposed to facilitate endotracheal intubation in extremely obese patients: The insertion of a single-use laryngoscope that is turned by 180° (i.e., Airtraq) until the pharynx is reached; the laryngoscope is then turned back to "normal" position. This quickened and facilitated intubation in obese patients; no differences were seen in lean patients [16]. Larger studies with more patients are not yet available.

Pharmacotherapy

Kinetics of many pharmaceuticals are modified in morbidly obese patients. Distribution volume differs from lean patients, because 60% of the excess weight is due to fat tissue and only 20–40% to lean body mass (LBM). For morbidly obese patients, LBM is calculated as following: Ideal body weight (IBW = 22 × (height in m²) plus 30% [33]. LBM and the amount of water are reduced in relation to total body weight (TBW). Obese patients also have an increased volume of extracellular fluid; their cardiac output is 25% higher to supply the "additional" tissue with blood. Reduced protein binding of pharmaceuticals is discussed. Uptake and elimination of inhalation narcotics is diminished due to impaired lung mechanics. These factors delay the elimination of pharmaceuticals, depending on liver and kidney function. In obese patients, renal blood flow is enhanced, which actually improves glomerular filtration rate and renal clearance. But this is only the case as long as there is no chronic kidney failure with severe proteinuria present [10, 25]. These problems must be taken into account when calculating pharmaceuticals for anesthesia. Data are scarce, but allow practical recommendations for pharmacotherapy.

There is no difference in pharmacokinetics of Remifentanil in obese or lean patients. Calculating the dosage with regard to the TBW will result in excessively high plasma levels of Remifentanil. This is why the amount given must be measured with regard to the IBW, not the TBW [15, 19, 37].

Fentanyl, sufentanil, and thiopentone must be dosed regarding the TBW. Propofol is dosed regarding to the IBW for induction and to TBW for maintenance. The muscle relaxants succinylcholine, atracurium, and cisatracurium are dosed regarding the TBW; vecuronium and rocuronium regarding to the IBW. There are no data concerning mivacurium; dosage calculation is recommended regarding to the TBW [15, 33, 37].

There are only few data concerning the administration of inhalation narcotics in morbidly obese patients available. Considering vital signs after termination of anesthesia and time spent in the recovery room, sevoflurane seems to be superior to isoflurane [43, 44].

In patients with a BMI of 44 and higher, Juvin and colleagues found faster recovery, less postoperative hypoxia, and quicker return of mobility after desflurane as compared to isoflurane and propofol anesthesia [28].

De Baerdemaker and colleagues reported more stable hemodynamics and better vital signs after termination of anesthesia in obese patients after desflurane compared to sevoflurane (De Baerdemaker et al. 2003); other authors however could not confirm this [3].

Some data concerning anesthesia in 145 patients undergoing laparoscopic gastric banding show benefits for a combination of inhalation anesthesia with desflu-rane and iv anesthesia with remifentanil [24]. One third of our patients suffered hypotension during the procedure, which was probably due to the extreme anti-Trendelenburg position that is required during surgery. This hypotension is aggravated through the creation of the penumoperitoneum and rise of the intraabdominal pressure up to 15 mmHg. Other authors noticed a similar impairment of hemodynamics during Sevo- or Desflurane anesthesia [14].

Summary

Morbidly obese patients are very high risk population for complications. Apart from planning airway management very carefully beforehand, the choice of the anesthetic procedure has first priority. In our clinic, we prefer elective nasopharyngeal fiber optic intubation to RSI for safety reasons. We combine desflurane and remifentanil (dosage regarding to the IBW and not TBW) as a standard method. We consider conventional intubation with intermittent mask ventilation unjustifiable for the sake of these patients' safety.

References

1. Adams JP, Murphy PG (2000) Obesity in anaesthesia and intensive care. Br J Anaesth 85:91–108
2. Altermatt FR, Muñoz HR, Delfino AE, Cortínez LI (2005) Pre-oxygenation in the obese patient: effects of position on tolerance to apnoea. Br J Anaesth 95:706–709
3. Arain SR, Barth CD, Shankar H, Ebert TJ (2005) Choice of volatile anesthetic fort he morbidly obese patient: sevoflurane or desflurane. J Clin Anesth 17:413–419
4. Baraka AS, Taha SK, Siddik-Sayyid SM, Kanazi GE, El-Khatib MF, Dagher CM, Chehade JMA, Abdallah FW, Hajj RE (2007) Supplementation of pre-oxygenation in morbidly obese patients using nasopharyngeal oxygen insufflation. Anaesthesia 62:769–773
5. Benoît Z, Wicky S, Fischer JF, Frascarolo P, Chapuis C, Spahn DR, Magnusson L (2002) The effect of increased FiO_2 before tracheal extubation on postoperative atelectasis. Anesth Analg 95:1777–1781
6. Berthoud MC, Peacock JE, Reilly CS (1991) Effectiveness of preoxygenation in morbidly obese patients. Br J Anaesth 67:464–466
7. Boyce JR, Ness T, Castroman P, Gleysteen JJ (2003) A preliminary study of the optimal anesthesia positioning fort he morbidly obese patient. Obes Surg 13:4–9
8. Brodsky JB, Lemmens HJM, Brock-Utne JG, Vierra M, Saidman LJ (2002) Morbid obesity and tracheal intubation. Anesth Analg 94:732–736

9. Buckley FP, Robinson NB, Simonowitz DA, Dellinger EP (1983) Anaesthesia in the morbidly obese. A comparison of anaesthetic and analgesic regimens for upper abdominal surgery. Anaesthesia 38:840–851

10. Casati A, Putzu M (2005) Anesthesia in the obese patient: pharmacokinetic considerations. J Clin Anesth 17:134–145

11. Combes X, Sauvat S, Leroux B, Dumerat M, Sherrer E, Motamed C, Brain A, D'Honneur G (2005) Intubating laryngeal mask airway in morbidly obese and lean patients. A comparative study. Anesthesiology 102:1106–1109

12. Coussa M, Proietti S, Schnyder P, Frascarolo P, Suter M, Spahn DR, Magnusson L (2004) Prevention of atelectasis formation during the induction of general anesthesia in morbidly obese patients. Anesth Analg 98:1491–1495

13. Cressey DM, Berthoud MC, Reilly CS (2001) Effectiveness of continuous positive airway pressure to enhance preoxygenation in morbidly obese women. Anaesthesia 56: 680–684

14. De Baerdemaeker LEC, Struys MMRF, Jacobs S, Den Blauwen NNM, Bossuyt GRPJ, Mortier EP (2003) Optimization of desflurane administration in morbidly obese patients: a comparison with sevoflurane using an 'inhalation bolus' technique. Br J Anaesth 91:638–650

15. De Baerdemaeker LEC, Mortier EP, Struys MMRF (2004) Pharmacokinetics in obese patients. Continuing Education in Anaesthesia, Critical Care Pain 4:152–155

16. Dhonneur G, Ndoko SK, Amathieu R, Attias A, Housseini LEL, Polliand C, Tual L (2007) A comparison of two techniques for inserting the AirtraqTM laryngoscope in morbidly obese patients. Anaesthesia 62:774–777

17. Dixon BJ, Dixon JB, Carden JR, Burn AJ, Schachter LM, Playfair JM, Laurie CP, O'Brien PE (2005) Preoxygenation is more effective in the 25° head-up position than in the supine position in severely obese patients. Anesthesiology 102:1110–1115

18. Edmark L, Kostova-Aherdan K, Enlund M, Hedenstierna G (2003) Optimal oxygen concentration during induction of general anesthesia. Anesthesiology 98:28–33

19. Egan TD, Huizinga B, Gupta SK, Jaarsma RL, Sperry RJ, Yee JB, Muir KT (1998) Remifentanil pharmacokinetics in obese versus lean patients. Anesthesiology 89:562–573

20. Ezri T, Medalion B, Weisenberg M, Szmuk P, Warters D, Charuzi I (2003) Increased body mass index per se is not a predictor of difficult laryngoscopy. Can J Anesth 50: 179–183

21. Farmery AD, Roe PG (1996) A model to describe the rate of oxyhaemoglobin desaturation during apnoea. Br J Anaesth 76:284–291

22. Frappier J, Guenoun T, Journois D, Philippe H, Aka E, Cadi P, Silleran-Chassany J, Safran D (2003) Airway management using the intubating laryngeal mask airway for the morbidly obese patient. Anesth Analg 96:1510–1515

23. Gander S, Frascarolo P, Suter M, Spahn DR, Magnusson L (2005) Positive end-expiratory pressure during induction of general anesthesia increases duration of nonhypoxic apnea in morbidly obese patients. Anesth Analg 100:580–584

24. Gervais HW, Korenkov M, Heintz A, Sauerland S, Junginger T, Schmidt A, David M, Baldering HJ, Kentner R (2011) Anästhesie zur Adipositaschirurgie - 145 konsekutive Fälle von laparoskopischem "Gastric banding" – eine retrospektive Prozessanalyse

25. Hall JE, Crook ED, Jones DW, Wofford MR, Dubbert PM (2002) Mechanisms of obesity-associated cardiovascular and renal disease. Am J Med Sci 324:127–137

26. Huang KC, Kormas N, Steinbeck K, Loughnan G, Caterson ID (2004) Resting metabolic rate in severely obese diabetic and nondiabetic subjects. Obes Res 12:840–845

27. Jense HG, Dubin SA, Silverstein PI, O'Leary-Escolas U (1991) Effect of obesity on safe duration of apnea in anesthetized humans. Anesth Analg 72:89–93

28. Juvin P, Vadam C, Malek L, Dupont H, Marmuse JP, Desmonts JM (2000) Postoperative recovery after desflurane, propofol or isoflurane anesthesia among morbidly obese patients: a prospective, randomized study. Anesth Analg 91:714–719

29. Juvin P, Lavaut E, Dupont H, Lefevre P, Demetriou M, Dumoulin JL, Desmonts JM (2003) Difficult tracheal intubation is more common in obese than in lean patients. Anesth Analg 97:595–600

30. Karkouti K, Rose DK, Wigglesworth D, Cohen MM (2000) Predicting difficult intubation: a multivariate analysis. Can J Anesth 47:730–739

31. Keller C, Brimacombe J, Kleinsasser A, Brimacombe L (2002) The laryngeal mask airway ProSealTM as a temporary ventilatory device in grossly and morbidly obese patients before laryngoscope-guided tracheal intubation. Anesth Analg 94:737–740

32. Langeron O, Masso E, Huraux C, Guggiari M, Bianchi A, Coriat P, Riou B (2000) Prediction of difficult mask ventilation. Anesthesiology 92:1229–1236

33. Lemmens HJM, Brodsky JB (2006) The dose of succinylcholine in morbid obesity. Anesth Analg 102:438–442

34. Livingston EH (2004) Procedure incidence and in-hospital complication rates of bariatric surgery in the United States. Am J Surg 188:105–110

35. Lumb AB (2007) Just a little oxygen to breathe as you go off to sleep… is it always a good idea? (Editorial) Br J Anaesth 99:769–771

36. Neumann P, Klockgether-Radke A, Quintel M (2004) Nutzen und Risiken der Beatmung mit positiv-endexspiratorischem Druck in der perioperativen Phase. Anästh Intensivmed 45:137–145

37. Ogunnaike BO, Jones SB, Jones DB, Provost D, Whitten CW (2002) Anesthetic considerations for bariatric surgery. Anesth Analg 95:1793–1805

38. Pelosi P, Croci M, Ravagnen I, Vicardi P, Gattinoni L (1996) Total respiratory system, lung, and chest wall mechanics in sedated-paralyzed postoperative morbidly obese patients. Chest 109:144–151

39. Pelosi P, Croci M, Ravagnan I, Tredici S, Pedoto A, Lissoni A, Gattinoni L (1998) The effects of body mass on lung volumes, respiratory mechanics, and gas exchange during general anesthesia. Anesth Analg 87:654–660

40. Rothen HU, Sporre B, Engberg G, Wegenius G, Reber A, Hedenstierna G (1995) Prevention of atelectasis during general anesthesia. Lancet 345:1387–1391

41. Rusca M, Proietti S, Schnyder P, Frascarolo P, Hedenstierna G, Spahn DR, Magnusson L (2003) Prevention of atelectasis formation during induction of general anesthesia. Anesth Analg 97:1835–1839

42. Shiga, T, Wajima Z, Inoue T, Sakamoto A (2005) Predicting difficult intubation in apparently normal patients. A meta-

analysis of bedside screening test performance. Anesthesiology 103:429–437

43. Sollazzi L, Perilli V, Modesti C, Annetta G, Ranieri R, Maria Taccino R, Proietti R (2001) Volatile anesthesia in bariatric surgery. Obes Surg 11:623–626

44. Torri G, Casati A, Albertin A, Comotti L, Bignami E, Scarioni M, Paganelli M (2001) Randomized comparison of isoflurane and sevoflurane for laparoscopic gastric banding in morbidly obese patients. J Clin Anesth 13:565–570

45. Voyagis GS, Kyriakis KP, Dimitriou V, Vrettou I (1998) Value of oropharyngeal Mallampati classification in predicting difficult laryngoscopy among obese patients. Eur J Anaesthesiol 15:330–334

46. Weiss M, Gerber AC (2008) Rapid sequence induction in children – it's not a matter of time (Editorial). Pediatric Anesth 18:97–99

47. Wender R, Goldman AJ (2007) Awake insertion of the fibreoptic intubating LMA CTrachTM in three morbidly obese patients with potentially difficult airways. Anaesthesia 62:948–951

48. Zander R (2005) Physiologie und klinischer Nutzen einer Hyperoxie. Anästhesiol Intensivmed Notfallmed Schmerzther 40:616–623

Further Reading

Lane S, Saunders D, Schofield A, Padmanabhan R, Hildreth A, Laws D (2005) A prospective, randomised controlled trial comparing the efficacy of pre-oxygenation in the 20° head-up vs. Supine position. Anaesthesia 60:1064–1067

Ogden CL, Carroll MD, Curtin LR, McDowell MA, Tabak CJ, Flegal KM (2006) Prevalence of overweight and obesity in the United States, 1999–2004. JAMA 295:1549–1555

Perilli V, Sollazzi L, Modesti C, Sacco T, Bocci MG, Ciocchetti PP, Tacchino RM, Proietti R (2004) Determinants of improvement in oxygenation consequent to reverse Trendelenburg position in anesthetized morbildly obese patients. Obes Surg 14:66–67

Wada DR, Bjorkman S, Ebling WF, Harashima H, Harapat S, Stanski DR (1997) Computer simulation of the effects of alterations in blood flows and body composition on thiopental pharmacokinetics in humans. Anesthesiology 87:884–899

Epilogue: Safety and Certainty in Bariatric Surgery

11

Michael Korenkov

Security is a situation free of unjustifiable risks of damage or one considered free of danger. With this definition security refers to the individual, other living beings, inanimate objects and systems, as well as to abstract entities.

(Wikipedia, The Free Encyclopedia)

Striving for safety in surgery is closely linked to uppermost medical rule "primum nil nocere." To achieve a situation of safety, various concepts have been developed for some time and have been implemented more or less.

In a discussion with my teacher and former superior Professor Hans Troidl, he used the terms "safety" and "certainty" as different aspects of safety. He defines "certainty" as the safety of choosing the appropriate therapy. "One can perform the wrong procedure with correct surgical technique," referring to surgery. "Safety" or "patients' safety" is safety while performing the procedure, meaning the avoidance of intra- and postoperative complications and an effective management of complications. "Safety" and "Certainty," combined with systematic aftercare are the conditions for the success of the surgical therapy of morbid obesity.

Due to the epidemic spreading of morbid obesity, bariatric surgery has developed immensely. New surgical techniques and medical instruments are developed and put to use. Evident knowledge is collected and analyzed, but just as all new fields, bariatric surgery has many gaps in evidence, which can have a negative influence on the outcome. So far there are no standardized safety algorithms in bariatric surgery.

The most controversial topic is the choice of procedure. Dividing bariatric procedures into restrictive, malabsorptive, and combined procedures is established. The most frequently performed procedures are the implantation of an adjustable gastric band and the proximal gastric bypass. Other procedures, such as sleeve gastrectomy or the duodenal switch have their place value, but are by far not as widespread. There is no surgical gold standard in bariatric surgery, which is why the choice of procedure is often based on varying and in part very subjective criteria. Factors as surgical preference, the patient's wish, local circumstances in the hospital, and new technical developments can all influence the choice of procedure (Fig. 11.1).

Table 11.1 is a simplified compilation of the advantages and disadvantages of the bariatric surgical procedures established today. Besides these features, the individual particularities of the patients and the qualification of the bariatric surgeon play an important role in choosing a procedure.

So far there are no valid classifications for obese patients requiring surgery. I use the terms "ideal patient," "problematic patient," and "critical patient." Criteria for this classification are BMI, age, and comorbidities. The "ideal" patient has a BMI of 45 or lower, is under 40 and has (almost) no comorbidities. The "critical" patient has a BMI of 60 and higher, combined with several preexisting diseases. Criteria for the "problematic" patient are somewhere in between.

M. Korenkov
Abteilung für Allgemein- und Visceralchirurgie,
Klinikum Werra-Meissner, Akademisches Lehrkrankenhaus der
Universität Göttingen, Elsa-Brendström-Straße 1,
37269 Eschwege, Germany
e-mail: michael.korenkov@klinikum-wm.de

Fig. 11.1 Influence of various factors on the choice of bariatric procedure

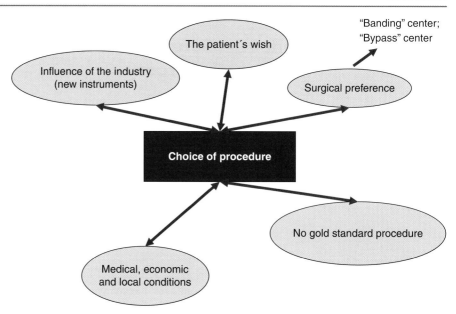

Table 11.1 Advantages and disadvantages of various bariatric procedures

Procedure	Advantages	Disadvantages
Gastric banding	– "Zero" mortality	– Not always efficient
	– Technically easy	– Expensive
	– Surgical steps standardized	– Aftercare
		– Late complications
	– Reversible	
	– Low perioperative morbidity	
	– In part outpatient treatment	
Gastric bypass	– Simpler aftercare	– Technically more difficult
	– Less late complications	– Mortality risk
	– Effective more often than gastric banding	– Irreversible
		– Higher perioperative morbidity
		– Lifelong substitution
Sleeve gastrectomy	– Technically easy	– Mortality risk low, but not zero
	– Simpler aftercare	– Irreversible
	– Less late complications	– Risk for postoperative complications: low, but not zero
		– Long term data concerning metabolism are not available
Duodenal switch	– Always efficient	– Technically the most difficult
	– Simple aftercare	– Highest mortality risk
	– Food ingestion not disturbed	– Serious postoperative complications
		– Irreversible
		– Metabolic dysfunction

For the "ideal" patient, restrictive and combined procedures can be chosen, whereas the "critical" patient can only receive a malabsorptive procedure.

Bariatric surgeons are divided into "polyvalent" and "monovalent" surgeons with regard to their services. The "monovalent" specialists master only one procedure (most frequently gastric banding) which is all they offer. This concept is a fact, in spite of its obvious shortcoming. There are "Clinics for Gastric Banding" that do not offer any other treatment at all.

Surgeons, who are not technically limited, will have to decide between gastric banding and gastric bypass most frequently. But even "polyvalent" surgeons are beginning to concentrate on one procedure only, i.e., gastric bypass. There are several reasons for this development, most of them of organizational and financial nature.

Another unresolved problem is the technical difficulty of the procedures ("safety"). Surgical techniques of the restrictive procedures (laparoscopic gastric banding, sleeve gastrectomy) are well standardized today; there are no basic technical divergences. But in contrast to the restrictive procedures, combined and malabsorptive procedures (gastric bypass, duodenal switch) have many different variations. Especially the gastric bypass is performed in many technical modifications. The influence of the variations on the outcome of gastric bypass surgery has not been clarified yet.

The influence of systematic aftercare on the results of bariatric procedures is just as significant as correct technique and strategy. There are no major disagreements concerning this matter. Troublesome and hardly feasible (at least in our country) is the problem of funding the concept.

Index

M. Korenkov (ed.), *Bariatric Surgery*,
DOI 10.1007/978-3-642-16245-9, © Springer-Verlag Berlin Heidelberg 2012

Printing and Binding: Stürtz GmbH, Würzburg